www.wadsworth.com

wadsworth.com is the World Wide Web site for
Wadsworth Publishing Company and is your direct
source to dozens of online resources.

At *wadsworth.com* you can find out about
supplements, demonstration software, and
student resources. You can also send e-mail to
many of our authors and preview new publications
and exciting new technologies.

wadsworth.com
Changing the way the world learns®

The Rehabilitation Model
of
Substance Abuse
Counseling

John J. Benshoff
Professor, Rehabilitation Counselor Training Program
Rehabilitation Institute
Southern Illinois University at Carbondale

Timothy P. Janikowski
Director, Rehabilitation Counseling Program
State University of New York

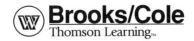

Brooks/Cole
Thomson Learning™

Australia • Canada • Mexico • Singapore • Spain • United Kingdom • United States

Acquisitions Editor: Eileen Murphy
Publisher/Executive Editor: Sean Wakely
Assistant Editor: Julie Martinez
Editorial Assistant: Annie Berterretche
Marketing Manager: Caroline Concilla
Project Editor: Marlene Vasilieff
Print Buyer: April Reynolds

Permissions Editor: Johee Lee
Production Service: Pre-Press Company, Inc.
Cover Designer: Yvo Riezebos
Signing Representative: Don Waller
Compositor: Pre-Press Company, Inc.
Printer/Binder: Webcom

For permission to use material from this text, contact us:
Web: www.thomsonrights.com
Fax: 1-800-730-2215
Phone: 1-800-730-2214

For more information, contact

Wadsworth/Thomson Learning
10 Davis Drive
Belmont, CA 94002-3098
USA
http://www.wadsworth.com

International Headquarters
Thomson Learning International Division
290 Harbor Drive, 2nd Floor
Stamford, CT 06902-7477
USA

UK/Europe/Middle East/South Africa
Thomson Learning
Berkshire House
168-173 High Holborn
London WC1V 7AA
United Kingdom

Asia
Thomson Learning
60 Albert Street #15-01
Albert Complex
Singapore 189969

Canada
Nelson/Thomson Learning
1120 Birchmount Road
Scarborough, Ontario M1K 5G4
Canada

Library of Congress Cataloging-in-Publication Data
Benshoff, John J.
The rehabilitation model of substance abuse counseling/John J. Benshoff, Timothy P. Janikowski.
p. cm.
Includes bibliographical references and index.
ISBN 0-534-34223-X (alk. paper)
1. Drug abuse counseling. 2. Substance abuse—Patients—Counseling of. 3. Rehabilitation counseling. I. Janikowski, Timothy P. II. Title.
RC564.B44 1999
362.29'186—dc21
99-050374

 This book is printed on acid-free recycled paper.

To
Sharon and Shauna and Linda, Alyssa, Alex, and Leah
You are our love and inspiration.

Contents

Preface

As rehabilitation counselor educators and as rehabilitation practitioners we have been undergirded in our work by the profound rehabilitation philosophic principles of intrinsic worth, capacity for change, self-determination, productive activity, and commitment. In this text we have tried to be true to that philosophy in its application to substance abuse treatment. Consequently we believe that substance abuse treatment should be holistic, individual, functional, in focus, and possess a strong emphasis on vocational issues. We do not view substance abuse simplistically. It has a complicated etiology and a complex course of involvement for most individuals. Correspondingly, recovery is not an event but a holistic, individualized, and functionally based evolutionary process.

In this text we trace the history of both rehabilitation and the substance abuse treatment movements, both of which are integral to the fabric of the 20th century. The first part of the text provides history and background and suggests a new paradigm combining rehabilitation and substance abuse treatment principles. Chapter 1, History and Background of Rehabilitation, chronicles the development and foundations of the rehabilitation movement, centering on issues such as federal legislation, rehabilitation philosophy, and sectors of rehabilitation practice. The chronology and heritage of substance abuse treatment are covered in Chapter 2, History and Background of Substance Abuse Treatment, also with an emphasis on history and legislation, philosophies of treatment, and the overlap with the rehabilitation movement. In Chapter 3, A Developmental-Environmental Model of Substance Abuse Rehabilitation, we argue for recognition of substance abuse as a disability, best treated with a functional assessment approach. The developmental-environmental realm of substance abuse is conceptualized with an emphasis on individualized, holistic rehabilitation.

The second part of the text is devoted to pharmacology. Chapter 4, Drugs and the Central Nervous System, examines the human nervous system, brain chemistry and neurotransmitters, and the impact caused by psychoactive drugs. The neurochemistry of addictions is examined. Chapter 5, Drugs of Abuse, focuses on stimulants, depressants, and hallucinogens.

As befits a text intended for counselor training, the majority of the book is devoted to the third part, Working with Clients. Chapter 6, Group Counseling, provides an overview of group counseling, examining group counseling models, leadership skills, group dynamics, and the advantages of group counseling. The contributions of peer self-help groups are introduced in Chapter 6. Chapter 7, Family Counseling, focuses on this increasingly vital and important part of substance abuse treatment. Topics include family systems theory and family counseling models, and discussions of Adult Children of Alcoholics (ACOA) concepts and codependency issues. Chapter 8, Treatment, discusses various modalities of treatment, including variations of detoxification, residential, inpatient treatment, outpatient and intensive outpatient treatment, and methadone maintenance. The section on each modality includes an analysis of the advantages and disadvantages of the modality. A significant portion of Chapter 8 is devoted to peer self-help groups, discussing Alcoholics Anonymous and similar groups, and groups that utilize different models and doctrines, including Women for Sobriety and Rational Recovery. We assert our belief that peer-self-help groups are not treatment but serve an extraordinarily important supportive, fellowship-based role in the recovery process. Chapter 9, Assessment, reviews the primary signs and symptoms of substance abuse, primarily from a DSM-IV perspective. The importance and significance of the intake process are reviewed, along with a discussion of standardized tests and their importance in the assessment process.

Chapter 10, Treatment Planning, Case Management, and Managed Care, begins with a review of treatment planning strategies in substance abuse facilities and rehabilitation programs, with an emphasis on the importance of individualized, comprehensive, and holistic planning. The sections on case management and managed care provide a background on case management practice and principles along with an analysis of the impact of managed care on substance abuse treatment.

Chapters 11 and 12 scrutinize issues related to subpopulations of individuals in need of substance abuse treatment. Chapter 11, Special Populations, looks at the distinctive treatment issues and needs of women, the elderly, members of ethnic minority groups, and gays and lesbians.

The last two chapters contain information not often seen in substance abuse treatment texts. Coexisting disabilities, discussed in Chapter 12, Substance Abuse as a Coexisting Disability, are an emerging and significant issue both for mainstream rehabilitation and substance abuse treatment. Recent evidence indicates that individuals with "traditional" disabilities have the same, and often higher, risks for substance abuse problems than members of the general population. Nevertheless, individuals with disabilities are underrepresented in substance abuse treatment populations, and modifications are required in treatment strategies to adequately serve these individuals. Chapter 12 reviews the evolution of coexisting disabilities as a construct and discusses the regulations and impact of the Americans with Disabilities Act. The functional limitations imposed by the coexistence of substance abuse and traumatic brain injury, mobility disabilities, sensory disabilities and mental illness are featured. Finally, Chapter 12 sets forth an empowerment model based on independent living concepts.

Chapter 13, Alcohol, Drugs, and Work, discusses the importance of work in the recovery process. Concepts of rehabilitation in recovery are emphasized with an examination of the importance of vocational functioning especially as it relates to self-esteem and self-identity.

We believe this text will be of value to substance abuse counselors and rehabilitation counselors serving both substance abusing and "traditional" rehabilitation populations. The basic substance abuse treatment information will be valuable to counselors, social workers, and other human service professionals. More important, the model incorporating substance abuse and rehabilitation ideas is unique to this book, and we believe it offers a fresh, vital perspective. Finally, the inclusion of issues related to coexisting disabilities, the importance of work, and the functional assessment approach to substance abuse covers important territory rarely seen in other training materials.

John J. Benshoff
Timothy P. Janikowski

List of Reviewers

The editors, authors, and publisher thank the reviewers of the manuscript for their helpful comments and suggestions:

Paul Alston
East Carolina University

Alan Davis
Montana State University-Billings

Dona Kennealley
University of South Dakota

Maureen C. Kenny
Florida International University

Eileen O'Mara
Hazelden Foundation

Beth Rienzi
California State University-Bakersfield

Amos Sales
University of Arizona

Meri Sahdley
University of Nevada.

1

History and Background
of Rehabilitation

HISTORY AND REHABILITATION LEGISLATION

Turn of the Century

Rehabilitation counseling, first an occupation and developing into a recognized profession, traces its history in the United States back to the early 1900s. This was a time of tremendous growth and transformation in the United States that proved to be formative for the future field of rehabilitation counseling as well. During a 30-year span (from about 1890 to 1920) significant societal changes were occurring in the United States: population size, urbanization, industrialization, medical and health practices, vocational education, and federal rehabilitation legislation. Each of these societal changes set the stage for the development of rehabilitation, and each will be briefly discussed.

During this 30-year period, the United States transformed itself from a primarily rural, agrarian society to that of an urban, industrialized one. The population roughly doubled during this time, increasing from about 50 million to 102 million people, largely due to massive immigration. Rapid growth coincided with a dramatic rise in the number of people living in cities (Tishler, 1971). In 1890 the ratio of rural to urban population was roughly 50–50, by 1920 it was 30–70. Urbanization caused a number of positive outcomes. Because of a centralized populous, people became better informed; there were significant increases in the numbers of newspapers and magazines that were widely read. The cities gave their citizens greater access to public education, resulting in a more literate population. Because people were living and working in groups, it became easier to organize and be heard as a group, and unions were created to protect workers and advocate for their rights. Accompanying these positive outcomes were negative realities. The concept of alienation became a major philosophical concern at this time because huge, impersonal cities had replaced the closely knit farming community (Nisbet, 1966). People labored alongside strangers and worked for indifferent employers. People flocked to the cities because of the lure of jobs, but the supply of jobs didn't always keep up with the demand. Therefore, for the first time in U.S. history, there were large numbers of urban unemployed.

The Industrial Revolution was sweeping over most of the Western world during this time that the United States' population was increasing and urbanizing. Industrialization resulted in marked changes in the nature of work and the roles of workers. People were required to work in groups, which was a marked change from the small villages and farm communities that had previously supplied employment. Workers were required to punch timeclocks; work for hourly wages; acquire specialized skills; and function within hierarchies with foremen, supervisors, and managers. For the first time social status was significantly affected by what one did for a living, rather than bloodlines or land holdings. What one did for a living was becoming more complicated and more closely tied to social class (Neff, 1977).

Prior to 1890, medicine was often ineffective. After this time, biological scientific techniques helped to develop medicines that could actually save lives. A few decades before this time, people commonly died of infections that resulted from injuries. Sulfa drugs and other antibiotics markedly increased the survival rate of injured people. Medical advances also contributed to an increase in the number of people with disabilities. In 1897 state legislatures first passed legislation for the treatment, care, and education of crippled [*sic*] children, and in 1902 the first public health hospital was founded and served as the precedent for federal government–supported health services (Wright, 1980). Also, there was more emphasis on preventive medicine, and improvements in sanitation resulted in people living longer and living with disability after an illness or disease. World War I, having ended in 1918, resulted in a large population of disabled men—men who were young and otherwise healthy. This group would normally have been in the early part of their productive years, but because of disability, they were faced with the possibility of being dependent on society for the rest of their lives. The American Medical Association responded by the creation of physiatry, or the medical specialization in physical medicine and rehabilitation (Wright, 1980).

Before the turn of the century there were few vocational education programs in public schools; those that did exist were usually for poor or disabled children. The sweeping changes stemming from industrialization made World War I the first technological war and resulted in the military's need for a skilled population of soldiers. Further, business and industry required a skilled workforce that could operate sophisticated equipment, using specialized skills. Hence, the needs of the military, business, and industry prompted the introduction of vocational education programs in the public school system curriculum. The Smith-Hughes Act was passed in 1917 to encourage the development of vocational education programs by making federal money available on a matching basis to states that was earmarked for vocational training or education. The concept of vocational guidance also began at this time. As jobs became more complex, it was clear that people needed a systematic approach to making vocational choices; worker abilities and aptitudes needed to be matched with more complex job demands. Frank Parsons, in 1896, established the Vocational Bureau in Boston, based on what became three central vocational guidance principles: (1) help the student get a clear understanding of himself or herself, (2) help the student acquire knowledge of work requirements and the conditions for success, and (3) integrate both sets of knowledge to select a proper fit between worker and job (Parsons, 1909). This basic approach is still used today in both the Trait-Factor Theory and the Theory of Work Adjustment (Isaacson & Brown, 1993) to help people with disabilities make appropriate vocational choices and plans.

Discussion Question: We are currently at the turn of the century and going through another revolution. What changes related to technology and the information age do you see as having the most impact on people with disabilities and their ability to work and be part of society?

Rehabilitation Legislation

The field of rehabilitation was essentially legislated into existence in 1918 with the Soldiers Rehabilitation Act. This act established the first national program for people with physical disabilities and is considered breakthrough legislation for, originally, veterans with disabilities and eventually for all people with disabilities. Disabled veterans of all prior wars were compensated through government pensions for their war-induced disabilities, with little or no effort to rehabilitate (vocational or otherwise) the disabled veteran (Rubin & Roessler, 1995). The Soldiers Rehabilitation Act placed the Federal Board for Vocational Education (FBVE; created by the Smith-Hughes Act of 1917) in charge of developing a national vocational rehabilitation program for all veterans with service-related disabilities. The service-related disabilities must have presented handicaps to employment; however, the veteran must not have been so disabled that employment wasn't potentially feasible (Oberman, 1965).

The Soldiers Rehabilitation Act was soon followed by the Smith-Fess Act (in 1920) that established a similar vocational rehabilitation program for civilians. Again, the FBVE was given responsibility for developing and running the program. Civilians who were 16 years old or older and had physical disabilities that impaired their ability to work were qualified for rehabilitation services. Again, one was not eligible for services if a disability was so severe that gainful employment wasn't possible. The emphasis of the early vocational rehabilitation program was on training, or the acquisition of skills to increase employability. Rehabilitation services could include vocational guidance (identification of a job goal), vocational education (training to acquire an occupational skill), occupational adjustment (help with functioning in a work setting), and placement (help identifying job openings and placing the client in a job). Physical restoration, physical therapy, artificial limbs, adjustment counseling, and similar rehabilitation services were not yet part of the rehabilitation process. The primary approach to rehabilitation was to "train around" the disability (Rubin & Roessler, 1995), for example, training someone who was blind to tune pianos or teach someone with paraplegia to type. The rehabilitation program was established on a national level by the federal government (via the FBVE) by providing funds to the States on a matching 50–50 basis to develop state programs that would meet federal guidelines. The matching funds were important financial incentives for the States to pass rehabilitation legislation and establish state offices. It was in this manner that the state/federal rehabilitation system was created; federal funds that matched state dollars were used to create state-run programs to assist with the vocational rehabilitation of people with disabilities. Such programs included the Division of Vocational Rehabilitation, the Department of Rehabilitation Services, and the Office of Rehabilitation Services that were created in various states.

Federal legislation in the 1930s and 1940s consistently supported vocational rehabilitation. The state/federal system was made a permanent program by the Social Security Act of 1935. Prior to this act, the state/federal rehabilitation program had to maintain its existence and secure funding through continued passage of bills through Congress. This law moved vocational rehabilitation from a temporary, experimental program to a permanent one that would need an act of Congress if it was to be eliminated. The Randolph–Sheppard Act, in 1936, made the federal government committed to support a stable market for goods produced by "the blind" by allocating funds for the development and expansion of facilities for people who were blind. The Wagner–O'Day Act, in 1938, made it mandatory for the federal government to purchase products from workshops for the blind; thus, even today, vending machines in federal buildings are typically serviced by people who are blind. The Barden-LaFollette Act, in 1943, expanded public rehabilitation beyond physical or sensory disabilities, recognizing for the first time both mental illness and mental retardation as disabilities eligible for services.

The next major piece of federal rehabilitation legislation passed was the Hill–Burton Act, or Vocational Rehabilitation Act Amendments, in 1954. These amendments increased the federal share of seed dollars by one-third (i.e., for every $2 spent by a state, the federal government would provide $3). It also required significant, overall increases in funding for the rehabilitation program. The federal government allocated $30 million for rehabilitation spending in 1955, $45 million in 1956, $55 million in 1957, and $65 million in 1958 (Oberman, 1965). This legislation began the "Golden Era" of rehabilitation, which lasted until about 1965. This time period was so named because of the steady and significant funding increases in client services, training rehabilitation personnel, and rehabilitation research (Rubin & Roessler, 1995).

Perhaps most important of all, the 1954 Amendments began the professionalization of rehabilitation counseling by providing grants to colleges and universities to prepare rehabilitation counselors at the master's degree level. Prior to this time, there were no standardized training programs available for rehabilitation counselors; in fact, those employed in the field were more appropriately labeled as rehabilitation workers, agents (Jaques, 1970), or advisors (Wright, 1980). The training of these rehabilitation workers, who had little previous experience or relevant education, was usually left up to each state agency or other rehabilitation employers (Wright, 1980). The establishment of graduate level training programs, beginning in 1954, ensured that rehabilitation counselors would have uniform education that resulted in necessary competencies. Today rehabilitation counselors have skills in counseling, assessment, case management, and job placement. Accredited rehabilitation counselor training programs typically require such course work as vocational development and job placement, counseling theories, counseling techniques, assessment, medical and psychosocial aspects of disability, case management, and supervised field experience (Linkowski & Szymanski, 1993). These courses, along with preservice field training, prepare professional rehabilitation counselors who have skills required to facilitate the rehabilitation of their clients with disabilities. Szymanski and Parker (1989) have demonstrated that rehabilitation counselors who have master's degrees are more effective than counselors with less training.

The Vocational Rehabilitation Act Amendments of 1965 increased the federal-state ratio of matching dollars to 75–25 (which was increased again in 1968 to 80 percent federal to 20 percent state dollars). Rehabilitation services were also made available to those who had "behavior disorders." *Behavior disorder* is a term coined by the successor of the FBVE, the Rehabilitation Services Administration (RSA); the behavior disorders designation was given to individuals with behavior-based problems who had been diagnosed by a psychologist or a psychiatrist. For the first time, rehabilitation services could be offered through the state/federal system to people with alcoholism and drug addiction, based on the behavior disorder classification. Services were also available to those with antisocial personality, sociopathy, and criminals with diagnosable behavior disorders.

The legislation with the broadest impact on the field of rehabilitation was the Rehabilitation Act of 1973. Its sweeping reform was due in part to its civil rights orientation. The act consisted of four sections:

Section 501   Mandated nondiscrimination by the federal government in its own hiring practices. The federal government, as an employer, had to submit affirmative action plans for hiring, placement, and promotion of people with disabilities. It was hoped that the federal government would prove to be a role model for private sector employers.

Section 502   Addressed concerns about accessibility, especially architectural barriers and their handicapping effect on people with disabilities. This section established the Architectural and Transportation Compliance Board to enforce accessibility standards.

Section 503   Prohibited discrimination in employment on the basis of physical or mental disability and required affirmative action on the part of all federal contract recipients and their subcontractors who received more that $2500 in federal dollars. This section affected about two million companies, usually defense contractors, space program contractors, construction companies, and other firms that sold equipment or supplies to the federal government (Bayh, 1979).

Section 504   Prohibited exclusion based on disability of an otherwise qualified person with a disability from participation in any federal or federal-sponsored program or activity, such as attending school (elementary, secondary, and postsecondary), day care centers, access to hospitals or public welfare offices (Bayh, 1979). This section emphasized accessibility of buildings and programs. A person with a disability cannot be found unqualified without considering whether a reasonable accommodation would render the individual qualified.

In addition to Sections 501–504, the Rehabilitation Act of 1973 gave support for rehabilitation research by establishing the National Institute of Handicapped Research (NIHR), which subsequently evolved into the National Institute on Disability and Rehabilitation Research (NIDRR). NIDRR is responsible for: (1) disseminating information on ways to improve the quality of life for people with disabilities; (2) educating the public about ways to provide rehabilitation to people with disabilities; (3) conducting conferences on rehabilitation research and engineering; and (4) producing and disseminating statistics on employment, health, and income of people with disabilities.

In addition to having a sweeping impact on discrimination and centralizing rehabilitation research, the Rehabilitation Act of 1973 regulated the daily practice of rehabilitation counseling in the state/federal system. It gave rehabilitation service priority to those people with the most severe disabilities and emphasized "consumer involvement." Consumer involvement meant that people with disabilities (i.e., the consumers of rehabilitation services) shared an equal role with the rehabilitation counselor in the development of rehabilitation plans. The Act mandated the use of Individualized Written Rehabilitation Programs (IWRP) for each rehabilitation client. The IWRP must specify vocational objectives and services provided to meet the objectives and how progress toward the objectives is to be evaluated.

The Rehabilitation Act of 1973 also broadened the definition of disability. The following criteria were to be used when determining the presence or absence of a disability:

1. The existence of a physical or mental impairment that substantially limits one or more of the major life activities

2. Having a record of such an impairment (e.g., recovering alcoholics or drug addicts, people with a history of mental illness, people with epilepsy who have been seizure free for years)

3. Being regarded as having such an impairment (e.g., having a disfigurement, obesity)

The Rehabilitation Act Amendments of 1978 was the next major piece of rehabilitation legislation to be passed. One of its primary objectives was the promotion of independent living. It authorized funds for independent living services to people with severe disabilities who may not have any vocational objectives. The intent of independent living services was to assist people with disabilities to gain maximum control over the management of their lives and to minimize reliance on others for self-maintenance. According to Wright (1980), independent living programming should consist of a three-level approach:

a. Prevention of Dependency, which entails early intervention designed to reduce or postpone dependency (e.g., teaching people with spinal cord injuries to prevent pressure sores or decubitus ulcers)

b. Rehabilitation for Independence, which provides special training for daily living skills, such as bathing, grooming, dressing, cooking, cleaning

c. Maintenance of Independence, which entails services designed to avoid relapses—hence, some services, like attendant care, may be needed for a lifetime

Independent living rehabilitation represents an expansion of support into life areas other than work. The Independent Living movement is based on other social movements in the 1960s and early 1970s, including civil rights, consumerism, decentralization, self-help, and deinstitutionalization (Independent Living Center Resource Handbook, 1993). Centers for Independent Living (CILs) were created to be community-based, nonresidential, private not-for-profit, consumer-controlled organizations. Consumer-controlled means that the majority of employees (and the boards of directors) are people with disabilities. The CILs' primary goals are the following:

a. Advocate for eliminating environmental, economic, human rights, and communication barriers that are detrimental to people with disabilities

b. Provide public education and increase awareness to dispel myths about disability and people with disabilities

c. Offer direct services that are designed to offer choices other than institutionalization and dependence (Independent Living Center Resource Handbook, 1993)

CILs are designed to respond to the needs of the local community of people with disabilities, so their operations vary from location to location. There are, however, four direct services usually offered.

1. *Information and referral.* Information is provided to help consumers (people with disabilities are *not* referred to as clients) self-assess their problems and situation. Consumers should then be in a better position to identify avenues that they may pursue, either through the CIL or other community resources, to achieve their goals.

2. *Peer counseling.* One-on-one or group interactions with other people with disabilities are used for self-exploration and help with self-advocacy. Peer counselors are selected by the CIL based on their life experience, communication skills, and identification with the CIL's goals; however, the counseling is supportive and nontherapeutic in nature.

3. *Skill training.* Skill training is more than the provision of information; it is the acquisition of specific skills or competencies in areas such as health maintenance, application and management of financial benefits, job development skills, household management, personal/interpersonal communication skills, and self-care in activities of daily living (e.g., bathing, dressing, transportation).

4. *Advocacy.* This is a service designed to help the consumer act on his or her own behalf to maintain or improve independent living goals. Advocacy services generally entail the provision of information about civil and human rights, services and benefits to which consumers are entitled, and assertiveness in interaction with the nondisabled community. Consumers learn how to appeal an agency decision, file a lawsuit, change guardianship, or take advantage of protection afforded by civil rights laws such as the Rehabilitation Act (1973) or the Americans with Disabilities Act (1990).

Although not formally rehabilitation legislation, the Americans with Disabilities Act (1990) is the highest-profile legislation affecting not only people with disabilities but employers and the general public as well. Like the Rehabilitation Act of 1973, the ADA is best conceptualized as a very significant piece of civil rights legislation. This legislation is currently in effect (until repealed or amended) and has three primary purposes:

a. Provide a national mandate for eliminating discrimination against people with disabilities

b. Provide enforceable standards against disability-based discrimination

c. Give the federal government a role in enforcing those standards (ADA Handbook, 1991)

The ADA defined disability using Section 504 of the 1973 Rehabilitation Act, but it added a category of disability for those with contagious diseases. The substantial population of people with Acquired Immune Deficiency Syndrome (AIDS) was nonexistent in 1973 when Section 504 was written, and this population was therefore given needed protection against discrimination. This extension of protection directly affects people who abuse intravenous (IV) drugs, given their relatively high rates of HIV infection and AIDS. A major contributor to the spread of AIDS is IV drug use in which contaminated needles are shared among drug users. In some parts of the United States, the use of infected needles is the number one cause of HIV contraction. Nationally, IV drug use is associated with 28.9 percent of all cases of AIDS ("Who Has AIDS," 1991). People with contagious diseases such as AIDS, however, are only protected under the ADA when they do not pose a direct threat to the health or safety of others. The ADA also explicitly excludes certain groups who might otherwise be considered disabled, including individuals who are currently using illegal drugs, transvestitism, exhibitionism, or other types of sexual behavior disorders, homosexuality, or compulsive gambling, kleptomania, and pyromania (ADA Handbook, 1991).

The ADA is organized into five sections or titles. These titles are briefly described below. Title I, the Employment Provisions, prohibits discrimination because of disability in hiring, job training, promotion, and firing. Although the ADA was passed in 1990, this section of the law wasn't implemented until 1992 in order to allow employers time to comply with the law. Essentially it required employers with 15 or more workers to make reasonable accommodations for qualified job applicants with disabilities if accommodation was not an undue hardship. Reasonable accommodations may include a variety of changes, such as physical modification of the workplace—ramps, adjusting table height, elevators; restructuring the job so the functions can be performed by the people with disabilities (e.g., having another employee deliver the mail if it is a nonessential job function); part-time or modified work schedules, or more or different breaks or rearranged hours; reassigning people with disabilities to vacant positions; provision of devices or equipment (e.g., providing a telephone handset amplifier for workers with hearing impairments or an extra-large computer screen for workers with visual impairments); modifying the job application process (e.g., giving a job application exam orally rather than in writing for those with dyslexia); modifying company policies (e.g., allowing people with disabilities to bring a guide dog into the workplace); or providing readers or interpreters (Americans with Disabilities Act Handbook, 1991). It should be noted that the employment provisions regarding reasonable accommodations do not apply to people who are drinking and taking drugs and have diagnoses of alcoholism or drug addiction—these two disability groups were specifically included in Title I. Employers may act against these employees if such action is consistent with the Drug-Free Work Place Act of 1988 (Shaw, MacGillis, & Dvorchik, 1994).

The courts will have the ultimate authority on deciding what is considered to be a reasonable or unreasonable accommodation. Private lawsuits may be filed by those who think they have been discriminated against. Some of the remedies sought by plaintiffs may include enforced hiring; job reinstatement; back pay; attorneys' fees; and compensatory and punitive damages, the ceiling of which is determined by the employer's size. Penalties are capped at $50,000 for employers with up to 100 workers to $300,000 for employers with more than 500 workers.

Title II, the Public Service Provisions, is an extension of Section 504 of the 1973 Rehabilitation Act. It prohibits discrimination against people with disabilities in state and local government programs and activities (e.g., it is prohibited to refuse public housing, use of a library, or admission to summer camp to someone based on disability), and people with disabilities must have equal access to the services and benefits of public entities, including access to buildings where services are provided. To comply with Title II, welfare offices must be accessible; public forums like city council meetings must provide interpreters; and telephones and bathrooms at public activities must be modified to be made accessible. This title also requires access to public transportation. All newly built buses used for public transportation on fixed routes must have wheelchair lifts. If new buses aren't available, the city or state must offer an alternative. Also, rail systems and subways must have at least one car per train that is wheelchair accessible.

Title III, the Public Accommodation Provisions, prohibits discrimination on the basis of disability in public establishments such as hotels, restaurants, theaters, lawyers' offices, auditoriums, laundromats, insurance offices, museums, parks, zoos, private schools, gymnasiums, daycare centers, banks, health care centers, and so on. All structural barriers must be removed, and reasonable accommodations must be made. Examples of Title III accommodations are adding grab bars to bathtubs, lowering telephone booths and drinking fountains, adding raised letter and braille markings to elevator control panels, providing braille bank loan application forms, adding flashing alarm lights in hotels, and so on.

Title IV, the Telecommunications Provision, requires that access to telephone and radio communications must be provided at a reasonable cost to those with hearing or speech impairments. Use of a telecommunication device for the deaf (a TDD is a device that uses a keyboard to transmit written messages over the phone, sometimes referred to as TTY or Teletype) for operator assistance must be given in relaying communication to third parties who use a conventional telephone. This is referred to as dual-party telephone relay services. Service must be comparable to the service available to nondisabled individuals (e.g., available 24 hours a day, no limits on length or location of calls, same fees for regular service).

Title V, the Miscellaneous Provisions, addresses procedural guidelines, litigation, and technical assistance for people with disabilities who wish to use the ADA to combat discrimination that they may have experienced. Title V states that, where appropriate, alternative means of dispute resolution, such as settlement negotiations, mediation, fact-finding, and arbitration, are encouraged to resolve disputes arising under this act (Americans with Disabilities Act Handbook, 1991).

The Rehabilitation Act Amendments of 1992 specified a rehabilitation philosophy consistent with the Americans with Disabilities Act, emphasizing the importance of respect and dignity of the individual in rehabilitation planning. This act affirmed the role of self-determination, personal responsibility, and informed choice of clients in pursuing meaningful careers. Along these lines, the act provided funds for demonstration projects to achieve high-quality placement outcomes for people with severe disabilities. The 1992 Amendments also established Rehabilitation Advisory Councils (RACs), bodies consisting of a majority of people with disabilities who help develop and steer rehabilitation agency policy and procedures in the States. These councils, which are organized separately in each state, may address such topics as eligibility determination; the extent of services; order of selection for services or prioritizing which consumers get served first; program evaluation and consumer satisfaction; and coordination of the relationships between the council, state agency, Independent Living Council, and centers for independent living throughout the state. The 1992 Amendments modified the eligibility criteria for services and reinforced the clients' involvement in their rehabilitation by specifying components of the Individualized Written Rehabilitation Programs (IWRPs). All IWRPs must be reviewed annually, and this review must involve consumers and/or their guardians. The 1992 Amendments also strengthened the experimental programs of transition (from school to work) services, on-the-job training, and supported employment services (jobs performed by consumers with the help of job coaches in a competitive work site), and continued support of research and development for rural areas, severe disabilities, personal care assistance, and underserved/minority groups.

Discussion Questions: What trends may be identified in rehabilitation legislation over the past 80 years? How has it shaped the profession of rehabilitation counseling? How have the lives of people with disabilities been affected?

THREE SECTORS OF REHABILITATION
COUNSELING PRACTICE

Rehabilitation counselors work in a wide variety of settings, including state agencies, rehabilitation facilities, hospitals, multidisciplinary clinics, private practice, private for-profit rehabilitation companies, employee assistance programs, and private industry. The varied work settings may be categorized under three broad headings: public sector, private not-for-profit sector, and private for-profit sector. Rehabilitation counseling, as it is performed in these three sectors, has much in common. In all sectors, rehabilitation counselors must be knowledgeable about medical and psychosocial aspects of disability and be able to use counseling theories and techniques when serving clients with physical, emotional, or cognitive disabilities.

Public Sector

Initially rehabilitation counselors were employed exclusively by the state/federal system, or public sector, that was created by the Soldiers Rehabilitation Act (1918) and Smith-Fess Act (1920). Rehabilitation counselors working in the public sector are state employees who function under federal guidelines that regulate the services that may be provided to clients with disabilities. Public sector rehabilitation counselors work with clients who qualify for, primarily free, services if they meet certain eligibility criteria. In some instances, clients may be required to assist in the payment for certain services (e.g., postsecondary education) if they have the financial means to do so. The eligibility criteria have been modified by legislation over the years. The most recent criteria are set out by the 1992 Rehabilitation Act Amendments and indicate that an individual is eligible for rehabilitation services under the following conditions:

1. He or she is an individual with a disability (meaning a physical or mental impairment that for the individual constitutes or results in a substantial impediment to employment).

2. He or she requires vocational rehabilitation services to prepare for, enter, engage in, or retain gainful employment (it is assumed that the individual can benefit, in terms of employment outcome, from vocational rehabilitation services).

Public sector rehabilitation counselors work with a variety of clients with disabilities that fall into three domains: physical (e.g., amputation, spinal cord injury, arthritis), emotional (e.g., schizophrenia, substance abuse, depression), or cognitive (traumatic brain injury, stroke, epilepsy). Public sector rehabilitation counselors tend to have large caseloads; it is not unusual for their caseloads to vary from 100 to 200 clients. Because they have large caseloads, they must prioritize their time and work more intensely with clients who are at critical phases in their rehabilitation (e.g., clients who are job ready). Clients may be at one of a number of phases or stages in their rehabilitation; these stages are categorized using "status codes." Cooper and Davis (1979) conceptualized the two-digit status codes in public rehabilitation to exist in three categories. The preservice status codes indicate the client's progress prior to the direct delivery of rehabilitation service. These codes are 00—Referral; 02—Application for Services; 06—Extended Evaluation; 10—IWRP Development; 12—IWRP Completed. The second category contains the service statuses: 14—Counseling; 16—Physical Restoration; 18—Training; 20—Job Ready; 22—Employed; 24—Service Interrupted. The third category of statuses is the closure statuses: 08—Ineligible for Services; 26—Successful Case Closure—Rehabilitated; 28—Not Rehabilitated from a Service Status; 30—Not Rehabilitated from Statuses 10 or 12.

Public sector rehabilitation counselors are allocated dollars in a yearly budget for which they are responsible; the sizes of these budgets vary depending on the size of caseloads, agency location, and state funding practices. Public sector rehabilitation counselors must choose which clients to fund, what services they will pay for, and when they will pay for services. Hence, public sector rehabilitation counselors exercise budgetary authority over their caseload as one form of caseload management authority (Roessler & Rubin, 1992). The services purchased may be anything, within reason, that is necessary to help clients achieve their rehabilitation goals. Typical public rehabilitation services include transportation, retraining, vocational testing, job-search clubs, medical evaluations, physical therapy, and so on. Because of the large size of public sector caseloads, much of the rehabilitation counselor's time is spent in case management activities (Rubin et al., 1984). Nonetheless, counseling, assessment, and job placement are the primary rehabilitation counselor's job functions (Vandergoot & Worral, 1979).

Private Not-For-Profit Sector

The second area of rehabilitation counseling practice is referred to as the private not-for-profit or nonprofit sector. Rehabilitation counselors who work in this sector are primarily employed in rehabilitation facilities that sell their services to public sector rehabilitation counselors and other referral sources capable of paying for their services (e.g., insurance companies). The three main types of rehabilitation facilities are rehabilitation workshops, comprehensive rehabilitation centers, and residential programs (Wright, 1980). Many rehabilitation facilities seek accreditation by the Commission on Accreditation of Rehabilitation Facilities (CARF). CARF was created in 1966 and is the body that sets and monitors quality standards for rehabilitation facilities and their staff. Although the private not-for-profit rehabilitation sector existed in the United States for many years (e.g., the Cleveland Rehabilitation Center was established in 1898), the public rehabilitation program largely ignored rehabilitation facilities until around World War II (Wright, 1980). Rubin and Roessler (1995) stated that rehabilitation facilities' ". . . widespread development had been restricted by the limited 'training around the disability' focus of state rehabilitation agencies" (p. 282). Rehabilitation facilities experienced rapid growth, however, after World War II. The facilities' nonprofit status means that they return all monies generated back to the facility and that they are tax-exempt entities.

Regarding rehabilitation workshops, the Rehabilitation Act Amendments of 1954 gave federal monies as seed money for rehabilitation facilities, and the number of new workshops doubled from 1950 to 1965 (Nelson, 1971). Although workshops serve the full range of the disabled population, clients with mental retardation, developmental disabilities, or chronic mental illness are their primary clientele (Wright, 1980). Rehabilitation counselors working in sheltered workshops provide services such as vocational evaluation, work adjustment training, and sheltered employment to people who are not able to function in competitive work environments. Today, workshops have expanded to include supported employment services, which entail placing clients into competitive job sites with the assistance of job coaches (Lam, 1986).

Clients of comprehensive rehabilitation centers comprise the entire spectrum of disabilities, often having more severe disabilities and more complicated rehabilitation prognoses (Wright, 1980). In comprehensive rehabilitation centers, the rehabilitation counselor is a member of an interdisciplinary rehabilitation team that includes physicians, psychologists, nurses, physical therapists, occupational therapists, and other health allied professionals. Comprehensive rehabilitation centers have a medical model orientation, with the rehabilitation team being headed by the physician. As a part of this team, rehabilitation counselors are typically engaged in vocational evaluation and counseling, rehabilitation plan development, and referral.

Residential facilities focus on community living issues for people with disabilities and include halfway houses, supported apartment living, and other community living situations. The rehabilitation services provided by residential facilities vary, depending on the needs of their clients and the resources of the particular community. Services may range from providing food and shelter, to behavioral-based programs in activities of daily living, to group therapy, to structured recreational activities. Richmond (1972) pointed out the following:

> An essential feature that distinguishes these (rehabilitation) residences from other housing, however, is the influence of the group in acting as an agent for change. . . . Techniques used by the staff may involve a range of treatment modalities including milieu therapy, behavior modification, and reality therapy. (p. 207)

The substance abuse treatment field has employed the residential approach to substance abuse treatment for many years. The rationale has been the importance of removing substance abusing clients from environments that reinforce drug use. The residential program then offers a milieu approach that would break the reinforcement cycle between the individual and his or her environment. Residential treatment programs for clients with substance abuse will be discussed in Chapter 8.

Private For-Profit Sector

The third major sector of practice in rehabilitation counseling is the private for-profit sector. Rehabilitation counselors in this sector market their rehabilitation services to third-party payers (e.g., insurance companies) and run rehabilitation businesses for a profit. This is the most recent sector (it did not exist before 1970), but it is also the fastest-growing area of rehabilitation practice (Matkin & Riggar, 1986). Today, private sector rehabilitation counselors are employed in very diverse settings, such as hospitals, multidisciplinary clinics, private practice, private-for-profit rehabilitation companies, outplacement counseling services, employee assistance programs, and private industry (Desmond, 1985; Garvin, 1985; Lemons & Sweeney, 1981; Lynch & Herbert, 1984; Matkin, 1983; Roessler, 1983; Scofield & Andrews, 1981; Shrey, 1979; Szymanski, 1984). The majority of private for-profit rehabilitation counselors work with workers compensation clients. These are people who were employed but were injured on the job, and their injuries resulted in long-standing problems that prevented them from returning to work.

Because of the varied settings in which they work, rehabilitation counselors in the private for-profit sector offer a multitude of services requiring divergent skills. In general, private for-profit rehabilitation counselors have smaller caseloads and work more intensely with their clients. Matkin (1983) believed that while there were differences between the private for-profit sector and the other sectors, these differences are transitory or specific to the idiosyncratic demands of each type of employment setting. He identified the most notable differences between the private and public sectors of practice as caseload size, disability type, client eligibility, rehabilitation goals and services, job placement, forensic involvement, case recording, funding sources, administration, and personnel hiring. Weed and Field (1994), however, identified a number of meaningful similarities between the two sectors, including a common rehabilitation philosophy; knowledge of medical, psychological, and vocational aspects of disability; skill in assessment or evaluation; familiarity with and use of occupational or world of work information; knowledge of community and assistive resources; ability to establish rapport (basic counseling skills); and rehabilitation plan development, implementation, and reporting.

Discussion Question: Because of differences in caseload sizes and work environment, would you expect substance abuse disability to be handled differently in the public sector than in the private for-profit sector? Justify your answer.

THE REHABILITATION PHILOSOPHY

A clear philosophy leads to consistency of practice and a straightforward link between the "means" and the "purpose" (Wright, 1980). An understanding of the rehabilitation counseling profession's values, outlook, or philosophy will aid in understanding rehabilitation counseling practice. The rehabilitation philosophy underpins practice with all clients. An entire book could be devoted to the philosophy of modern rehabilitation practice. For the purposes of this textbook, however, five major concepts of the rehabilitation philosophy will be presented: intrinsic worth, capacity for change, self-determination, productive activity, and commitment.

Intrinsic worth of the client implies that rehabilitation counselors have value and respect for clients. Clients, regardless of their abilities or disabilities, deserve respect and dignity based on their inherent worth as individuals (Arokiasamy,

1993). Putting this principle into practice, rehabilitation counselors ought to focus on assets and strengths of their clients, rather than dwelling on their limitations. The importance of the client's intrinsic worth and client primacy in the rehabilitation process is clearly spelled out in Cannon 2 of the rehabilitation counseling code of ethics:

> Rehabilitation counselors shall respect the integrity and protect the welfare of people and groups with whom they work. The primary obligation of rehabilitation counselors is to their clients, defined as people with disabilities who are receiving services from rehabilitation counselors. Rehabilitation counselors shall endeavor at all times to place their clients' interests above their own (Commission on Rehabilitation Counselor Certification, 1987).

Capacity for change implies that, regardless of how longstanding or severe a client's problems are, the client is capable of changing past patterns of behavior and creating new, more functional behaviors. This principle is related to intrinsic worth because even a client who does deplorable things (e.g., abandons his or her family, steals, sells drugs), has the capacity for positive change that justifies the counselor's efforts to facilitate rehabilitation. This concept is especially important for working with clients who are frustrating or appear to be fixed in a current lifestyle or situation, which is often the case for clients with substance abuse problems. If the counselor cannot fully believe that the client is capable of change, the counselor should strive to recapture this belief or refer the client to another professional. When a counselor believes that the client is incapable of change, it is inevitable that this belief will be communicated to the client, with the result that the client may internalize this belief and give up on himself or herself. Fortunately, the reverse may also be true, and the counselor's belief in the client's capacity for change can empower the client to become more functional and effective. Personal responsibility for change is important for clients because rehabilitation counselors are only able to facilitate the change process. Clients are ultimately responsible for the time, energy, and effort necessary to change their behavior, participate in their rehabilitation, and achieve their goals.

Self-determination implies that rehabilitation counselors believe that client involvement is absolutely necessary for attainment of rehabilitation goals. People with disabilities are responsible for themselves and their outcomes and have an absolute right to participate in identifying goals and developing plans designed to achieve those goals. This philosophical principle is manifested by the clients' involvement in the development of their rehabilitation plans. Client self-determination is necessary for clients to have a stake in the "ownership" of their rehabilitation plan. Rehabilitation plans will have a higher probability of success if clients have fully participated in identifying goals and developing plans because client time, energy, and effort will be necessary to follow through with the most critical aspects of their rehabilitation program.

Productive activity acknowledges that people with disabilities, like everyone else, live within a larger society that serves to meet many of their needs and, in turn, influences behavior through social norms and mores (Neff, 1977). Because we are social animals, everyone is motivated to belong to a group, to be full members and contribute to the good of their community or society. In re-habilitation, productive activity often takes the form of work, which is usually the ultimate rehabilitation outcome. Having a job, obtaining an income from productive activity, fosters independence rather than dependence, which is fos-tered by entitlement programs. Work has many psychological advantages; in fact, it is often recommended as treatment for people with depression and other forms of mental illness (i.e., work therapy). Benefits from employment, aside from wages necessary for economic survival, certainly include such things as value and worth from others, positive self-esteem, contribution to the self-concept, and a sense of belongingness to a larger group (Neff, 1977).

The philosophical principle of *commitment* means that rehabilitation coun-selors believe that they can be effective facilitators in the rehabilitation process and that the process will result in positive change. Hence, assessment, counsel-ing, planning, service coordination, job placement, and similar services may all be combined, and this approach will result in effective rehabilitation programs and successful outcomes for clients. Commitment to the rehabilitation process also means that rehabilitation counselors persevere, do not give up on clients, and continue on in the face of rehabilitation plan setbacks and failures. Glasser's (1967) concepts regarding commitment are consistent with the reha-bilitation philosophy. Behaviors and rehabilitation plans may fail, but clients will not if they persevere. Giving up is seen as inconsistent with rehabilitation because it destroys the client-counselor relationship, damages the client's sense of self-worth, and cuts off client alternatives. If rehabilitation plans fail, the committed rehabilitation counselor will help the client cycle back to any one of the earlier steps in the rehabilitation process, identify errors or problems, modify the plan, and begin again.

Discussion   Use the 12 Steps of Alcoholics Anonymous to operationalize a
Question: substance abuse treatment philosophy. In what ways is it similar
                  to and different from the rehabilitation philosophy?

TERMINOLOGY AND
IMPORTANT CONCEPTS

The language and terminology of a field are important to understanding its concepts and approach toward problems. Hence, these terms and concepts are basic to rehabilitation and will be used throughout this textbook.

Disability: A disability is any medically diagnosable (by a physician, psychi-atrist, psychologist, or similarly qualified professional) physical, cognitive, or emotional condition that is chronic or permanent in nature (i.e., a nontempo-rary condition). This condition must result in a limitation of function that causes a handicap or multiple handicaps. For example, for a drinking problem to be considered a disability, it must be diagnosed by a qualified professional, usually using the Diagnostic and Statistical Manual-IV (DSM-IV) criteria of Alcohol Dependence (303.90). The functional limitations associated with this condition may be persistent or recurrent physical or psychological problems that are likely to have been caused or exacerbated by alcohol (DSM-IV, 1994).

Functional limitation: Limitations in physical, behavioral, cognitive, or emotional function that result from disability are referred to as functional limitations. Functional limitations exist in such areas as mobility (e.g., inability to walk resulting from the disability of spinal cord injury), communication (e.g., inability to hear conversational speech resulting from deafness), sensory acuity (e.g., finger numbness resulting from peripheral neuropathy), atypical appearance (e.g., having a missing limb due to traumatic amputation), and pain (chronic leg discomfort resulting from a herniated disc in the lower spine) (Wright, 1980). While medical diagnosis and prognosis are the primary concerns of physicians and other medical professionals, functional limitations are the primary concerns of rehabilitation counselors.

Handicap: Handicaps are the barriers to achieving goals that are created by functional limitations imposed by a disability. They are the actual obstacles that a person with a disability encounters in the pursuit of life goals, no matter what the source (handicaps are usually thought of as existing in one's environment). The nature of a handicap depends on the context; for instance, the amputation of a little finger for a bus driver is probably not handicapping, but it can be substantially handicapping to a concert violinist. Other handicaps are more universal and include such things as a lack of ramps to get into buildings, inaccessible public transportation, television programs without closed captioning, employer bias in hiring practices, and negative societal attitudes toward people with disabilities. Historically, it has been the practice to use the terms *disability* and *handicap* interchangeably. Given these definitions, however, it is clear that an important distinction exists: People have *disabilities,* while environments impose *handicaps.*

Rehabilitation: The classic definition of rehabilitation comes from a symposium of the National Council on Rehabilitation held in New York in 1942 (Wright, 1980). This definition was adopted by the International Labor Office, established in 1973, and still applies to today's rehabilitation counselor. Rehabilitation was defined as "The restoration of the handicapped [*sic*] to the fullest physical, mental, social, vocational, and economic usefulness of which they are capable" (p. 1). This sweeping definition is idealistic and should be considered the ultimate goal of rehabilitation counseling. Similarly, Arokiasamy (1993) defined rehabilitation as ". . . a holistic and integrated program of medical, physical, psychological, psychosocial, and vocational interventions that empower a disabled person to achieve a socially meaningful and functionally effective interaction with the world and a requisite level of personal autonomy" (p. 84). In practice rehabilitation professionals help clients identify obtainable life goals and assist in the process by planning and providing or coordinating services designed to achieve those goals.

Rehabilitation process: The rehabilitation process is conceptualized as a planned and ordered set of activities that are designed to help clients identify an appropriate goal or goals, activating client movement toward that goal, and achieving the goal in a timely manner. According to Roessler and Rubin (1992), rehabilitation goals should be identified with the collaboration of the client and his or her family, while services and practice management procedures are set by the rehabilitation counselor, and case coordination is conducted in conjunction with external community service personnel. The rehabilitation process is conceptualized as a sequential progression of steps:

1. Intake
2. Evaluation/assessment
3. Eligibility determination (public sector only)
4. Counseling and rehabilitation plan development
5. Plan implementation and provision of services
6. Placement and follow-up

   (Monitoring and problem solving performed continuously throughout the entire process)

Rehabilitation program or plan: The rehabilitation plan or program is created by the rehabilitation counselor and his or her client as a service strategy. The development of an Individualized Written Rehabilitation Program (IWRP) was mandated by the 1973 Rehabilitation Act for all rehabilitation counselors and clients in the state/federal sector. Because of the utility of individualized and formalized (written) plans, they are regularly used by all rehabilitation counselors regardless of the sector in which they work. The 1992 Rehabilitation Act Amendments identified the minimum, essential components of an Individualized Written Rehabilitation Program as (1) a statement of the long-term rehabilitation goals for the client and the intermediate rehabilitation objects that are logically tied to attaining the goals; (2) a statement of the particular rehabilitation services to be provided; (3) a method of accountability to determine whether or not the intermediate and long-term goals are being attained; and (4) information from the client that indicates the nature of his or her involvement in choosing among the possible goals. Most recently, legislation has changed the IWRP to the designation IPE (Individual Plan for Employment).

Vocational rehabilitation: The International Labor Office (1973) defined vocational rehabilitation as "The continuous and coordinated process of rehabilitation which involves the provision of those vocational services, e.g., vocational guidance, vocational training and selective placement, designed to enable a disabled person to secure and retain suitable employment" (p. 4). Therefore, vocational rehabilitation uses vocational counseling theories and approaches to assist clients in identifying a suitable vocational goal and development and implementation of a plan to achieve the vocational goal. The typical services provided in vocational rehabilitation counseling are work adjustment training, vocational evaluation, job-seeking skills instruction, job placement, and placement follow-up to maintain employment.

SUMMARY

Chapter 1 presented an overview of the history and practice of rehabilitation counseling for the nonrehabilitation counseling student or professional. The overview was intended to provide a foundation necessary for understanding the application of rehabilitation counseling principles and practices in the context of substance abuse treatment. Historically, the stage for the emergence of the rehabilitation counseling was set during the turn of the century when the United States was being transformed by industrialization, increases in population, urbanization, developments in medical and health practices, and vocational education.

Federal legislation was seen as initiating the development of rehabilitation in the United States, beginning with the Soldiers Rehabilitation Act of 1918. When compared to other professions, rehabilitation counseling has had a relatively brief history. The occupation was created in the 1920s, and professionalization began after the Rehabilitation Act Amendments of 1954 provided funding for graduate-level training programs. The most recent piece of federal legislation, having the broadest impact on people with disabilities, was the Americans with Disabilities Act of 1990.

Federal legislation will continue to be passed and influence the field of rehabilitation counseling; however, its impact may be lessened by the expansion and diversification of the field. Rehabilitation counseling has organized itself into three distinct sectors of practice: public, private not-for-profit, and the private for-profit sectors. The marked expansion of rehabilitation counseling, especially in the private sector, has resulted in rehabilitation counselors being employed in a wide variety of sites, such as hospitals, multidisciplinary clinics, private practice, private for-profit rehabilitation companies, outplacement counseling services, employee assistance programs, and private industry.

Chapter 1 also included a discussion of the primary tenets of rehabilitation philosophy. The principles of client intrinsic worth, capacity for change, and right to self-determination were presented, along with the importance that rehabilitation counselors place upon productive activity and commitment—both to the client and the rehabilitation process. A clear understanding of the rehabilitation philosophy is hoped to lead to consistency of practice and a straightforward link between the means and purpose of rehabilitation counseling.

Finally, basic rehabilitation terms and concepts were introduced to provide the reader with a clearer understanding of the meanings of disability, functional limitation, handicap, rehabilitation, rehabilitation process, rehabilitation program or plan, and vocational rehabilitation. These concepts will applied to discussion of substance abuse treatment throughout the rest of this text.

2

Drug and
Alcohol History

ALCOHOL AND DRUGS
IN THE 18TH AND 19TH CENTURIES

The history of drug and alcohol use, abuse, dependency, and treatment is a pastiche of cultural influences, morality standards, legal and bureaucratic regulatory activities, business conditions, and clinical/professional developments. It is notable that an initial problem of George Washington's presidency was the Whiskey Rebellion of 1790 that merged business interests, morality concerns, and regulatory policy (Doweiko, 1996). Alcoholism as a social issue surfaced in the 1830s and 1840s when religious groups opposed alcohol inebriation, starting the first temperance movement and laying the foundation for the development of the Moral Model of alcohol use (Fisher & Harrison, 1997; White, 1997). Shortly afterwards, the American Association for the Study and Cure of Inebriety was founded, public and private for-profit inebriate asylums were opened, and a variety of medical and patent medicine cures were developed for the treatment of alcoholism. In 1876 the *Journal of Inebriety* began publication to disseminate treatment and research findings about inebriation treatment (Kinney & Leaton, 1995). Ironically, many patent medicines touted as inebriation cures contained mixtures of alcohol and opium or alcohol and cocaine. The first notion of alcoholism as a disease caused by inherited characteristics or environmental/developmental influences appears in the 1870s, giving rise to a network of more than 500 alcoholism treatment centers (White, 1997). As the 19th century progressed, temperance philosophies gave way to prohibitionist sentiments voiced by groups such as Women's Christian Temperance Union (WCTU) and the Anti-Saloon League (Jung, 1994). The industrial revolution and America's shift from a rural-based, agrarian economy to an urban-based, industrial economy contributed to the growth of this prohibitionist sentiment. Employers supported prohibitionist stances, often as a matter of paternalistic company policy. Many industrialists of the 19th century held conservative Protestant religious views that they were not reticent to impose upon their employees. More importantly, the development of mass production, assembly line business practices, and sophisticated but dangerous machinery altered the face of the industrial environment. Absences or accidents caused by drunkenness resulted in lost productivity and lost revenue. Business sentiments were not always driven by concern for the worker. In the coalfields of the 1890s mules were used to haul coal from the mine to the surface, and the job of leading the mules was very important and very dangerous. Accidents involving the mules usually brought mining to a halt. Companies learned quickly that many accidents were related to alcohol consumption, and miners in charge of the mules were subject to immediate termination of employment if they reported to work in an intoxicated condition. However, the company's concern was not for the miner but for the mule. Training a mule to enter the mines was troublesome, and a mule lost in an accident was difficult to replace; conversely, miners were easily trained and replaced.

The shift from a temperance, controlled use philosophy to a prohibitionist model marked a shift in public perception of alcoholism as a moral failing or medical problem to that of alcohol consumption as socially proscribed behavior. Thus, the notion of criminalization of drug-taking behavior was born.

Alcohol was not the only drug of concern in the 19th century. Marijuana was cultivated for its hemp fibers and for its medicinal and intoxicating purposes. Evidence shows Washington grew hemp at Mt. Vernon, and large hemp plantations were mainstays of the southern rural economy until it became cheaper to grow and process cotton with the invention of the cotton gin. Worldwide, marijuana has been cultivated for at least 5000 years (Abadinsky, 1997) for both its industrial and intoxicating uses. The honeycomb and honeywood of the Old Testament Song of Solomon are probably marijuana; Brecher (1972) refers to pharmacological and historical records revealing marijuana cultivation and use by the ancient Greeks, Persians, Chinese, and Native Americans. He notes that the Spaniards introduced marijuana to the New World during their explorations and conquests in South America during the 1500s. Others have asserted the drug was first introduced to the Western Hemisphere through the Brazilian slave trade in the 1600s. Technically termed *cannabis sativa,* the word *marijuana* comes from the Spanish word *maraguango,* meaning "a substance that causes intoxication."

The isolation of cocaine from the coca bush and the discovery of its use as a therapeutic agent is generally attributed to German scientists working about the middle part of the 19th century. Cocaine use as coca leaf chewing among South American indigenous peoples dates back centuries. For the Incas, the coca bush was of divine origin (Abadinsky, 1997), and coca chewing was a rigidly controlled practice more highly honored than the possession of gold or silver. Following the Spanish conquests, the Spaniards took control of the coca practices, and consequently controlled the populace. Rather than reserving the drug for ceremonial or royal uses, the Spanish made the drug available to slaves to boost stamina and suppress hunger and fatigue. Interestingly, neither Incan nor European accounts record any evidence of cocaine addiction among indigenous users, either before or after Spanish occupation. Coca chewing never caught on among the Spaniards or other European groups, probably because it was regarded as a heathen practice.

By the latter half of the 19th century the medicinal qualities of cocaine were established, as was a growing awareness of the abuse potential of the drug. Medicinal use of cocaine had been introduced to Europe as Mariani's wine, an elixir containing wine and coca leaves (Brecher, 1972), and reportedly Pope Leo XIII and other Christian ascetics used Mariani's wine to overcome hunger and fatigue during fasting and arduous rituals. Other famous boosters of Mariani's wine included Gounod, Massente, Thomas Edison, the kings of Sweden and Norway, the prince of Wales, and the czar of Russia (Brecher, 1972; Goldberg, 1997). In this country cocaine became a constituent of many popular patent medicines and was an ingredient of the popular soft drink Coca-Cola™. Before inventing Coca-Cola™, Atlanta resident John Styth Pemberton marketed several patent medicines including the cocaine-laced *French Wine Coca—Ideal Nerve and Tonic Stimulant.*

Sigmund Freud's encounter with cocaine is well documented in the psychology literature. Freud's adherence to cocaine stemmed from his self-treatment of his own digestive problems and depression; he recommended it as a treatment for morphine addiction also (Goldberg, 1997). Freud prescribed the drug for a variety of ailments suffered by friends, family, colleagues, and patients, but he recanted his support when a colleague suffered a cocaine psychosis while under Freud's care.

The use of opium (*Papaver Somniferum*) as either medicine, religious ritual sacramental element, or recreational drug dates back to the Stone Ages. The dried juice of the opium poppy capsule was introduced to the United States by many routes in the 19th century. Opium in medicinal form came to this country from Europe about the time of the Revolutionary War. In 1799 an opium alkaloid, morphine, was extracted by a German pharmacist (Abadinsky, 1997). Mistakenly thought to be nonaddictive and with few side effects, morphine became the principal component of many patent medicines. Chinese immigrants in the 1850s introduced recreational use of opium in the form of opium smoking, and in the last half of that century operated legal commercial opium smoking establishments known popularly as "opium dens," which were regarded much like saloons (Abadinsky, 1997). Indeed, Brecher (1972) calls the 19th century "a dope fiend's paradise" (p. 3). Opium and morphine were available as prescription and patent medicines dispensed by physicians and pharmacists, general stores, mail order houses, opium dens, drugstores, and itinerant sales agents. Among the ailments treated by opiate-laced compounds were toothaches, "women trouble," diarrhea and dysentery, pulmonary disorders, pain, and consumption (tuberculosis). Morphine was used on a large and indiscriminate scale during the Civil War. So many Civil War veterans became dependent on the drug, used to treat pain, fatigue, and dysentery, that the phrase "Soldiers Disease" entered the lexicon to describe opiate addiction. Toward the end of that century heroin was isolated by European scientists as an antidote for morphine or opium addiction. The addicting qualities of opium and its derivatives were well known in the 19th century, and individuals with opiate dependency problems faced a certain amount of social approbation. This was especially the case for individuals whose dependence resulted from recreational rather than medicinal use. Importantly, however, addiction was not met with the legal or moral sanctions present in today's society (Brecher, 1972). Addicts participated in the community, raising children, working, attending school and church, and interacting with the rest of society. The acceptance of addicts as community members rather than as social pariahs forestalled the development of a deviant addiction subculture, isolated and cut off from the support systems of family and community.

Most regard inhalant and hallucinogen use as products of modern chemistry; however, inhalant use has been documented throughout recorded history. Inhalation as a practice to ingest intoxicating substances has been recorded among ancient Babylonians, Scythians, Egyptians, Africans, and the indigenous peoples of North and South America (Goldberg, 1997; Inaba & Cohen, 1989). The first manufactured, synthetic inhalant was most likely nitrous oxide, invented by English chemist Sir Humphrey Davy in 1776 (Goldberg, 1997). Still in use today as a minor anesthetic, nitrous oxide was and is abused for its euphoric effects, although much of its use and abuse has been traditionally limited to groups who have easy access to the drug (i.e., health care providers). Other inhalants with a long history of abuse include ether and chloroform, but again, users have tended to be individuals with access to these drugs (Brecher, 1972). Problems related to inhalant abuse of volatile solvents such as gasoline, paint thinner, glue, and hair spray do not appear in the professional literature until the latter half of the 20th century. However, it is likely individuals had discovered the intoxicating effects of volatile solvent inhalation long before.

Hallucinogens were not invented by Timothy Leary and his colleagues during their experiments with LSD during the 1960s, although this is the time when hallucinogenic chemicals first attracted widespread attention. In truth, hallucinogenic substances were in use in North and Central America during pre-Columbian times, both for ceremonial purposes and intoxication. According to Doweiko, the indigenous people of Central America have a history of hallucinogenic mushroom use (*Amanita muscaria*) dating from 1500 BC. Further, he asserts peyote use among the Native American population of the America Southwest and Northern Mexico may date back 7000 years. Peyote continues to play an important ceremonial role in the rituals of the Native American Church of the United States (Hanson & Venturelli, 1995). While little recorded use of hallucinogenic substance use by European settlers in the New World exists, it is known they were aware of the properties of Jamestown weed. Named for the first colony of English settlers in the United States, this substance is also called jimsonweed or locoweed.

THE LEGISLATIVE ERA—1900 TO 1936

By the turn of the century several forces began to coalesce to deal with growing social problems related to drug and alcohol abuse. The Anti-Saloon League had been founded in 1893 and was a growing political force, successful in mobilizing a number of groups, notably the Protestant church and its hierarchy, toward the goal of national prohibition (Abadinsky, 1997). Professional groups such as the American Medical Association began to advocate for greater regulation of patent medicines, a sentiment echoed by the popular media. Populist and Progressive political factions began to call for government intervention to protect the safety, welfare, and opportunities of the citizenry overall and the workforce in particular (Rubin & Roessler, 1995). In 1906 Upton Sinclair published his exposé of the Chicago meat-packing industry, *The Jungle* (Fishbein & Pease, 1996), describing the filth, disease, and unsanitary practices of that industry. Public uproar and response were immediate and vocal; meat sales plummeted. In response to these forces, Congress passed the Pure Food and Drug Act of 1906. The act did two fundamental things: it established the Food and Drug Administration as a federal regulatory body, and it required all packaged foods and drugs, including patent medicines, to carry a label listing their ingredients. For the first time, the quantity of opium, cocaine, and other drugs contained in patent medicines was regulated. Fishbein and Pease assert that patent medicine use declined by a third following passage of the act and promulgation of ingredients. Additionally, overall opiate addiction rates fell, as other Americans began to control their drug consumption.

The same political factions that supported the Pure Food and Drug Act also motivated changes in the workplace during the first decade of the 20th century. Before 1900 workers who were injured on the job had limited recourse; they could sue their employers for damages and compensation but most often lost because the system was stacked in favor of business and industry (Jenkins, Patterson, & Szymanski, 1992). The public demand for protection from unsafe working conditions and the establishment of just compensation resulted in the development of workers' compensation laws by the federal government and by the states. For the first time workers suffering on-the-job accidents were granted a degree of compensation. To be sure, compensation varied from state to state, and many occupations were excluded from coverage. Nonetheless, workers and families were protected from sure poverty resulting from workplace-caused disability. Alcoholism and drug addiction were not covered disabilities under this legislation, but workers who were involved in alcohol and drug-related accidents were eligible for compensation, especially if the accident was caused by a fellow worker who was intoxicated.

Worldwide concern was growing for drug- and alcohol-related problems also. Many European countries had vast colonial empires, especially in Asia and the South Pacific, and opium consumption was a growing concern. In part this was a consequence of imperialistic practices; missionaries and other prohibitionist forces were calling for the eradication of drug abuse that they cited as the cause of ignorance, poverty, disease, and despair (Abadinsky, 1997). Others were less beneficent in their view of drug consumption; local laws regulating opium smoking in the United States were passed only after it was discovered that white Euro-Americans were becoming addicted; Chinese addicts were viewed as disgusting and immoral (Fishbein & Pease, 1996). African Americans were depicted as intemperate consumers of cocaine who became crazed, violent, and licentious when under the influence of the drug. While some forces were seeking to control drug consumption, other forces, notably business and colonial expansionist groups, fought against regulation. Portugal, Holland, Persia, and Russia were concerned with maintaining their profitable opium poppy trade, and Germany sought to protect its burgeoning pharmaceutical industry (Abadinsky, 1997). In the United States, sentiment was divided. Pharmacist members of the American Pharmaceutical Association favored patent medicine regulation, while commercial members (drugstore owners and manufacturers) did not; southern politicians objected to any form of federal regulation of drugs on states-rights platforms. Globally, the United States was seeking to improve trade relations with China and promised to help with its severe internal opium addiction problem (Abadinsky, 1997). Ironically, many scholars believe China's opium problems can be traced directly to earlier British colonial and commercial interventions.

In 1913 the Hague International Opium Convention agreements calling for controls on opium, morphine, and cocaine abuse were ratified by the U.S. Congress (Abadinsky, 1997), and the next year the Harrison Narcotic Act of 1914 was passed. "The chief proponent of the measure was Secretary of State William Jennings Bryan, a man of deep prohibitionist and missionary convictions and sympathies. He urged that the law be promptly passed to fulfill United States obligations under the new treaty" (Brecher, 1972, pp. 48–49). This was not an unusual position; many national leaders seemed more interested in imposing America's will and sense of morality about drug abuse on other nations than with dealing with domestic drug abuse problems.

Taken at face value, the Harrison Act was not a prohibitionist act but an act designed to regulate the orderly and safe marketing of opium, morphine, and cocaine. Under the law, individuals who were in the business of dispensing drugs covered in the act were required to register annually with the federal government and pay an annual fee of $1. Subsequent regulations promulgated by the Department of the Treasury, the responsible federal agency, limited registration to medical professionals and established the practice of maintaining records of all drugs that were dispensed (Abadinsky, 1997). Cocaine, opium, and morphine were removed from patent and over-the-counter medicine and could be prescribed by physicians only. In turn, the physicians were deluged by demands for prescriptions from individuals who had become addicted to previously legal pharmaceuticals and subjected to unprecedented scrutiny by Treasury agents. The law limited the prescribing of opiates to valid pharmacological treatment of disease in a time when addiction of and by itself was *not* considered a disease. In effect, the ability of physicians to prescribe opiates was removed, creating and initiating the underground market for opiate drugs that persists to this day. Addiction was transformed from a medical or moral problem to a criminal problem, and thousands of addicts and physicians were incarcerated for violations of the Harrison Act. Federal narcotics farms were established to "treat" individuals prosecuted under the act.

In 1919 the ultimate goal of the Prohibitionists was achieved with the passage of the 18th Amendment to the Constitution. Popularly known as the Volstead Act, the amendment banned the manufacture and sale of beverages containing alcohol. As was the case with the Harrison Act, previously legal activities became illegal at the stroke of a pen. The Volstead Act was more influential and widesweeping, however. It criminalized alcohol dependence and abuse behaviors, but it also criminalized alcohol use behaviors. Responsible businesses were forced to close down, and the market for certain farm products (grapes, hops, barley) virtually evaporated. Despite the total ban on alcohol, people still drank, got drunk, became alcoholic, and had alcohol-related accidents and died. Often alcohol-related accidents and illnesses were a result of consuming home-brewed alcohol (home brewing was legal), moonshine, or alcohol from questionable sources, since saloons and taverns were closed. During Prohibition drinking patterns shifted from beer drinking to hard liquor consumption, based on simple economics. Hard liquor was easier to transport illegally. Prohibition marked the emergence of organized crime as the principal supply and control force for illegal alcohol and was the forebearer of the role of crime in illegal drug distribution. In fact, "Marijuana, a drug little used in the United States, was first popularized during the period of alcohol Prohibition . . . and ether was also imbibed" (Brecher, 1972, p. 266). Control of alcohol-consuming behaviors shifted from social and religious mechanisms to law enforcement. The country soon recognized that the losses caused by Prohibition outnumbered the gains, and the 21st Amendment repealed Prohibition, granting power to the individual states to opt to be wet or dry. In 1966 Mississippi was the last state to abolish statewide prohibition of alcohol. However, individual governmental entities (counties, cities, townships) retain the right to impose local sanctions against the manufacture, distribution, or consumption of alcohol.

Discussion Question: What are some local legal sanctions against alcohol consumption?

The ostensible purpose of The Marijuana Tax Act of 1937 was to regulate the medical use and dispensing of marijuana, then a drug included in the *United States Pharmacopeia*, the standards for drug preparation and dispensation. In reality, passage of the act was a direct result of a public campaign and resultant hysteria that equated marijuana use with cocaine or opium use (Abadinsky, 1997). Cultural implications came into the arena: many southwestern states had established antimarijuana laws to control marijuana use among Mexican immigrants, who were believed to participate in violent crime because of marijuana ingestion. Abadinsky writes that Harry Anslinger, commissioner of the Federal Bureau of Narcotics from 1930 to 1962, orchestrated a presentation before Congress that typified marijuana as a drug whose evils caused moral, mental, and physical decay and suggested it was a scourge on society. Anslinger's campaign was successful, and marijuana legally became regarded as a narcotic, a status it maintained until 1972. Opposition to the act came from two unlikely groups, the American Medical Association and the manufacturers of birdseed. Brecher (1972) suggests the AMA took a rational approach. Few physicians prescribed *cannabis,* and to impose a tax and regulatory restrictions would impose an unnecessary burden to medical practice. Moreover, the AMA argued for maintenance of the pharmacological status of marijuana to permit its continued use and to study additional uses. Finally, the AMA argued that regulation of the medical profession was apt to have little impact on illegal recreational use of marijuana. Marijuana was removed from the *Pharmacopeia* and still has very limited medical use, despite evidence of its value in treating diseases such as glaucoma and the side effects of chemotherapy. Birdseed manufacturers opposed the bill with the argument that canaries would sing less sweetly if deprived of birdseed that included marijuana. In the end the act contained provisions permitting sterilized marijuana seeds in domestic birdseed.

Using the same model as the Harrison Act, medical practitioners, growers of marijuana, distributors, and importers were charged a fee, a tax was placed

on marijuana itself, and possession of marijuana was made illegal. Consequently, payment of the tax was tantamount to admission of possession of an
illegal substance, a clear violation of constitutional protections against self-in-
crimination (Hanson & Venturelli, 1995). Marijuana was later classified as a
Schedule I drug (as it still is today), a classification reserved for drugs with the
highest abuse potential and whose possession, use, and sale are punished with
the most stringent measures. In response to the federal legislation nearly all of
the states adopted marijuana prohibitions that equated marijuana with heroin
and were often more draconian in their penalties than the federal law.

Discussion   Should the use of marijuana be legalized for medical purposes?
Questions: What are the potential benefits and hazards of such legislation?

Noticeably absent from all of the antidrug and antialcohol laws were provisions for treatment, and treatment did not exist in any organized form. The
hospitals and asylums for the inebriated of the 19th century failed to survive
for a number of factors, according to White (1997). They failed to develop a
solid core technology and were unable to display sound evidence of successful
outcomes. They were expensive and appealed to the upper socioeconomic
class, excluding others. In addition, they failed to generate a unitary foundation of support, existing on the fringes of medicine, religion, charity, business,
and science. Finally, criminalization of drug- and alcohol-consuming behaviors resulted in closing of many treatment facilities. By 1920 White notes there
were 22 hospitals serving individuals with alcoholism problems, down from a
peak of over 500 in the latter part of the 19th century. Federal leadership in
antidrug and alcohol legislation effectively wrested control and responsibility
for intervention from the states. Consequently, local drug and alcohol problems were ignored or shunted off to an overloaded and underequipped federal
bureaucracy. This federal legislation established a model of drug and alcohol
restriction based on interdiction, control, and punishment—a federal policy
philosophy that persists and is dominant to this day. Service provision was
shifted to the states, a responsibility they mostly ignored, or to private charitable groups and health care organizations. Finally, the drug and alcohol policies
adopted in the early part of this century stigmatized a number of groups creating lasting impressions. Passage of legislation was often accomplished by
linking ethnic groups with drug types: the Chinese with opium; African
Americans with cocaine and marijuana; and Mexicans with marijuana. After
laws were enacted, individual users became stigmatized with stereotypic labels
that often had no basis in reality.

TREATMENT EMERGES: THE SIXTIES

In America, little concern about drug or alcohol problems was evident during
the forties and fifties. World War II raged from 1941 to 1945, diverting public
attention. Drug or alcohol use and abuse that might have harmed the war effort were considered unpatriotic yet socially sanctioned. Fears that military

personnel returning from the war might have addiction problems either from indiscriminate use of analgesic medication or from exposure to foreign cultures failed to come to fruition. The late forties and fifties were periods of industrial growth and prosperity unmatched by any other time in history. A few companies began to realize that alcohol problems resulted in productivity losses in the workplace, and a handful of employee assistance programs were begun. Most Americans were pursuing the American dream, with little interest in or tolerance for what might be perceived as deviant behavior. Federal drug control policy was firmly in the hands of Harry Anslinger and the Federal Bureau of Narcotics, and drug addiction reached all-time recorded lows, especially during the war years. Scarcity of opium was one reason for the decline, however. Most opium products went to the war effort for medicinal purposes, and when foreign-grown opium supplies were cut off, Congress passed the Opium Poppy Control Act of 1942, reestablishing the right of U.S. farmers to grow opium poppies (Hanson & Venturelli, 1995). Ironically, agricultural conditions for growing opium poppies in the United States never permitted a very productive or high-quality yield. Anslinger was instrumental in getting a number of federal laws (Boggs Act; Narcotic Control Act of 1956) passed, broadening the drug-control powers of the federal government and increasing the severity of punishment for narcotics and marijuana possession and use (Abadinsky, 1997; Hanson & Venturelli, 1995). State legislatures conformed to these trends by stiffening state and local drug-control regulations.

Emergence of the Drug Culture

If the fifties marked a decade of complacence and avoidance of drug and alcohol use and abuse, the sixties ushered in a decade of public drug use unlike any seen prior. Marijuana, previously driven underground by the Marijuana Tax Act of 1937, reemerged as a recreational drug, first used by the "beatnik" culture and adopted by the later "hippie" culture. Doweiko (1996) asserts marijuana became and remains the most popular recreational drug in the United States, Great Britain, and Germany. Marijuana use became so widespread by the mid-seventies that it was touted as one of California's largest cash crops; legalization was discussed openly in the popular media and politically advocated by NORML, the National Organization for the Reform of Marijuana Laws (Connor & Burns, 1995).

LSD (lysergic acid diethylamide) was popularized by the counterculture and by such diverse groups as researchers Drs. Timothy Leary and Richard Alpert of Harvard, the creative film community in Hollywood, and a group of psychiatrists and psychologists experimenting with hallucinogenics for the treatment of severe mental disorders (Abadinsky, 1997). The drug was popularized by the media and entertainment communities and vilified by the drug control bureaucracy. Apocryphal stories abounded about its pleasures and its dangers. In one instance the director of a state agency for the blind asserted the agency was treating a dozen young men because they had stared at the sun while under the influence of LSD, irrevocably damaging their retinas. Others hailed LSD for its mind-liberating properties and its ability to allow the user to find and know fundamental truths (Fishbein & Pease, 1996). "Psychedelic" entered the lexicon to describe both the effects of the drug and the counter-culture that grew around it. Alarmed by the popularity of LSD and other emerging drugs, Congress gave the Food and Drug Administration the power to regulate the development of new pharmaceuticals (Stevens, 1987). The American Medical Association editorialized against LSD in 1963, the same year Alpert and Leary were fired from Harvard. Shortly afterwards the United States placed LSD on the controlled substance list through the Drug Abuse Control Amendments of 1965, and Sandoz Pharmaceutical Laboratories ceased further research on the drug (Abadinsky, 1997; Fishbein & Pease, 1996; Hanson & Venturelli, 1995). Because of these restrictions and because of user concerns about adverse reactions, LSD consumption dropped dramatically. To-day the drug is enjoying a rebirth of popularity, although at lower-dosage lev-els than in the 1960s.

Heroin was the opiate drug of choice of the sixties, and its use became pandemic (Wilson, 1990). Interdiction efforts to control importation of heroin were largely unsuccessful; as Turkish supplies were cut off, Mexican supplies flourished. When Mexican poppy fields were eradicated, the source of supply shifted to Southeast Asia. "The Vietnam War was an important landmark for heroin use in the United States. It was estimated that as many as 40 percent of the U.S. soldiers serving in Southeast Asia at this time used heroin to combat the frustrations and stress associated with this unpopular military action" (Han-son & Venturelli, 1995, p. 238). The number of soldiers who continued to use heroin after their return home was only about 7 percent of the total veteran population, but they contributed significantly to the continued escalation of the heroin problem (Golding, 1993). By 1972 estimates placed the heroin ad-diction population at a half-million (Wilson, 1990), with the majority of ad-dicts injecting heroin intravenously.

Cocaine use remained quiescent through the sixties and much of the sev-enties until it was popularized by shifts in societal trends. Connor and Burns (1995) suggest that cocaine's association with money, glamour, discos, and the yuppie lifestyle moved its use from the sidelines of the drug culture to what Haaga and Reuter (1995) described as "epidemic proportions." A number of other factors contributed to the surge in cocaine use. Before 1980 treatment professionals and researchers considered cocaine a benign drug of limited abuse and no dependence potential (Davison & Neale, 1986). Almost no treatment services were available for individuals with cocaine problems (Washton & Gold, 1987), and cocaine was not classified as a dependence-causing drug by the third edition (1980) of the *Diagnostic and Statistical Man-ual of Mental Disorders* of the American Psychiatric Association. It was common for treatment professionals to minimize the impact of cocaine use, and substance abuse treatment textbooks of the seventies and early eighties rarely discussed cocaine treatment. Users were mainly limited to individuals seeking a stimulant rush, a marked contrast to the sedating, mellowing effects sought by heroin or marijuana users. As long as cocaine was available only in powder form and mainly ingested through nasal inhalation, users, society, and treatment professionals perceived few problems, especially concerning addiction (Rosenhan & Seligman, 1995). The invention of cocaine in a smokable form, first as freebase cocaine and later as crack cocaine, changed everything. Powder cocaine is alkaloid cocaine bound to (usually) hydrochloride salt. In this form it easily crosses mucous membrane barriers and readily dissolved in the blood for transportation to the brain (Siegel, 1987). Cocaine alkaloid is destroyed by heat, and the practice of sprinkling cocaine on marijuana cigarettes to create a dual-enhanced effect was futile. Freed of its hydrochloride base, however, cocaine is highly volatile, delivering a large amount of the drug to the brain in a few seconds (Jones, 1987). The very immediate, intense, and euphoric gratification contributed to the popularization of crack cocaine. No longer did users need to wait the two- or three-minute time lapse between snorting powder cocaine and the euphoric effect on the brain. The AIDS fear of the early eighties also contributed to the growth of crack cocaine. The appeal of intravenous drug use dropped dramatically when AIDS was linked to using unsafe needles. Crack cocaine use is often linked to unsafe heterosexual or homosexual sex practices, however, and many users may have traded one form of AIDS risk for another (Robe, Russell-Einhorn, & Baker, 1986; Wetli, 1987). Finally, the price of crack cocaine dropped substantially below powder cocaine, and it could more easily be transported, delivered in smaller doses, and concealed from the police and other authority figures. In many ways crack cocaine distribution was done in textbook marketing style. A heterogeneous population of individuals who wanted and needed the drug was created quickly. The product itself was low priced, easily consumed, and resulted in near instant gratification, and it appeared to have few dangerous side effects such as an overdose, disease contraction through dirty needles, or septal perforation, a danger of intranasal ingestion of powder cocaine.

The dependence-inducing properties of crack cocaine became quickly apparent. Compulsive, repetitive use takes over the life of the individual addicted to crack cocaine, resulting in mounting legal, vocational, marital, occupational, physical, and emotional health problems (Benshoff & Riggar, 1990; Extein & Dackis, 1987). Indeed, the dangers posed by cocaine dependence caused a rethinking and reshaping of the clinical issue of addiction. Formerly, addiction was understood as compulsive use and defined by the physical consequences of withdrawal and tolerance. Addicts are driven to use, and discontinuation of the addicting drug leads to physical discomfort. Eventually, greater quantities of the drug are required to achieve the desired effect. This model of addiction works well to explain the addictive properties of alcohol, the opiate drugs, and even coffee and cigarettes. However, it did little to explain cocaine addiction. Individuals quickly became compulsive users, but tolerance seemed to vary (Jones, 1987; Winger, Hofmann, & Woods, 1992), and withdrawal included none of the florid physical symptoms of heroin withdrawal. Fishbein and Pease (1996) assert that acute tolerance to crack cocaine develops very rapidly. Since the euphoric effect of crack may last only 20 minutes or so, the user feels compelled to repeat the dosage; however, each successive dose results in gradually decreased euphoric responses. If the user can abstain for 24 hours, acute tolerance will disappear. Chronic users quickly become dependent on the drug and sensitized to its effects. Withdrawal from cocaine may be more a psychological process than a physiological one. Rather than the total body discomfort of withdrawal from alcohol or opiates, the individual addicted to cocaine appears to suffer withdrawal at the neurological cellular level. Withdrawal symptoms include lethargy, depression, irritability, sleep disturbances, and intense cravings for the drug (Benshoff & Riggar, 1990; Fishbein & Pease, 1996; Winger, Hofmann, & Woods, 1992). Robertson (1989) introduced the phrase "cocaine anhedonia" to describe the intense feelings of depression, lack of motivation, paranoia, and feelings of worthlessness accompanying cocaine withdrawal. In addition, he suggests failure to understand the dynamics of withdrawal leads to early termination from treatment and abrupt relapse. Controlling the psychological aspects of withdrawal during the first few days of treatment is crucial. Individuals addicted to cocaine seem to have significantly higher rates of self-discharge from treatment against staff advice than their peers addicted to opiates or alcohol.

Legislative Changes

Rather than relying on control through interdiction or taxation, the sixties saw movement toward reduction in use, abuse, and dependency through legislation, research, and treatment. One of the first legislative efforts designed to make treatment available on a widespread basis was the Community Mental Health Center (CMHC) Act of 1963 (Godley, 1996). This act provided funding for a network of 760 community-based mental health programs across the country. Utilizing sliding scale fees, services were offered to individuals based on their ability to pay. In order to qualify for the community mental health center designation and federal funding, programs had to offer a comprehensive array of services, including inpatient and outpatient counseling, community education through consultation and education, crisis services and case management. Consequently, CMHCs were some of the first facilities to provide publicly funded treatment to individuals with dependence problems, and they became home to drug and alcohol treatment-specific programs funded under later legislation. The deinstitutionalization movement was another force driving the establishment of community mental health centers. Prior to the CMHC act, large government hospitals served as the principal service delivery sites for individuals with severe mental illness. Individuals could be and were confined involuntarily for extended periods, often on the word of mental health or rehabilitation professionals. The deinstitutionalization movement sought to abolish involuntary hospitalization and to require states to treat individuals with severe mental illness in the community. While this movement made significant gains in protecting the rights of individuals with mental illness, economic resources were not shifted from large institutions to the community programs, and the community health center movement has failed to reach its potential.

Discussion   What is the role of the Community Mental Health Center in
Questions: your community? How extensive is the array of offered services?
Who is served?

In 1970 Congress passed the Comprehensive Alcohol Abuse and Alcoholism Prevention, Treatment and Rehabilitation Act, popularly known as the
Hughes Act, named for chief sponsor Senator Harold Hughes of Idaho (Dickman & Challenger, 1988). The act created the National Institute of Alcoholism and Alcohol Abuse to support, through funding and leadership, efforts
in alcohol research, treatment, prevention, and public education. Hughes was
a recovering individual and sought to create both treatment opportunities and
protections for discrimination for individuals with alcoholism (Kinney &
Leaton, 1995). For the first time in federal legislation, the Hughes Act advanced the notion that alcoholism was a disease, amenable to treatment.

In 1971 the Comprehensive Drug Abuse Prevention and Control Act was
passed by Congress, consolidating the policies and procedures of more than 50
pieces of legislation. Although less liberal than the original legislation sent to
the Hill by President Nixon, the act called for expanded treatment services for
drug abuse in Public Health Service Hospitals and federally funded community mental centers and established the Commission on Marijuana and Drug
Abuse to study the effects of drugs of abuse other than alcohol and tobacco
(Hanson & Venturelli, 1995). In addition, the act created the Drug Schedules, a
system of classification of drugs according to their accepted medical use and
their potential for abuse. The schedules are divided into five categories ranging
from Schedule I drugs, which have no currently accepted medical use in the
United States and the highest abuse potential, to Schedule V drugs, with little
abuse potential and current medical use. Schedule I drugs are available for research purposes under tightly controlled conditions. Among the Schedule I
drugs are heroin, peyote, marijuana, and LSD. Schedule II drugs have high
abuse potential that may lead to severe psychological or physiological dependence and extremely restricted current medical use in the United States. Cocaine, methadone, amphetamines, PCP, morphine, and raw opium are Schedule
II drugs. Substances in Schedule III include anabolic steroids, codeine and hy-
drocodeine with aspirin or Tylenol, and certain barbiturates. These drugs are
regarded to have moderate or low risks of physiological dependence and high
risk of psychological dependence. Schedule IV drugs have low abuse potential
and may have the risk of limited physiological or psychological addiction. The
benzodiazepines (e.g., Valium, Librium, Xanax, Ativan, etc.), barbiturates not
listed in other schedules, and Darvon are listed in Schedule IV. The act codifies
record keeping and prescription and dispensation requirements for physicians
and pharmacists. The Schedule V category encompasses over-the-counter
medications containing codeine and other drugs regarded to have limited
abuse potential and dependence-causing potential. Drugs in Schedules II
through IV are available through physician prescription only, whereas Schedule V drugs can be dispensed by a pharmacist under heavily regulated standards. The schedules are controlled and monitored by the Drug Enforcement

Administration of the Department of Justice, which replaced the Treasury Department's Bureau of Narcotics in 1973 (Hanson & Venturelli, 1995). The Comprehensive Crime Control Act of 1984 amended the Comprehensive Drug Abuse Prevention and Control Act, giving the administrator of the DEA the power to place a substance in Schedule I in the interest of public safety. This legislation came in direct response to growing public fears about the dangers of designer drugs.

The Drug Schedules classify drugs according to legal criterion, not pharmacological standards, and reflect the beliefs, attitudes, and opinions of lawmakers and not pharmacological realities. Consequently, benzodiazepines, capable of producing severe, difficult to treat addictions, are in Schedule IV, while marijuana resides in Schedule I.

Discussion   Do the Drug Schedules reflect our current understanding of
Questions: drugs, their abuse potential, and their use? What would you
                 change?

In 1971 Nixon's Special Action Office for Drug Abuse Prevention monitored and coordinated drug abuse prevention and treatment efforts among the states, giving way to the National Institute on Drug Abuse (NIDA) (Hanson & Venturelli, 1995). Like its sister organization, NIAAA, NIDA-funded programs promoted and conducted research and education and provided a national leadership role. The director of NIDA became the chief advisor to the president on drug abuse treatment efforts.

The Hughes Act and the Comprehensive Drug Abuse Prevention and Control Act required states to establish a mechanism for receiving federal funding and ensuring its appropriate distribution to local service providers. States were required to monitor program activities and to establish program credentialing standards also. In response, the various states established Single State Authorities (SSAs) to oversee drug and alcohol services delivered at the local level, often by Single County Authorities (SCAs). In the early days of program funding, three parallel funding streams existed, controlled by three bureaucracies but often serving the same clients or at least clients from the same families. A mother might be in treatment funded by community mental health center dollars, while dad was being seen in an alcoholism clinic funded through NIAAA, and the children were seen in NIDA-funded programming. Most states administered separate drug, alcohol, and mental health systems, although funding services at the local level might be unified or in competition. Even today most states operate separate mental health and drug and alcohol bureaucracies, and many states did not combine their state drug and alcohol agencies until well into the eighties. In 1973 NIAAA, NIDA, and NIMH (the National Institute of Mental Health) were placed under the auspices of the Alcohol Drug Abuse and Mental Health Administration (ADAMHA), a part of the Department of Health, Education and Welfare. The ADAMHA Reorganization Act of 1992 created the Substance Abuse and Mental Health Services Administration (SAMHSA) in the Department of Health. This new federal bureaucracy incorporated the programs of NIAAA, NIDA, and NIMH and assumed lead federal responsibility for prevention and treatment of mental health problems and substance abuse and dependency prevention and treatment (Hanson & Venturelli, 1995).

Discussion   How are drug and alcohol and mental health services
Question: administered and provided in your state and area?

In the late sixties, Dole and Nyswander published a series of articles advocating the use of methadone maintenance as a treatment modality for heroin addiction (Bratter, Pennacchia, & Gauya, 1985). Public Health Service hospitals had shown little success in treating heroin addiction, and other treatment models, notably therapeutic communities, were in their infancy. In response to the need for programming, the Congress passed the Methadone Control Act of 1972. The act established controls on the prescribing and dispensing of methadone partly to prevent its diversion as a street drug. Dole and Nyswander's vision was that of methadone as a biological curative, and they rejected the need for additional psychological intervention. However, recent research suggests that individuals on methadone maintenance derive substantial benefits from concurrent psychotherapeutic intervention (O'Brien, Woody, & McLellan, 1995).

The federal legislation of the sixties and seventies can be credited with providing the impetus and funding for a broad network of treatment facilities for drug and alcohol problems. From 1969 to 1974 the number of federally funded drug rehabilitation programs increased from 16 programs to 926 programs, and funding increased from about $80 million to $800 million (Abadinsky, 1997). Data are sketchy, but there is no doubt that the numbers of alcoholism treatment programs grew at the same or even faster rates. Initially the states or local municipalities administered most treatment programs with direct state funding. However, it soon became apparent that the demand for services far exceeded the supply ability of state and local government. Private not-for-profit treatment centers began to contract with state government to provide services on a grant basis at first and later on a fee-for-service basis. No doubt motivated by the financial success of nonprofit agencies, for-profit organizations began to provide alcoholism and drug dependency treatment services in the early eighties. These programs accepted clients funded through state mechanisms and negotiated with private insurance carriers to establish fee-for-service arrangements to serve clients with insurance coverage. Within a 15-year period, from 1969 to 1984, the substance abuse treatment industry grew from a handful of facilities and programs to a major health care sector with hundreds of facilities housing thousands of treatment slots and employing thousands of employees. Regulation of this rapid growth could be termed spotty at best. Some states established sophisticated program monitoring and evaluation systems, while others lagged behind. Both the Joint Commission on Accreditation of Healthcare Organizations (JCAHO) and the Commission on the Accreditation of Rehabilitation Facilities (CARF) established voluntary accreditation standards for facilities. In fact, the initiation of standards for mental health and substance services resulted in the Joint Commission on Accreditation of Hospitals, re-configuring itself as the Joint Commission on Accreditation of Healthcare Organizations. In many locales a two-tiered system of treatment developed. Individuals with insurance coverage or financial resources had a range of treatment choices; individuals with no financial resources were eligible to receive services in state-run or nonprofit state-funded programs only. Often private for-profit programs charged what the market would bear, and treatment costs exceeded $500 per day in the late eighties. For-profit companies developed elaborate marketing strategies to attract clients, including television, newspaper, and magazine advertising campaigns. The funding base or proprietary status of a program seldom correlated directly with the quality of care delivered. Many small local programs offered excellent care provided by dedicated, diligent, and compassionate professionals, and many larger, proprietary programs provided excellent care as well. However, while the substance abuse treatment industry mushroomed, it failed to develop a sound base of scientifically measurable clinical strategies. Outcome measures were nonexistent or methodologically unsound. Many programs routinely reported success measures based on samples of discharged clients who could be found. Clients lost to the address rolls of treatment programs or who had ceased participation in aftercare were not included in outcome samples. Unfortunately this group of clients is the group most likely to have relapsed.

Other ethical issues began to plague the treatment industry. Marketing promises were either overstated or delivered in misleading ways. The clinical needs of clients were subverted to the financial needs of programs. Nonprofit, grant-funded programs admitted and retained clients to meet state-mandated numeric quotas; for-profit programs admitted and retained clients based on insurance coverage. Both groups abandoned clients when the funding ended. Finally, the substance abuse treatment community failed to monitor and respond to the external political and social environment; as a result, the nineties saw a dramatic decline in the number of nonprofit and for-profit treatment programs. Entire chains of proprietary facilities closed or reorganized to provide other services, including mental health care and pain management.

Discussion Question: Discuss some of the issues related to the rapid growth and development and equally rapid decline of the substance abuse treatment industry. Consider these issues: client services, staffing, administration, outcomes, treatment modalities.

Involvement of Business and Industry

Employee assistance programs are established by employers to help employees whose job performance has declined because of alcohol or drug dependence, family difficulties, mental health problems, and similar life disruptions (Desmond, 1985). American companies have long recognized that on-the-job problems, including lost productivity and job performance, were affected by non-job–related factors but did little to address these problems until recently. Data reveal that alcohol and drug consumption workplace problems annually cost American employers more than $80 billion in lost productivity due to death or injury (U.S. Department of Health and Human Services, 1995). Nearly half of all industrial fatalities and injuries can be traced to alcoholism or alcohol consumption (Bernstein & Mahoney, 1989). Absenteeism rates for workers with alcohol and drug abuse or dependency problems are 3.8 to 8.3 times higher than the general population. They use significantly more sick leave benefits and are five times more likely to file workers' compensation claims (Backer, 1988; Bernstein & Mahoney, 1989). In addition, Bernstein and Mahoney suggest that nonalcoholic members of families where alcohol dependency is present use ten times as much sick leave in comparison to the general population.

Alcohol-related problems were the first to be confronted by business and industry. Kemp (1985) traces the beginning of programs to the World War I era when the R. H. Macy Company and the Northern State Power Company of Minneapolis established programs to assist employees with alcohol problems. The next phase of recorded employee support program development took place in the 1940s when Eastman Kodak, DuPont, Consolidated Edison, and Western Electric developed company Occupational Alcoholism Programs (Trice & Schonbrunn, 1988) in response to alcohol problems emerging in the workforce. During the World War II years production demands and the composition of the pool of job seekers forced companies to hire marginal employees who often had histories of drinking problems. Moreover, after the war, some veterans developed alcohol problems because of war experiences or as a coping mechanism to deal with memories of the war or the stresses of returning home. In order to deal with these emerging problems, early programs offered assistance to employees, although solely for alcohol-related difficulties. These programs were often administered through the company medical department. The company medical director served as the gatekeeper to employment, and alcoholism was viewed as an illness, responsive to treatment. Volunteers in many companies, frequently recovering individuals, spearheaded efforts to help co-workers with alcoholism problems. About 100 companies had occupational alcoholism programs in place by the early sixties (Kurtz, Googins, & Howard, 1984), although often these programs were not acknowledged by the company as a formal part of the employee benefits program. While medical departments or AA volunteers were willing to recognize alcoholism as a disease, many administrators still viewed it as a moral failing or were loathe to admit the presence of alcoholism problems among the workforce.

Discussion Question: What are the implications of offering alcoholism intervention services and supporting alcoholism treatment services for employees?

Paul Roman summarized the guidelines for occupational alcoholism programs in an article in 1981. He argued that it was a valid and desirable

function of business and industry to intervene when individuals are dependent on alcohol and when that dependence resulted in impairment of job
functioning. Second, he felt treatment in a professional setting was not always required; some individuals could succeed using behavioral self-control
strategies, including participation in AA programming. Finally, Roman argued that ". . . the workplace provides structures for effective early intervention, including confrontation and crisis precipitation to produce behavioral
change" (p. 245). Supervisory identification and confrontation were key
components of the alcoholism intervention process.

In 1962 a corporate decision by the Kemper Group to expand its services
to employees with problems other than alcoholism and to families of employees ushered in the beginning of the "broad-brush" era of Employee Assistance
Programs (Dickman & Challenger, 1988). In contrast to OAPs, employee assistance programs took a more holistic approach, emphasizing concern for a variety of behavioral problems experienced by employees and their families.
Along with these shifts, EAPs came increasingly under the control of personnel departments, and some began to offer treatment services within the
company. The growth of EAPs was slow during the 1960s, but in 1972 a
tremendous surge in EAP programming developed. One provision of the
Hughes Act included funding for two employee assistance consultants per
state. Known as the "thundering hundred," these individuals set out to introduce the EAP model to large and small companies throughout the country.

Other forces were at work promoting business and industrial approaches
to alcoholism problems. The National Council on Alcoholism (NCA) was
founded in 1944 by Marty Mann, the first woman to become sober through
AA (National Council on Alcoholism and Drug Dependence, 1997a). Created
to serve as an advocacy group for individuals with alcoholism and with the
mission of educating the country about the impact of alcoholism, NCA became increasingly involved with workplace alcoholism efforts in the sixties.
In 1971 these efforts contributed to the formation of ALMACA, the Association of Labor-Management Administrators and Consultants on Alcoholism.
Now known as the Employee Assistance Professionals Association, ALMACA
brought together employee assistance professionals, treatment providers, recovering individuals, human resource staff, and educators in a loose coalition
aimed at promoting professional and industrial awareness of workplace drug
and alcohol problems and the potential of the employees' assistance movement.
University programs at Cornell University and The Center of Alcohol Studies
at Yale University were promoting greater business and industrial involvement
in alcoholism problems at this time also.

The stigma attached to alcoholism declined during the sixties and seventies,
prompting more individuals to admit their problems and encouraging more
companies to begin offering EAP services to serve employees. In part, the reduction in the stigma associated with alcoholism can be attributed to the social
fabric of the times. In addition, stigma reduction occurred as a result of the increasing acceptance of alcoholism as a treatable illness by the established medical
community. By the mid-eighties, estimates of the number of companies offering

employee assistance services ranged from 5000 (Forrest, 1985) to 9000 (Beale, 1984), with corporate EAP programs mostly found in larger companies (Burke, 1988).

The earliest employee assistance programs were company-run Internal Programs. As the name implies, these programs serve employees of the host company and are administered as part of the corporate entity. Some company programs are Union Programs, serving only members of a particular union within a company. In the early days of the EAP movement, the adversarial nature of management-labor relations often led to problems in the implementation of EAP services. Rank-and-file employees saw company-sponsored internal programs as little more than tools of management aimed at terminating employees with troublesome work records. Conversely, management perceived union programs as efforts to save the jobs of substandard employees. Often, neither side trusted the other, as illustrated by the experiences of the authors' colleague. He was hired as the first employee assistance program coordinator of a major Fortune 500 company. Charged with providing employee assistance services to the labor force, he soon discovered that everyone from labor avoided him, even to the point of refusing to eat lunch with him in the employee cafeteria. Why? It seems the program was conceived by management, and our colleague was hired without the knowledge and consent of labor. Word spread quickly through the labor grapevine that this was not an individual to be trusted.

In another work setting the union labor-management contract included a provision for mandatory treatment and suspension of disciplinary activities for employees whose job performance problems could be traced to alcoholism problems. Union members, including some union leaders, exploited this provision to protect the jobs of employees whose job problems were related to poor performance and not alcoholism. Individuals were referred to treatment services but had no legitimate history of alcohol problems.

According to Burgess, Fried, and Benshoff (1989) one of the employee assistance program's most important tasks is working with both labor and management in a coordinated, collaborative effort. Communication lines must be established with both groups, and training activities must include both labor and management representation.

Many smaller companies are unable to afford internal EAP services. Two models have been developed to meet their needs: consortium programs and external programs. Consortium programs serve a group of companies with a common interest. In some situations, companies may join forces based on geography; in others, companies from a particular industry or trade group may band together. In the Midwest a group of companies manufactures specialized steel piping for the oil and gas drilling industry in plants ranging from Chicago to New Orleans. None of these companies can separately afford the costs of in-house EAP services, but by joining together they can establish an EAP program for employees and assure that the program is staffed by personnel sensitive to the needs of their unique industry.

External programs are private proprietary or nonprofit companies that sell employee assistance services to companies on a fee-for-service basis or on a

capitated basis, charging a fixed dollar amount based on the number of employees working for a company. External model programs are most apt to employ counselors trained at the master's level according to research conducted
by Hosie, West, and Mackey (1993).

Obtaining the cooperation of industry and business supervisors is a significant challenge faced by all EAP providers and especially by external providers
(Burgess, Fried, & Benshoff, 1989). Supervisory referral has been a constant of
the EAP process, dating from the OAP era (Roman, 1981). However, the
quantity and quality of supervisory referrals are dependent on several factors.
The length of supervisors' job tenure is positively related to the number of and
frequency of EAP referrals (Gerstein & Bayer, 1988). Supervisors who participate in referral training are more likely to make more EAP referrals (Gerstein
et al., 1988), and they are more likely to refer employees with severe problems
rather than employees with minor problems (Gerstein & Bayer, 1991; Hartog,
Hickey, Reichman, & Gracin, 1993). According to Burgess, Fried, and Benshoff
(1989) the trust that exists between supervisors and the employee assistance
program is a key factor in referrals. Supervisors who are not well acquainted
with EAP personnel and EAP practices, a situation common to external
EAPS, appear less likely to make referrals and may engage in codependency
behaviors with the troubled subordinate (Shaw, MacGillis, & Dvorchik, 1994).
Internal programs are less likely to encounter this problem if they maintain an
active presence on the job site and are seen as approachable and receptive by
supervisory personnel (Burgess, Benshoff, Early, & Taricone, 1990; Shaw,
MacGillis, & Dvorchik, 1994).

By 1991 as many as a third of U.S. companies had active employee assistance programs, but lingering questions remain about their effectiveness and
their penetration rates in the workforce (Shaw, MacGillis, & Dvorchik, 1994;
Gerstein & Bayer, 1988). A number of studies have attempted to evaluate the
effectiveness of EAP programs with mixed results, but the variability and complexity of programs make precise evaluation difficult. The National Council
on Alcoholism and Drug Dependence (1997c) asserts that employee assistance
programs save employers millions of dollars annually through reduction in
lost-time injuries and illnesses, increased productivity, and fewer grievances and
disciplinary problems. Generally, the data reveal that it is less costly to rehabilitate an employee with a personal problem than it is to ignore the problems until it becomes necessary to engage in a protracted and litigious disciplinary
process. Workers with drug or alcohol problems report having more jobs and
more job turnover than workers from the general population (U.S. Department of Health and Human Services, 1996). When the costs of recruiting,
training, and equipping a replacement employee are considered, the savings
resulting from employee assistance programs grow dramatically. Myers and
Myers (1985) note that employee assistance programs frequently serve a risk
management function, protecting employers from safety violations, lost productivity, work quality deficiencies, and criminal behavior caused by troubled
employees. However, they caution that employee assistance programs can create employer liabilities for misdiagnoses, inequitable treatment, violations of
confidentiality rights, and excessive treatment costs. The best strategy to reduce

any liability threat to employee assistance programs is to operate a well-organized, well-integrated, and, well-coordinated program (Burgess, Fried, & Benshoff, 1989; Myers & Myers, 1985).

THE DISEASING OF
ALCOHOLISM AND ADDICTION

The growing popularity of AA as a resource for individuals with alcoholism problems and the concerted efforts of the National Council on Alcoholism to increase public and professional awareness of alcoholism problems paralleled steps taken by the medical profession in the 1950s and 1960s. In 1952 the American Medical Association issued its first of a series of definitions of alcoholism, and in 1954 the New York City Medical Society on Alcoholism was founded (National Council on Alcoholism and Drug Dependence, 1997a). It later became the American Society of Addiction Medicine (ASAM). Later in that decade the American Hospital Association passed a resolution aimed at preventing discrimination against alcoholics in member institutions

In 1952 E. M. Jellinek published a landmark article setting forth a linear model of the progression of alcoholism. According to Jellinek, alcoholics progress through four distinct phases: the prealcoholic phase, the prodromal phase, the crucial phase, and the chronic phase. Central to Jellinek's model were his beliefs that alcoholism as a disease is characterized by loss of control, specific symptomotology, and fatality if not interrupted by treatment (Doweiko, 1996). Jellinek believed that individuals with alcoholism problems differed from other members of society. The social drinking that characterized the prealcoholic phase is not simply drinking to be sociable and pleasant. Instead, it includes a stress or tension relief element not seen in the drinking of members of the general population. In the prodromal phase the individual has increased the amount and frequency of alcohol consumption and has begun to experience a variety of neurological, cognitive, and emotional disturbances. According to Jellinek this stage is characterized by blackouts, preoccupation with obtaining and drinking alcohol, secretive drinking, and increased guilt and anxiety about drinking behavior and its consequences. Physical dependence, including the emergence of tolerance and withdrawal symptoms, signal the initiation of the crucial phase. "Other symptoms of this third stage of drinking are a loss of self-esteem, a loss of control over one's drinking, social withdrawal in favor of alcohol use, self-pity, and a neglect of proper nutrition" (Doweiko, 1996, p. 216). The crucial phase is typified by the emergence of severe physiological and psychological problems. For Jellinek this was the stage of total lifestyle deterioration, including lowered social status and social participation, the development of specific physical problems highlighted by motor tremors, a total obsession with drinking, and loss of tolerance for alcohol related to organ damage.

Jellinek followed and expanded on this work with the *Disease Concept of Alcoholism*, published by the College and University Press. Clinging to his beliefs about the primacy of alcoholism as a fatal disease with specific symptoms and a distinct progression, Jellinek postulated the existence of five types of alcoholics. Alpha alcoholics have a pure psychological dependence on alcohol but do not suffer any physical consequences from their drinking. The individual who *must* drink three beers with dinner each evening would fall into Jellinek's categorization of an alpha alcoholic. Jellinek believed that individuals could be alpha alcoholics throughout their lives, never progressing to other stages or developing alcohol-related physical symptoms. Individuals falling into the beta alcoholic classification display physical complications related to alcohol consumption, including gastrointestinal disorders, alcohol-related cardiac myopathy, cirrhosis of the liver, and others. Individuals in this group exhibit psychological dependence but not physical dependence and progress into gamma alcoholism with continued drinking. Gamma alcoholics have a plethora of physical symptoms, including tolerance, withdrawal, obsessive craving, and loss of control over drinking. They are unable to abstain from drinking for any length of time and develop significant medical problems related to their consumption. Unlike individuals in the previous category, delta alcoholics display few physical symptoms or medical complications related to their uncontrolled drinking, yet they, too, develop tolerance and experience withdrawal when they stop alcohol consumption. Delta alcoholics maintain a steady state of drinking and a steady state of mild intoxication. While Jellinek suggested these individuals are unable to control their drinking, it appears they control their drinking at a level greater than that experienced by the general population. A more recent term to describe these individuals might be functional alcoholics. Binge drinkers are epsilon alcoholics. Their drinking is characterized by extended periods of sobriety interrupted by periods of uncontrolled, significant alcohol consumption. The epsilon category is Jellinek's least well-developed categorization.

Jellinek's model became the underpinning of the American alcoholism treatment movement. It set forth, in linear fashion, a model easily understood by individuals with alcoholism and their families and established a framework for diagnosis and treatment. Although Jellinek focused solely on alcoholism in his model, it became the paradigm for all forms of dependency treatment, including heroin and cocaine dependency treatment.

Discussion Question: Discuss the implications of the linear structure of Jellinek's models.

Discussion Question: Discuss the relevance of Jellinek's model to heroin and cocaine dependency.

In 1990 the board of directors of the National Council on Alcoholism and Drug Dependence Inc., and the American Society of Addiction Medicine collaboratively approved the following definition:

Alcoholism is a primary, chronic disorder with genetic, psychosocial, and environmental factors influencing its development and manifestations. The disease is often progressive and fatal. It is characterized by continuous or periodic: impaired control over drinking, preoccupation with the drug alcohol, use of alcohol despite adverse consequences, and distortions in thinking, mostly denial. (National Council on Alcoholism and Drug Dependency, 1997b)

This definition is notable for its inclusion of multiple etiological factors and the incorporation of multiple characteristics of alcoholism. Consequently, it goes beyond Jellinek's formulation of alcoholism as a unitary, linear process to a depiction of alcoholism as a complex mechanism with circular patterns of development. The insertion of the word "often" before "progressive" and "fatal" is an important distinction of this definition. Its use implies a growing recognition that some individuals may spontaneously recover from alcohol dependency through little-understood, self-devised intervention and treatment strategies. Nevertheless, the use of the words "progressive" and "fatal" stress the persistence over time of alcoholism and its cumulative effects and the reality that alcoholism is related significantly to higher fatality rates from secondary illness, disability, accidents, and violence (National Council on Alcoholism and Drug Dependence, 1997b).

Discussion Question: Create a definition for dependence that encompasses all forms of substance dependence.

The American Society of Addiction Medicine is an association of physicians specializing in the treatment of addictions. Its mission includes promoting high-quality patient care for individuals with substance dependency and increasing physician and medical student understanding of addiction through its program of continuing education (American Society of Addiction Medicine, 1997). Membership in the society is obtained by passing a national certification examination. One of the most significant contributions of ASAM is the Patient Placement Criteria, designed to establish parameters for decisions about placement in various levels of care. The criteria specify four levels of care and indicators for admission to each level. Level I: Outpatient Care is the least restrictive care setting and is intended for individuals who have minimal withdrawal needs and risks; an existing support system or the social skill necessary to develop one; no concurrent psychiatric, behavioral, or emotional problems; no risk of harm to self or others; and a willingness to cooperate in treatment and maintain abstinence. In order to remain in Level I care, individuals must not demonstrate signs of acute intoxication, must be making progress in resolving emotional issues, must be making progress on achieving goals and objectives, and should not be abstinent but mentally preoccupied with the use of substances.

Level II: Intensive Outpatient/Partial Hospitalization Treatment encompasses treatment services provided on an outpatient basis at least nine hours per week. Individuals needing this more intense level of service typically demonstrate minimal withdrawal symptoms; the ability to self-detoxify; the inability to remain emotionally stable over a 72-hour period; spouse or child abuse related to dependence; behavioral or emotional problems requiring monitoring; mild risk of injury to self or others; likelihood of relapse; and an unsupportive work environment and/or family environment. The need for continued stay in the level of care is indicated by inability to maintain behavioral stability for a 72-hour period of treatment; continued emotional or behavioral disorders despite demonstrated improvement in other areas; improvement in risk of self-injury or harm to others; an ability to begin to take responsibility for recovery but with a need for clinical motivation. Other need factors include failure to understand work stressors; failure to cope with stressors at home; insufficient functional ability to prevent relapse outside a structured milieu; and failure to have or develop social skills and a social network.

Admission to Level III: Medically Monitored Intensive Inpatient Treatment requires individuals to demonstrate a risk of severe withdrawal syndrome as measured by the Clinical Institute Withdrawal Assessment-Alcohol or one of several behavioral indicators linked to excessive drug or alcohol consumption over an extended time. Additionally, the individual must demonstrate signs of possible health damage if alcohol or drug use is continued; emotional or behavioral symptoms interfering with abstinence; moderate risk to self or others; stressors related to losses at home or work; history of violent or disruptive behavior when intoxicated; or coexisting personality or psychiatric disorders requiring continuous intervention. Other risk factors necessitating admission to this level of care include inability to control drug use, especially when drugs are present; inability to relate drug use to adverse consequences; a home environment not conducive to treatment success; inability to remain drug free long enough to benefit from Level I or Level II treatment; logistic problems preventing participation in Level I or II (i.e., rural environment; no transportation); and holding a safety-sensitive occupation where continued drug or alcohol use poses a threat to public safety and welfare.

Individuals who are eligible for admission to Level IV: Medically Managed Intensive Inpatient Treatment are in need of acute medical care based on their current compromised medical status or their history of continued extensive use of sedative hypnotics or alcohol. These individuals may display severe acute withdrawal problems necessitating medical support, including life support, recent head trauma or loss of consciousness, coexisting medical problems requiring inpatient care, or previous detoxification failures at Levels I through III. Individuals exhibiting serious behavioral or emotional problems including alcoholic hallucinosis, toxic psychosis, extreme depression, mental confusion, or uncontrolled behavior endangering self or others are candidates for Level IV admission. Other unique considerations for Level IV admission include pregnancy, long-term dependence on high doses of benzodiazepines, and severe opiod withdrawal characterized by severe physical symptoms and the need for acute nursing care. Continued stay Level IV criteria include withdrawal symptoms requiring 24-hour management; biomedical problems that interfere with

dependency treatment; continuing emotional or behavioral problems preventing transfer to less restrictive environments; and the continued presence of a
major psychiatric disorder that is being treated actively.

The ASAM criteria contain two vital features: They specify the criteria required for admission to a level of care, and they specify the criteria required to
remain in a given level of care. At first glance, this is a simple notion. However, it
is a notion foreign to the manner in which dependency care has been offered
historically in this country. By emphasizing individual needs, individual problems, and individual progress, the ASAM criteria dictate a length of stay based on
individual client recovery and the achievement of treatment goals and objectives
and not a predetermined length of stay or preprogramed number of sessions.
Termination from a particular level of stay is bidirectional. Individuals who are
successful in a treatment modality can be discharged to a less intensive, less restrictive modality based on their individual progress; individuals who are unsuccessful
can be referred to a more intensive treatment milieu based on a clinical determination. Consequently, the ASAM criteria require treatment providers to develop
treatment plans neither based on 28 days of stay nor on completion of a module
of outpatient programming but on the basis of client progress and client need.

THE REAGAN-BUSH YEARS: POPULISM
AND GOVERNMENT INTERVENTION

The heightened attention given to drug and alcohol use, abuse, and dependency in the 1960s and 1970s, along with the emergence of crack cocaine,
spawned a resurgence in government drug control efforts and populist anti-
drug and antialcohol measures. Per capita alcohol consumption reached an all-
time high in 1980, catalyzing several forces into action, according to the
National Council on Alcoholism and Drug Dependence (1997a). At the grass
roots level, Mothers Against Drunk Driving was founded to advocate for reform and stiffening of drunk driving penalties. The moving and graphic testi-
mony provided to the federal congress and state legislatures and grass roots
lobbying efforts culminated in the adoption of strict drunk driving laws in virtually every state. This effort followed closely on the heels of the work of the
Parent Resources Institute on Drug Education (PRIDE) to counter the
emerging adolescent drug problem. In 1986 the Partnership for a Drug Free
America, a coalition of advertising, publishing, and media groups launched the
most comprehensive public service advertising campaign against drug and alcohol abuse ever (Backer, 1995). Nearly every potential drug-using element of
society received attention from Partnership ads. Early in the campaign the
Partnership emphasized fear as a tactic to gain attention and make an immediate impression generating the now famous, or infamous, fried egg commercial
("This is your brain on drugs . . ."), later turning to more sophisticated ads targeting minority groups, working groups, attitude change, and increased awareness of the effects of drugs (Backer, 1995; Pisani, 1995).

The federal block grant program of 1982 transferred responsibility for drug and alcohol treatment programming entirely to the states at a time when treatment demands and treatment resources were bourgeoning. That same year former First Lady Betty Ford acknowledged publicly her dependency struggles, and the Betty Ford Center in Palm Springs, California was renamed in her honor. Other important treatment and prevention efforts of the early eighties included the "Just Say No" Campaign of First Lady Nancy Reagan; the formation of the Children of Alcoholics Foundation; and the emergence of a certification examination for addiction medicine specialization in California (National Council on Alcoholism and Drug Dependence, 1997a).

Federal legislation concerning drug and alcohol issues took a decidedly legalistic, control-oriented turn during the eighties. Prior to 1984 each state had the power to establish the minimum alcohol possession and consumption age. While many states specified 21 as the legal drinking age, other states allowed alcohol consumption at age 18 for all forms of alcohol, and still other states permitted consumption of certain types of alcohol-containing beverages at that age. Trying to achieve a nationwide drinking age of 21, the federal government passed the National Minimum Age Drinking Act in 1984. This act did not take away the right of the states to establish the minimum legal drinking age. Instead, it linked federal funding for highways to compliance with a 21 drinking age. States that adopted a 21 drinking age were eligible for continued receipt of federal highway dollars, and failure to adopt the 21 minimum age resulted in loss of federal highway monies. Despite initial protests about the infringements on states' rights, all of the United States and its territories soon adopted an alcohol possession and consumption age of 21.

Discussion Questions: What should be the criteria for possession and consumption of beverages containing alcohol? Who should have the power to set those criteria?

Continuing the theme of increasing governmental control and regulation of drugs, the Anti-Drug Abuse Act of 1988 declared the intention to create a drug-free America by 1995 and created the Office of National Control Policy led by a director appointed by the president (Abadinsky, 1997). Popularly known as the U.S. "drug czar," the director has a broad range of powers and influence covering such diverse issues as treatment, prevention, interdiction, domestic law enforcement, and international strategies (Office of National Drug Control Policy, 1997). Interestingly, the Office acknowledges that addiction to drugs is a disease and calls for both treatment availability and stringent legal sanctions to protect the public and force individuals into treatment.

It is ironic that both the Reagan and Bush presidencies were marked by efforts to decrease the role and involvement of the federal government in the day-to-day lives of Americans, except where drugs and alcohol were concerned. In 1988 the federal government mandated warning labels on all alcoholic beverage containers. This legislation followed on the heels of President

Bush's 1987 declaration of a War on Drugs and the 1988 adoption of workplace drug testing requirements for individuals in federally regulated, safety sensitive positions, including nuclear power plant workers, interstate commerce truck drivers, and railway workers. The legislation led to the implementation of drug testing standards by nonsafety sensitive private industry employers for preemployment screening, random screening, screening for probable cause, and routine medical screening (Blum, 1989). Additionally, many states developed legislation permitting drug-testing programs for the private sector and for public sector employees (Angarola & Rodriguez, 1989). Initially, state-mandated drug testing was limited to safety sensitive positions such as police officers, firefighters, and correctional employees. Recently, however, mandatory drug testing has expanded to include human service workers, including counseling professionals, most frequently in agencies serving children. Ackerman (1995) notes that, except for closely supervised work settings such as the military, drug testing alone has done little to prevent drug abuse or addiction.

Discussion Questions: Should professionals employed in counseling agencies be required to participate in drug testing for drugs and alcohol? What sanctions should be imposed on individuals who test positive? What other employee groups should be tested?

Reflecting mounting concerns for the social and health costs of alcohol consumption, federal legislation mandated the warning labels on all alcoholic beverages beginning in 1989. Pregnant women, drivers, and operators of dangerous machinery were particular targets of this campaign. Warning labels and public media campaigns may not be the answer, however. The Centers for Disease Control reported in 1997 that the number of pregnant women who consumed alcohol on a frequent (more than seven drinks per week or more than five drinks at a single sitting in the past month) basis during pregnancy jumped at a fourfold rate between 1991 and 1995. In 1991 only .08 percent of pregnant women reported drinking frequently, but in 1995, 3.5 percent (about 140,000) of pregnant women reportedly were frequent consumers of alcohol, according to CDC data.

The Americans with Disabilities Act departed from the control emphasis of federal legislation by extending rehabilitation eligibility protection to individuals who are dependent on alcohol and individuals recovering from drug dependence. Feldblum (1991) illustrates the distinction drawn between alcohol and drug dependency. Individuals with alcohol dependency are protected by ADA with no regard to their current alcohol-consumption status. A strict interpretation of the law would suggest that they could be drinking actively or they could be abstinent or in some in-between status. Conversely, individuals with a history of drug dependence are not eligible for services unless they have completed or are completing a supervised program of drug rehabilitation or are otherwise regarded as rehabilitated *and* are drug free. ADA is silent with respect to what is considered a supervised rehabilitation program, failing to specify if supervised rehabilitation implies participation in a licensed or otherwise credentialed program or if less structured alternatives are acceptable. The notion of being otherwise regarded as rehabilitated is even more vague. Would an individual who achieved recovery through a self-designed program of participation in peer self-help programming through Narcotics Anonymous be regarded as otherwise rehabilitated? Would an individual who achieved recovery status through participation in transcendental meditation be regarded as rehabilitated?

Discussion   What minimal standards, if any, should be established in order
Question: to meet a criterion of rehabilitated for an individual with a
                 history of drug dependence?

While it protects the rights of individuals with drug and alcohol dependency disabilities, the Americans with Disabilities Act does not supersede drug-free workplace laws, and drug testing as a condition of employment is permitted as long as the testing is equally applied to all applicants. Individuals with concurrent psychoactive substance dependence problems and other disabilities are protected by ADA as long as they refrain from the resumption of illegal drug use. For example, an individual with a concurrent visual impairment disability and a history of drug dependence is protected by ADA; however, ADA protection is lost if that individual resumes the illicit use of drugs even though the visual disability remains (Rehabilitation Research and Training Center on Drugs and Disability, 1996).

Because ADA is either vague or silent on its standards for rehabilitation of individuals with drug and alcohol dependence disabilities, provisions for eligibility and receipt of rehabilitation services have been left to the various state rehabilitation agencies. Consequently, provisions vary from state to state and often from local office to local office. Despite the language contained in the Americans with Disabilities Act expressly protecting individuals with alcohol dependencies at any stage of their dependency, many states have adopted formal or informal rules for participation in the state rehabilitation system. A period of sobriety, typically a year or two, may be required for eligibility or participation in Alcoholics Anonymous, or formal treatment programming may be required through the IWRP process. Other states have been more liberal in their interpretation, however. In other locales, individuals with an extensive history of recovery from alcohol or drugs may be regarded erroneously as not having a disability. Although ample evidence suggests that many participants in the state-federal rehabilitation system have concurrent drug and alcohol problems that often interfere with successful rehabilitation, states have been slow to implement training in drug and alcohol dependency for state VR counselors (Benshoff, Grissom, & Nelson, 1990; Moore & Li, 1994). Additionally, changes in the Social Security law in 1997 reversed some of the gains made in inclusion of individuals with drug and alcohol problems in the rehabilitation caseload. The Social Security Administration dropped nearly 200,000 individuals with primary diagnoses of alcohol or drug dependence from the Social Security disability roles. However, many individuals reapplied for Social Security disability benefits, often citing alcohol-related or drug-related problems (e.g., diabetes, pulmonary problems) as their primary disability.

Discussion   Discuss the pros and cons of psychoactive substance dependence
Question: as a disability covered under the Social Security Administration.

THE CURRENT SITUATION: IS IT DIFFERENT FROM THE PAST?

In the new millennium, examining recent situations and the lessons of history to develop a framework for providing psychoactive chemical dependency intervention and treatment is essential. One of the first considerations must be the expanded compendium of drugs and alcohol available for use, abuse, and dependency. Unlike previous times, concerns about drugs and alcohol no longer focus on the societal impact of a single substance or class of substances. The emergence of synthetic drugs, preprocessed drugs (i.e., crack cocaine), alcohol and drugs targeted at specific groups, and use of commonly available volatile solvents as hallucinogenics have outpaced the understanding of drug actions and reactions and treatment knowledge. The American treatment model for dependency centers around the treatment of sedative-hypnotic drugs, alcohol, and the opiates, using a paradigm of peer self-help of questionable universal value. This is not to suggest that disease model treatment or Alcoholics Anonymous are valueless. Quite the contrary. The disease model and AA have made significant contributions to the understanding of dependency and to the recovery of many individuals, and they will continue to do so. However, the problems presented by individuals dependent on stimulant drugs, volatile substances, prescription medications, or a concurrent mixture of sedative-hypnotics and stimulants may differ significantly from alcoholism or heroin addiction. Logically, treatment strategies to improve problems must go beyond a one-size-fits-all mentality to a focus on individual problems and individual needs, which may include traditional treatment strategies as one portion of the rehabilitation plan.

Besides expansion of the drug and alcohol menu, increased and more sophisticated targeting of consumers for particular attention has materialized, especially by the manufacturers of licit drugs and alcohol. Examples of this phenomenon include marketing malt liquor toward the African-American community and targeting women and younger drinkers with advertising campaigns for wine coolers and other "flavored" alcoholic beverages. Natural drugs have been touted as safe and effective wellness strategies and as treatment for several, often stress-related, conditions. The use of melatonin as a stress reducer and sleep aid is an illustration of this trend. Public perception, shaped by advertising, is that natural drugs have few side effects and low abuse potential. However, since natural drugs are largely unregulated by either the pharmaceutical industry or state or federal government, their dangers and abuse potential are unclear and unknown until a fateful event occurs. For many years L–tryptophan, an over-the-counter medication, was used to treat sleep disturbances in individuals recovering from alcoholism because of its low abuse potential and seeming safety (Smith, 1982). Then in 1989 an outbreak of eosinophilia myalgia syndrome traced to L–tryptophan consumption killed several people and sickened many others. In a still controversial move, the Food and Drug Administration removed L–tryptophan from the market, citing its dangerous side effects (Fishbein & Pease, 1996).

The population of individuals comprising the abusing and dependent group has also changed. Overall drug use among adolescents has been in a declining trend. Nevertheless, the average age of first use has been dropping also, and earlier use may lead to abuse earlier and dependency. Young adolescents may lack developmental skills required to self-monitor and self-regulate psychoactive substance use, and they may never develop a sense of "normal" drug and alcohol use through positive personal experience.

Women are increasingly identified as problem drinkers or drug users. Unlike the heroin dependency problems of the 1960s and 1970s that were mostly a male phenomenon, crack cocaine is much less gender specific, and women comprise a significant part of the crack cocaine dependent cohort. The numbers of women identified with alcohol abuse and dependency problems have increased in recent years, as have the number of women entering treatment. Treatment resources remain more limited for women and fail to address a number of important needs, such as child care, pregnancy, financial and insurance resources, victimization from sexual abuse (Glover, Janikowski, & Benshoff, 1995), and the dual struggle many women encounter trying to overcome dependency and developing a sense of personal autonomy (McBride, 1990).

Another growing cohort within the psychoactive substance abuse and dependence population is the group of individuals experiencing concurrent problems with dependence and another disability (Moore & Li, 1994). Often members of this group receive both dependence treatment service and services from the state-federal or private rehabilitation systems but with almost no coordination or integration of services (Backer & Newman, 1994). This is not a new event. Concern for individuals with dual disabilities has been voiced for a number of years, but little was accomplished until recently, sparked by state initiatives, federal grants, and grassroots efforts from consumers and professional groups. Anecdotal and empirical evidence suggests that many individuals seen in community mental health centers have dual substance dependency and mental health problems (Aleisan & Firth, 1990), and there is increasing evidence of the frequent coexistence of abuse/dependency with physical disabilities, sensory disabilities, and learning disabilities.

Along with changes in the types and kinds of drugs and alcohol available for abuse and dependence, and changes in at-risk populations, changes in the context of psychoactive drug dependence are evident. The violence related to the consumption and distribution of illicit drugs, notably cocaine and crack cocaine, is unprecedented in history. Huge sums of money, increased use of technology by drug traffickers, and the porous nature of international boundaries have coalesced to create a drug distribution system little affected by even the most arduous control efforts. On the domestic scene, gangs, both as drug distribution points and as havens or surrogate families for individuals raised in dysfunctional families or dysfunctional circumstances, present challenges for communities and professionals. The threat imposed by HIV continues into the nineties. While the most obvious threat is from HIV contraction through dirty needles, a more subtle but equally dangerous threat is posed by the disinhibiting effects of crack cocaine and alcohol. In the past, drug or alcohol use presented dangers but not the risk of disease-borne fatality both for user and offspring.

Current cultural responses to dependence are in the direction of less tolerance, as suggested by demands for stiffer DUI laws, more restrictions on tobacco and hard liquor advertising, stiffer prison sentences, and more harsh correctional policies. Treatment trends have been toward briefer lengths of stay and more emphasis on intensive outpatient programming instead of inpatient treatment. The societal forces driving these changes are a consequence of failed policies in the past, but many new policies and procedures have little empirical evidence supporting them.

SUMMARY

Alcohol and drug problems have been part of society through the ages. In the 19th century alcoholism surfaced in the United States as a social issue attacked through a moral model in an ill-defined treatment system focusing on inebriation. The Temperance Movement arose along with the Industrial Revolution, ultimately giving way to the Prohibitionist Movement of the early 20th century. Marijuana, cocaine, and opiates were all introduced to the U.S. culture, not as illicit drugs but as substances with legitimate commercial, medicinal, or recreational uses.

The first part of the 20th century encompasses the Legislative Era and included the passage of the Pure Food and Drug Act of 1906, the Harrison Narcotics Act of 1914, the Volstead Act (Prohibition), and the Marijuana Tax Act of 1937. Many laws were driven by populist sentiment or irrational fears and resulted in the first examples of criminalization of addictive behavior.

Treatment emerged in the 1960s, initially centering on alcoholism treatment and spurred by growing public need and demand for services and by a number of federal laws. The Community Mental Health Center Act of 1963 established a network of community-based mental health facilities. The Comprehensive Alcohol Abuse and Alcoholism Prevention, Treatment and Rehabilitation Act and its sister legislation created federal support for research, treatment, and prevention. Many public facilities were established, followed quickly by private, for-profit agencies. While treatment flourished for a number of years, the treatment community failed to develop a sound philosophical and theoretical basis for treatment and failed to respond to political and economic pressure. Consequently, dependence treatment has experienced and continues to experience profound changes.

Business and industry concern for alcoholism problems surfaced just after World War II with the development of occupational alcoholism programs. Employee assistance programs broadened both the types of problems concerning companies and the scope of services available to employees. The broadbrush approach brought a concept of multiple solutions for multiple problems to the workplace. Key forces working along with business, industry, and labor organizations included the National Council on Alcoholism, the Association of Labor-Management Administrators and Consultants on Alcoholism, and the federal government. Several models of EAP service delivery arose, including internal programs, union programs, consortium programs, and external programs. Communication and cooperation have been central to the success of all EAP programs.

The diseasing of alcoholism and addiction gathered impetus with the publication of Jellinek's classic work and was given added support through the American Medical Association and the National Council on Alcoholism. Consequently the disease model became the dominant treatment model for all forms of abuse and dependence in the United States. More recently, the patient placement criteria of the American Society of Addiction Medicine have sought to establish a more systematic and clinically driven model for evaluating treatment placement and treatment progress.

Populist, grass roots movements have continued to alter the landscape of drug and alcohol abuse and dependence prevention and treatment. Groups such as MADD, SADD, and the Partnership for a Drug-Free America, made significant contributions. Continued federal legislative activity established a national minimum drinking age and vigorously continued to wage war on drugs. The Americans with Disabilities Act (ADA) recognized drug and alcohol dependence as disabilities, although with differing eligibility characteristics. ADA fostered the recognition of coexisting disabilities as a significant problem in rehabilitation.

Problems facing the rehabilitation of individuals with drug and alcohol abuse and dependence problems included an expanded menu of drugs and alcohol, including a shift away for sedative-hypnotic drugs, implying the need for a new treatment model and the need for more individualized treatment. Both licit and illicit suppliers of drugs and alcohol have attempted to target consumer groups, and rates of consumption appear to be rising among adolescents, women, and people with disabilities. Changes in the context of use, abuse, and dependence suggest the importance of taking a multifaceted approach to both prevention and rehabilitation.

3

Conceptualizing Substance Abuse and Dependence: A Rehabilitation Perspective

CHAPTER 3 OUTLINE

OVERVIEW OF ADDICTION TREATMENT
AND REHABILITATION

Throughout history in the United States, there seems to have been at least three major views toward alcoholism and addiction that have influenced how alcoholics and addicts have been treated by our society. The oldest notion is that addiction, of any type, is a form of moral failing, comparable to stealing, lying, or promiscuity. Addiction and other unacceptable behaviors weren't tolerated by decent society, and people with these problems were subjected to social ostracism, imprisonment, or other forms of punishment. Around the turn of the century, public sentiment shifted somewhat, and the popular attitude was to view the drug itself as the problem, as typified by the popular slogan "the demon rum." This attitude logically led to governmental attempts to protect the public by banning access to alcohol (Prohibition in 1919) and drugs (Harrison Narcotics Act, 1914). Most recently (since about the 1940s, at least) public attitudes shifted to the notion that alcoholism and addiction were diseases, something beyond the control of the individual. As with any disease, the proper way to address the problem is to seek medical treatment.

The "modern era" of substance abuse treatment can trace its roots to when Alcoholics Anonymous (AA) was founded by Bill Wilson and Bob Smith in 1935. This was soon followed by E. M. Jellinek postulating the disease concept of alcoholism in an 80-page research article published in 1947. This work was based on a survey of 158 questions that were taken by AA members and was later followed by a landmark book, *The Disease Concept of Alcoholism*, in 1960. In 1956 the American Medical Association officially recognized alcoholism as a disease, and the substance abuse treatment began to grow markedly in the 1960s and 1970s with insurance coverage paying for substance abuse treatment because of its disease status. Prior to the 1960s, substance abuse treatment, as a fee-for-service entity, was virtually nonexistent. Most treatment programs for individuals with alcoholism problems were based in hospitals and offered detoxification services, followed by outpatient therapy and referral to Alcoholics Anonymous. A number of specialized treatment services utilizing AA-based concepts for long-term treatment typically offered services on a free or low-cost basis. Often residents of these programs were supported through family contributions, private charitable contributions, or work performed at the facility because public financing or insurance financing of treatment was virtually nonexistent.

As indicated in Chapter 2, a number of developments in the 1960s contributed to the rapid rise of the addictions treatment field that is in place today. The crucial milestones in the growth of the alcohol/drug treatment field include the passage of the Hughes Act and creation of the National Institute of Alcoholism and Alcohol Abuse and the National Institute of Drug Abuse (today a program overseen by Substance Abuse and Mental Health Services Administration (SAMHSA)); the expansion of the National Council on Alcoholism; the advent of methadone clinics for treating heroin addiction; passage of the Federal Narcotic Rehabilitation Act, designating opioid addiction as a disease, rather than a crime; the rise of Employee Assistance Programs in business and industry; and third-party (insurance company) payment for alcohol and drug treatment (Dickman, 1985; Winger, Hofmann, & Woods, 1992). Today, about 9 percent of U.S. adults meet diagnostic criteria for alcohol dependence (alcoholism) and the less severe medical disorder of alcohol abuse. Of these, more than 500,000 Americans were treated in 1993 in more than 8000 inpatient and outpatient alcohol treatment programs in the United States.

What exactly is the "traditional treatment model"? From the 1960s to the present, most substance abuse treatment consists of the applications of the concepts of AA, most notably the 12 Steps, a self-help mentality, and an emphasis on abstinence. The primary components of traditional substance abuse treatment planning typically involved these tasks:

1. Confronting the client's denial of substance abuse or dependence
2. Educating him or her about the disease concept of addiction
3. Inpatient counseling based on the 12-Step model (AA) of substance abuse
4. Referral to a 12-Step program, such as AA or Narcotics Anonymous (NA), for follow-up or aftercare

The treatment goal for all clients was always the same: lifetime abstinence from alcohol or psychoactive drugs (Morgan, 1996), and anecdotal reports state that millions have been saved (currently there are about 1.5 million AA members in 115 countries). Tremendous social and political pressure has been exerted to apply AA/disease model and abstinence concepts to *all* substance abuse treatment (Haskell, 1993). Blum and Roman (1987) reported that 93 percent of all treatment centers in the United States incorporate a 12-Step treatment approach. This model has had its detractors; Peele (1990) refers to it as the "one size fits all" approach. Hence, clients are forced into a treatment approach with little or no alternatives being offered. The lack of alternatives and flexibility of treatment has been identified as one source of client resistance or lack of motivation for treatment.

Rehabilitation Field

The growth, development, and professionalization of the rehabilitation field proceeded quite separately from the chemical dependency field. The rehabilitation movement began with legislation in the early 1900s; prior to that, people with disabilities often relied on family or charities for survival. The United States' federal government mandated vocational rehabilitation services for veterans in the Soldiers Rehabilitation Act in 1918 (also known as the Smith-Sears Act). Basically, in order to qualify for assistance with vocational education, the person must have had a vocationally handicapping disability resulting from military service. The Civilian Rehabilitation (Smith-Fess) Act of 1920 provided rehabilitation services for the general population and set up the state/federal system using matching funds for states as an incentive to initiate rehabilitation programs. Disabilities at this time were usually physical in nature, and substance abuse or addiction was not addressed. Several amendments were made in the 1920s, 1930s, and 1940s to expand rehabilitation services and increase funding. Arguably the most important was the 1935 Social Security Act making the state/federal rehabilitation system permanent. In 1954 Vocational Rehabilitation Act Amendments (Hill-Burton Act) provided money for research and demonstration and professional preparation of rehabilitation counselors, resulting in the beginning of professionalization of the field.

The rehabilitation field continued expansion in the 1960s, benefitting from President Johnson's war on poverty. During this expansion period, disability groups were widened from a focus on physical or cognitive disabilities to include mental illness and substance abuse, alcoholism, and addiction. Although substance abuse was recognized as a disability, its treatment or rehabilitation was left up to the just emerging chemical dependency treatment field. The common practice was to refer substance-abusing clients to a treatment facility, instructing them to come back when they were "clean and sober."

So what we see are two parallel fields that historically had little organized or coordinated contact with one another. Rehabilitation counseling had begun its professionalization earlier (1950s), with substance abuse just now requiring certification credentials and college degrees. Despite rehabilitation's recognition of substance abuse and addiction as a disability, it has been slow to serve this population and reluctant to carve out a niche in what has been seen as a separate, though related, field.

DISABILITY AND HANDICAP CRITERIA

There has been hesitancy by some in the rehabilitation field to view alcohol and drug addiction as a disability, based on the notion that these were behavior problems under the control of the individual and therefore not permanent disabilities. Once the alcohol- or drug-using behaviors were altered by the person, all disabling aspects of the condition would disappear. This brings up the question "Is alcoholism or addiction a bona fide disability?" A systematic examination of the condition clearly demonstrates that it is. The eligibility criteria of a disabling condition used by the state/federal rehabilitation system are as follows:

1. A disability is any medically diagnosable (by a physician, psychiatrist, psychologist, or similarly qualified professional) physical, cognitive, or emotional condition that is chronic or permanent in nature (i.e., a nontemporary condition).

2. This condition must result in a limitation of function that causes a handicap or handicaps that prevent the person from achieving goals in a number of life areas.

3. There must be some reasonable expectation that the person could benefit from rehabilitation.

Alcohol or drug problems (to be considered a disability) must be diagnosed by a qualified professional, usually using the Diagnostic and Statistical Manual-IV (DSM-IV) criteria of Psychoactive Substance Abuse or Dependence. If not, then we may be dealing with something like heavy drinking or problematic use—a rehabilitation issue but not a disability.

1. The functional limitations associated with this condition may be persistent or recurrent physical or psychological problems that are likely to have been caused or exacerbated by alcohol (DSM-IV, 1994). These limitations occur in important life areas familiar to rehabilitation counselors: family, social, vocational, educational, and activities of daily living (ADL) functioning.

2. Clearly, people benefit from treatment and rehabilitation services: The functional limitations associated with substance abuse/dependency become more manageable when use is curtailed or eliminated. Despite high relapse rates (near 75 percent), recent research shows that most people improve after treatment (Project MATCH, 1997). All substance abuse clients would probably benefit from traditional vocational and psychosocial rehabilitation services because of the interruption and dysfunction that occurs in these life areas—most notably the educational and vocational realms.

ADA Definition

Affirmation of alcoholism and addiction as disabilities is found in the Americans with Disabilities Act (1990). It formally recognized substance abuse and dependence as a qualified disability. However, there are restrictions on its recognition when it comes to alcohol and illicit drugs.

ADA defined *disability* using Section 504 of the 1973 Rehabilitation Act:

a. A physical or mental impairment that substantially limits one or more of the major life activities

b. A record of such an impairment (e.g., recovering alcoholics or drug addicts, people who have recovered from mental illness, people in remission from MS, etc.)

c. Being regarded as having such an impairment (e.g., obesity as a disability has been upheld in a 1993 case, or if an employer or agency thinks you're an addict or alcoholic)

d. Added to this definition was those with a contagious disease (most notably referring to AIDS, which didn't exist in 1973). People with contagious diseases are only protected when they do not pose a direct threat to the health or safety of others. Also, ADA does not cover less socially acceptable behaviors related to homosexuality, transvestitism, exhibitionism or other sexual behavior disorders, compulsive gambling, kleptomania, and pyromania.

Qualifiers

The ADA makes important distinctions between illicit drug use and alcoholism or alcohol abuse (Shaw, MacGillis, & Dvorchik, 1994).

Illicit drug users (as found on Schedule I to V of the Controlled Substance Act, 1990) are explicitly excluded from coverage under the ADA if they are currently using and not under the direction of a doctor. If they are no longer using and have successfully completed or are currently in treatment, they do qualify as disabled.

Alcohol abuse and dependence are not specifically defined, addressed, or excluded from the ADA. Therefore, although one interpretation is that employers and others can't discriminate against those who abuse alcohol, it does go on to indicate that employers may discipline workers who violate policies that conform to the Drug-Free Workplace Act (1988). Basically, anyone who uses alcohol on the job or is under the influence on the job may be fired without protection under the ADA (as long as the policy applies to all employees). On the other hand, if no work-related use occurs or has been documented, the person may not be fired or otherwise disciplined. Job applicants who are regarded as alcoholics or alcohol abusers must be treated like any other disability group, and nondiscrimination practices must be followed (Shaw et al., 1994). Alcohol or drug testing is not viewed as medical testing and therefore not addressed or covered under the ADA. Then case law or the Omnibus Transportation Employee Testing Act of 1991 governs whether employers can perform or require drug or alcohol testing.

FUNCTIONAL LIMITATIONS

Now that we all recognize alcoholism and drug addiction (and perhaps alcohol and drug abuse as well) as bona fide disabilities, we need to analyze them as we would any other disability by exploring their functional limitations.

Disease vs Symptom

A lot of debate and energy have been directed toward the question "Is alcoholism or addiction a disease?" From a moral and political perspective the answer to this question has meaning. Morally, the disease relieves or at least reduces the blame and stigma associated with alcoholism or addiction. Disease may happen to anyone, regardless of moral character or willpower. From a political perspective, big money is involved: Insurance companies are willing to reimburse for medical treatment for a disease, but they won't pay a dime to help amoral or weak-willed people who make poor lifestyle choices.

The first researcher to make a strong argument for the disease concept was E. M. Jellinik, a respected scientist who first postulated the concept in 1947. The disease concept considers the damage done by heavy alcohol consumption as a product of the disease and the person and holds that a minority of people are allergic to drinking—a biological vulnerability places them at risk once alcohol enters their bloodstream. For these people, to start drinking is to start down a fatal alcoholic road that for many follows this sequence:

1. First, what looks like normal, social drinking
2. Then, heavier and more frequent drinking (insidious and inevitable)
3. Drunken bouts, secret drinking, morning drinking
4. Blackouts of memory from the night before. It begins to take more and more liquor to get drunk, and attempts to stop are potentially life-threatening (tolerance and withdrawal).
5. Crucial symptom develops—loss of control. At this point, whenever the person takes a drink, the alcohol automatically triggers an inability to control drinking, and drunken bouts become the rule.
6. There follows an inevitable deepening slavery to alcohol that wrecks social life, brings ruin, and culminates in death.

Characteristics of the Disease

The American Medical Association defines alcoholism as a primary, chronic disease with genetic, psychosocial, and environmental factors influencing its development and manifestations. The disease is often progressive and fatal. It is characterized by continuous or periodic impaired control over drinking, preoccupation with the drug alcohol, use of alcohol despite adverse consequences, and distortion in thinking, most notably denial (Morse & Flavin, 1992). This definition is commonly applied to other drugs by simply substituting the word "addiction" for alcoholism and "drug use" for drinking. Some of the terms used in this definition require further clarification.

Primary disease: Refers to alcoholism as an entity unto itself and not a symptom of something else (e.g., you don't develop alcoholism because of a traumatic childhood—although trauma may be a triggering event in someone who has the genetic risk factors).

Progressive disease: Refers to the course of the disease as characterized by deteriorating physiological and psychological functioning; it gets worse over time.

Chronic disease: Refers to alcoholism as a disease that will not disappear of its own accord—in fact, relapse is expected. With abstinence as the only acceptable pattern of treatment, remission will occur. The disease will manifest itself, however, whenever the person begins drinking or using drugs again.

Fatal disease: The disease, if not arrested and sent into remission by abstinence, will result in death. Death may occur from the direct result of drinking or drug use (e.g., cirrhosis of the liver, overdose, stroke brought on by increased blood pressure) or more commonly by indirect causes such as trauma occurring while under the influence (e.g., motor vehicle accident) or lifestyle dangers (e.g., gunshot wounds related to drug deals).

The disease is treatable and has a very favorable diagnosis with abstinence. Treatment options typically include inpatient, outpatient and intensive outpatient, dominated by the AA model that requires the individual to do the following:

- Accept the label "alcoholic" or "addict"
- Admit loss of control of use
- Express a desire to quit drinking or using drugs
- Become and remain abstinent from all forms of alcohol or mood altering drugs

The Functional Limitations Approach

From the rehabilitation counselor's perspective, whether alcoholism or addiction is a disease is a secondary issue. As with all disabilities, the most important question is "What are the functional limitations of alcoholism or addiction?" Functional limitation is "The hindrance or negative effect in the performance of tasks or activities, and other adverse and overt manifestations of a mental, emotional, or physical disability" (Wright, 1980, p. 68). According to Wright (1980), "For rehabilitation the issue is not a medical condition but the resulting limitation in functioning, in a life adjustment context" (p. 84).

There are a number of reasons why focusing on the functional limitations of substance abuse/dependence is preferable to focusing on disease or a diagnostic label.

1. This approach takes into account the wide variation that exists among people with the same disabilities. This individualized approach is especially relevant for substance abuse/dependence because there is marked variation in how it affected development and current function in vocational, educational, family, financial, and other realms.

2. Focusing on functional limitations is more empirical because it deals with observable behaviors, rather than inferred psychological processes. Therefore, the problems are easier to identify and modify as a result of counseling (Crew & Athelstan, 1984).

3. Functional limitations are logically linked to the rehabilitation goals and eventual rehabilitation outcome, which gives a clear structure to rehabilitation planning designed to address functional limitations. Failure to address vocational, educational, or developmental issues is closely linked to relapse.

4. Functional limitations require an individualized assessment of the person, reducing the chances of stereotypical thinking and treating all clients alike.

5. Medical or psychological diagnostic models provide limited information about the individual's ability or capacity to participate in life activities.

6. Most medical or psychological classification systems are specific problem oriented and have little to no correlation with observable behaviors and no examination of client strengths. Consequently, there is little opportunity to observe and evaluate behavioral change.

7. Little or no information is provided in traditional classification schemes about developmental, sociocultural, or environmental conditions that impede or enhance performance.

DEVELOPMENTAL-ENVIRONMENTAL REALM

In 1993 Hanoch Livneh and Robert Male created a classification system composed of six functional realms aimed at describing completely the possible manifestations of functional limitation and capacities encountered by individuals with disabilities. The intention of their model is to create a more complete and utilitarian system for examining limitations and capacities in terms of their impact on the individual and the performance of life activities. Table 3.1 illustrates their six functional realms.

Table 3.1 Livneh and Male Classification System

Functional Realm	Context
Physical-Structural	Structural and physical abnormalities
Physical-Neurological	Physical functioning affected by neurological problems
Cognitive-Processing	Neurological structural abnormalities and diminished cognitive abilities
Cognitive-Affective	Neurological structural abnormalities resulting in impaired judgment, attention, concentration, chronic pain, etc.
Social-Structural	Impairments in social functioning resulting from structural (i.e., physical) or environmental conditions
Social-Affective	Impairment in social functioning grounded in affective issues

While Livneh and Male's model offers a comprehensive examination of the issues confronting individuals with "traditional" disabilities, it falls short in its lack of analysis of the functional limitations and functional capacities possessed by individuals with substance abuse and dependence disabilities. Many individuals with substance abuse problems also have coexisting disabilities and consequently possess limitations in the areas identified by Livneh and Male. For example, an individual with coexisting traumatic brain injury and substance abuse problems might typically have limitations in cognitive, structural, or social realms accounted for by the traumatic brain injury. That same individual might have other problems created by the substance abuse disability, which may exacerbate the overall disabling condition. Unfortunately, Livneh and Male's classification system fails to address the problems created by and inherent in the disability of substance abuse.

Do unique characteristics that typify substance abuse as a disability exist? If the problems commonly related to substance abuse are examined, two central themes emerge: Individuals with substance abuse and dependence problems exhibit a variety of personal development problems and experience a variety of environmental problems. Using the Livneh and Male model, these individuals can be conceptualized as experiencing limitation and capacities in the developmental-environmental realm. The realm includes those personal attributes, behaviors, and characteristics that occur as a result of pathological psychological, behavioral, or personal development, or as a result of the individual's interaction with the environment. This model is not a causal model, nor is it a certainty model, but it might best be described as a relation-risk factor model. Developmental or environmental problems do not cause substance abuse problems, nor do developmental or environmental problems always lead to substance abuse or dependence. Rather, clinical evidence and data suggest that individuals with developmental-environmental problems appear to be at much higher risk for the acquisition of drug and alcohol problems, and both treatment and recovery are fraught with more pitfalls and setbacks.

Developmental Issues

It is readily acknowledged that substance abuse and dependence have a significant impact on individual development. Individuals in treatment often report relationship problems, self-esteem and self-concept difficulties, feelings of isolation and loneliness, and loss of control, not only of drinking and drugging behaviors but a total loss of the ability to control and direct their own lives. Clearly these are individuals with significant personal development issues. Many individuals begin their substance abuse careers as adolescents, and the developmental problems they encounter as adults may be easily traced to their failure to accomplish the normal developmental tasks of adolescence. In his classic model, Erickson (1963) views adolescence as a time of identity formation and establishment of an understanding of self in relation to others and to society at large. Individuals leave behind the dependence of childhood as they struggle to achieve a sense of the independence of adulthood. For nearly all individuals, this is a time of great turmoil and tribulation filled with experimentation with new roles, developing new identities, and responding to the reaction of peers, siblings, parents, teachers, and others. Additionally, growth spurts, body transformations, hormonal variations, and emotional upheaval compound the struggle, and successful struggle becomes more difficult when drugs and alcohol enter the picture. For nearly all adolescents, some experimentation with alcohol and drugs is a normal part of the adolescent struggle as they shift away from conformity to parental authority and toward conformity with peer pressure and their demands (Santrock, 1990).

Discussion   Identify the conformity demands of parents and peers. Are they
Questions: similar? How do they differ? Do peers exhibit only negative
                 conformity demands?

Indeed, although politically incorrect, it might be argued that some level of experimentation is an important and necessary element of adolescent adjustment. The prevalence of experimentation is clearly seen in the data: Federal studies consistently reveal that 98 percent of high school seniors experiment with one of the "gateway" (alcohol, marijuana, or tobacco) drugs. The vast majority of teenagers experiment briefly with drugs and alcohol and then move on to other issues and concerns. Three groups are worthy of concern, however. Some individuals develop severe abuse or dependence problems by going beyond experimentation. Another problem group includes those individuals who turn to drugs and alcohol as a means of coping with the problems of adolescence. Finally, the emergence of gangs and concurrent drug- and alcohol-related behaviors is especially troublesome with regard to individual development. Data reveal that teenage drug use declined for a number of years until an upsurge that began in the early 1990s. Alcohol use has remained more or less steady through the years, although the same data reveal that the age of first teen drug or alcohol use is declining. The earlier onset of drug and alcohol use, and the earlier potential onset of drug and alcohol problems, is particularly troubling from a developmental perspective. Young teenagers may have less physical ability to cope with the potential ravages of alcohol and drug abuse and certainly have fewer developmental skills to cope with abuse-related problems. In any case, adolescents who abuse alcohol and drugs are less likely to achieve important developmental milestones, often resulting in severe deficits in adult functioning. Erickson would suggest they suffer from identity confusion and alienation, whereas Havighurst (1948) would question their ability to be independent and capable of displaying socially responsible behavior.

Developmental deficits are not limited to the psychological milieu. According to Jean Piaget's schema of intellectual development, individuals go through a "progressive unfolding of conceptual and thought processes" (Vinacke, 1968, p. 390) en route to full intellectual development. Clearly the cognitive impairment powers of drugs and alcohol can affect full intellectual development. As will be seen later, a significant environmental concern arises in this area also. Vocational development appears to be also impeded by adolescent drug and alcohol abuse. Super (1957) suggests that adolescents progress through a series of discrete vocational development stages, culminating in adopting a career direction and beginning the career by implementing a vocational preference and appropriate first job. Super argues that vocational development is not an isolated event or series of events. Rather it is closely aligned with, and should be viewed as one element of, the total self-concept. If the individual fails to achieve appropriate developmental personality milestones, it follows that vocational milestones and vocational progress will be effected. Indeed, many young adults seen in treatment have limited work histories characterized by frequent job changes, lack of progression beyond entry-level positions, or no legitimate job history at all. This is also an area of environmental concern.

Most developmental theories focus on childhood and adolescent development with little or no consideration of adult events or activities and their impact on development, and the assumption seems to be that once developmental milestones are achieved, regression to an earlier developmental state is not possible. However, when adults with substance abuse problems are examined, it becomes clear that nearly all adults with substance abuse problems rely on or exhibit developmentally inappropriate or regressed strategies and behaviors. Certainly the overwhelming reliance on defense mechanisms (i.e., denial, repression, rationalization, etc.) by adults with dependence problems points to developmental regression. These adults may have successfully negotiated childhood and adolescent stages, only to experience developmental loss as a result of their drug or alcohol dependence. Many adults with substance abuse problems fail to participate in normal social and vocational events and relationships of adulthood. Often their social circle is limited to other substance abusers, and nonusing friends and acquaintances are avoided or dropped; similarly, social activities are confined to events where drug or alcohol consumption is the centralizing theme or will at least be possible. The Alcoholics Anonymous precept calling for individuals in recovery to seek "new playmates and new playpens" speaks directly to this developmental concern, and many treatment centers urge individuals in recovery to be aware of social relationships and activities to prevent relapse.

Alcoholism has been called the lonely disease, reflecting the isolation experienced by many individuals with alcoholism. That isolation from friends, family, society, and the world of work results in not having a sense of what is normal, a common concern of individuals in treatment. This lament is heard from individuals whose substance abuse dates from their teenage years and from those who acquired substance abuse problems as adults. Isolation occurs as a result of stigma, too. Individuals with substance abuse problems are clearly stigmatized by society, both as individuals and as part of a culture seen as deviant by society: In effect they get the message that they are not normal.

Women with substance abuse problems are often doubly or triply stigmatized and regarded as abnormal. Historically, women with substance abuse problems have been regarded as promiscuous and wanton; more recently women who abuse crack cocaine are seen as unfit mothers. Some Alcoholics Anonymous members have been known to look unfavorably on drug users, especially illicit drug users, and of course, society in general is more tolerant of alcohol abuse than drug abuse. Parents, upon learning that their teenage child has an alcohol problem, often breathe a sigh of relief that "it's not a drug problem, thank God." Some drug use is regarded as so deviant that society does its best to remove the abuser from participation in society, as is seen in the disproportionately severe prison sentences given to individuals convicted of crack cocaine use compared to sentences for powder cocaine use. This hierarchy of stigma also exists within members of the drug culture. For example, individuals within the drug culture look down on individuals who smoke crack cocaine ("pipers") as the lowest form of drug user. Inhalant use among teenagers is seen as exceptionally deviant and abnormal, as seen in the case study.

Institutionalization itself may be another factor contributing to the feeling of not understanding what it is to be normal. People who grow up in institutions or who are confined to institutions as adults often fail to develop a sense of normal drug-consuming and alcohol-consuming behaviors. For example, many children with congenital or early onset disabilities are educated in residential schools where they are unable to observe normal adult drinking behaviors or to participate in normal adolescent drug and alcohol exploration behaviors. Individuals incarcerated as adults (especially young adults) may develop a skewed view of the appropriateness and reality of drug use and abuse. Prisons rarely are a place of rehabilitation; rather they often are a training ground for illicit behavior.

The Juvenile Prison Drug Program

The task was to evaluate the drug treatment program within a model juvenile correctional facility located in the suburbs of one of the largest cities in the country. The evaluator was shocked to discover that the client caseload consisted nearly entirely of white males from rural counties in the state, not the minority, inner-city males who seemed to be the center of attention in the newspaper headlines and on the evening news. Interviews with each client revealed that nearly all were incarcerated for inhalant substance abuse offenses, typically involving gasoline, paint thinner or glue sniffing, and in one case, air freshener sniffing. The evaluator's reaction was one of puzzlement: In the hierarchy of drug-related crimes, inhalant abuse seemed to be insignificant compared to crimes related to crack, heroin, or methamphetamine abuse. Certainly inhalant abuse rarely, if ever, made the headlines. Exploring the situation further, the evaluator discussed the issue with program staff and probation and parole officers. Everyone agreed that the "drug crimes" committed by the clients were insignificant compared to the violent crimes committed by inner-city youth high on crack.

After much interviewing and discussion, a hypothesis and a consensus finally emerged. It appeared that the inhalant-sniffing behavior exhibited by these youth was so deviant and so far outside the definition of normalcy that the juvenile criminal justice system's response was to remove them from the society. Many of the youth who were interviewed indicated a history of concurrent alcohol problems that were treated relatively lightly by the court and social systems in their rural counties. However, a significantly more stringent response occurred upon arrest for inhalant abuse-related crimes, resulting in incarceration and referral for drug treatment. Another hypothesis emerged with respect to inner-city youth and crack or heroin dependence. While these activities were seen as illegal and inappropriate, they were not seen as remarkably deviant because of the users' low socioeconomic and minority status. Crack and heroin dependence appeared to be within the boundaries of "normal" illicit drug-taking behavior for inner-city youth and less likely to elicit a referral for drug treatment.

Developmental problems do not require institutionalization to eventuate: They occur for many individuals raised in traditional two–parent households and are also seen among adult children of alcoholics. Their developmental problems attest to the negative developmental influence of growing up in a home where one or both parents has an alcoholism problem. Victimization by violence, either as a child or an adult, can result in developmental issues affecting drug or alcohol abuse behaviors. The majority of women seen in treatment centers report childhood incest victimization (Glover, Janikowski, & Benshoff, 1996); the relationship between domestic violence and alcohol or drug abuse seems quite clear. Often the perpetrator of violence is high or intoxicated, and often the victim is under the influence also. An effort to ascribe causality or blame is neither appropriate nor warranted in these situations. Although they may be predisposing, drugs and alcohol do not cause violent events, nor should the victim of physical or sexual violence be blamed for his or her drinking behavior. Instead, the realities of developmentally based problems should be addressed as part of the intervention and treatment process.

Environmental Issues

The environment can be a hostile place for individuals with substance abuse and dependence problems. As it is conceptualized in this model, the environment includes vocational and educational settings, the community, institutions and care-providing organizations, and economic issues. Vocational issues are perhaps the most often neglected or overlooked elements of recovery in substance abuse treatment programs, often because substance abuse counselors have little training or background in this area. Sadly, a typical entry in the case file on vocational problems may be limited to "has a job to return to" or "unemployed." While some clients are referred to treatment by employee assistance programs and do have a job to which they will return, many clients enter treatment with very deficient or nonexistent work histories. Typically, they have engaged in a series of entry-level jobs, have experienced frequent job loss, or have no verifiable work history whatsoever. No matter the situation, vocational status is a central component of normal adult functioning and for many people serves as the central definer of their self-concept. Logically, then, vocational concerns must be addressed during the treatment process and in the recovery program. To do less is to be short-sighted or even unethical, but many treatments fail to include vocational counseling or even to address vocational issues as a fundamental part of treatment. Since vocational issues are so intimately and intricately linked to adult functional status, is there any wonder that relapse is more common among individuals who are underemployed or unemployed?

At a minimum, substance abuse treatment programs should include as part of the intake and assessment process an evaluation of the client's vocational history, and treatment plans should include any needed interventions, including services provided directly by the agency as well as referrals to other agencies. Recovery will not be successful if treatment fails to implement strategies to deal with vocational deficits. Even clients with successful work histories should be encouraged to examine vocational issues during treatment. It is easy to assume that clients referred by employee assistance programs will have no trouble reintegrating into the workforce or to assume that no vocational problems exist. In reality, the very fact that a client has been referred by an employee assistance program is a tacit indicator that some level of job performance problems existed prior to treatment. Is does not matter if those problems were identified by the employer or by the employee. The employee will be returning to a work environment that will treat the employee differently, in most cases, and the employee will, in all likelihood, view the work environment differently.

The Case of Harvey

Harvey was a skilled and highly experienced finish carpenter referred to treatment for a long-term alcoholism problem. His employer became concerned when he disappeared from the job in late afternoons and when customers began to complain about shoddy work. Finally, he was arrested for driving under the influence while behind the wheel of a company truck. Contacted by the employee assistance program, Harvey disclosed a history of progressive drinking problems and agreed to enter an intensive outpatient program in his community. Near the end of treatment he expressed some anxiety about returning to work. Upon questioning by his counselor, Harvey revealed that his work crew also functioned as his social network. He related that the crew always ate lunch together and nearly always ate in a local bar. Afternoon beer breaks were a frequent occurrence, accounting in part for his (as he put it) "lost" afternoons. Finally, he noted that the work crew played softball and golf together and bowled together during the winter. Harvey did concede that he was the only member of the work crew who had developed an alcohol problem, although he thought others "might be on the way." Harvey's anxiety about returning to work had nothing to do with his ability to do his job or with his employer's reaction. Instead, he was concerned about how he would fit into the social life of the job and about how he would deal with the reactions of his colleagues to his newfound and much enjoyed recovery status.

Discussion Question: Discuss strategies that will be important for Harvey to adopt in the recovery process.

Individuals entering the workforce for the first time following treatment may need to learn specific vocational environment skills in order to be successful on the job. Analysis of job failures among welfare to workfare participants revealed that new workers did not fail at their jobs because of vocational skill deficits but that job loss was usually related to lack of awareness of workplace standards and ethics, nonworkplace demands that interfered with the job, limited external resources, and troubles dealing with authority figures (*U.S.A. Today,* March 1997). They lost their jobs because they failed to come to work every day or came late too often; family demands (especially child care) interfered with employment, and no outside resources existed to meet those demands; and reasonable and normal orders and directives from supervisors were not followed and were actively challenged and defied.

Often *economic environmental problems* arise from and are linked to vocational problems, and many individuals with substance abuse problems fail to develop or maintain economic skills. Interestingly, individuals who sell drugs as part of their dependence often have a history of making large amounts of money, albeit illegally, and this income is a powerful disincentive to treatment and recovery. The more common scenario, however, tends to involve situations in which individuals have a history of making little or no money or spending all their money on drugs, and have limited or no money management skills. Individuals who are employed often have economic problems, generally centering around credit problems. Frequently all of their disposable income and their necessary income has gone for drugs or alcohol, and many are one step away from bankruptcy, with implications for treatment and recovery. A two-tiered drug and alcohol treatment system has evolved in this country, and the majority of clients are eligible for only lower-tier programs. Because of economic problems, treatment participation is limited to crowded publicly funded programs, with no opportunity for treatment in higher-cost, more comprehensive private programs. The economic ranking of programs does not imply quality of care, however. Many public programs offer comprehensive state-of-the-art services, and some private programs offer a limited range of services. Increasing demands for accreditation and licensure and insurance company/managed care regulations have narrowed the gap between public and private providers. Economic difficulties are often more specific to the client than general to the system and may differ according to locale or situation. For example, economic problems may mean that the client cannot afford a car, which is not much of a problem in an urban environment with available public transportation. However, this is a major problem for treatment and recovery program access for individuals who live in rural areas. Child care costs can keep women out of treatment, but this is not typically seen as a problem for men. Economic problems do not go away just because a person enters treatment, and money management, credit development, and budgeting skills should be part of treatment planning for many individuals.

Discussion Question: Identify other economic problems typically confronting individuals with substance abuse problems. How would your own eonomic situation change if you had alcohol or drug problems?

Many individuals with substance abuse problems have educational deficits because of faulty interactions with the *educational environment*. If substance abuse begins during the adolescent years, this faulty interaction is often attributable to removal from or dropping out of the educational system. There is some evidence that the process is not as simple as just indicated, nor is it specific to individuals who leave school early for whatever reason. Mounting data suggest that learning disabilities are related to drug and alcohol problems in a very hidden way and in a way that has harmed the treatment and recovery process of many individuals. Learning disabilities were first recognized as a distinct disability in the late 1970s, and it was only after that time that individuals began to receive remedial support during their school years. Even today, most support for learning disabilities problems ends with high school graduation, and virtually anyone who graduated from high school prior to 1980 never participated in programming for learning disabilities. Consequently, it is possible, and likely, that many individuals in their late thirties and older enter treatment with undiagnosed and untreated learning disabilities. For example, Rhodes and Jasinski (1990) found that 40 percent of adult clients in treatment for alcoholism had indicators of undiagnosed learning disabilities. Other adults in treatment may have hidden educational deficits that have a relationship to the development of alcohol or drug problems and that impede the treatment process, as illustrated in the case of Homero.

The Case of Homero

Homero was admitted to inpatient treatment for alcoholism on a referral from his company physician. He was the foreman in charge of all operations at a huge assembly plant in the next community, a job he had held for the past five years. Homero went to work for the company just after high school graduation and steadily progressed through the ranks from laborer to assistant machine operator to machine operator to night shift foreman to general foreman. He boasted proudly that he could operate any machine in the plant during his intake interview. Upon admission his prognosis was listed as good, based on strong family and employer support, a cooperative attitude, and a relatively short history of alcohol dependence. Shortly thereafter, Homero began to experience problems. The psychologist revealed that he was uncooperative, failing to complete paper and pencil tests as scheduled. His counselor stated that he refused to turn in his written assignments from the group, and he refused to read aloud from the Big Book in Step group. His social worker related that he refused to write his family history. In staff review, the consensus was that Homero was inexplicably uncooperative, defiant, and irresponsible. After much discussion, the clinical director asked if Homero could read and write, a suggestion greeted with much derision. "Of course, he can read and write. He manages all of the activities in a multimillion-dollar plant."

As it turned out, Homero was functionally illiterate. His reading level was at about the second or third grade level, and he was not able to comprehend the reading and writing activities of the treatment program. Moreover, he related that his alcohol problems began when he was promoted to general foreman and left the plant floor for the plant office, and they grew worse as the plant increasingly modernized and computerized.

Clearly Homero's case presents a situation in which difficulties with his educational environment led to alcohol and treatment problems. He is not alone. Many individuals labeled "uncooperative defiant" or just "not getting it in treatment" may in fact be suffering from educational deficits that catalyze drug or alcohol problems and impede progress in treatment and recovery.

Discussion Question: What strategies should be used to meet Homero's needs in treatment?

The *social environment* can exacerbate or even serve to create drug and alcohol problems. Peer and family influences are well recognized for their powerful influence on drinking behaviors, both among adults and adolescents, and typically can be thought of as exerting forceful developmental influences. However, the social environment itself as seen in the day-to-day interactions with and associations with other individuals is problematic itself. A social network limited to other individuals with drug and alcohol problems is a network that is ultimately destructive. It is isolated from the mainstream activities of society and presents the individual with the fewest opportunities for growth and development. If it is true that you are known by the company you keep, then individuals with substance abuse problems are in a dire situation if their social network is limited to other abusers. The alternative social reality often seen in substance abuse is social isolation. Often abusers are estranged from family and friends and operate outside the usual social boundaries of society, with few resources for support, encouragement, and advocacy, and strong feelings of rejection and societal separation. Fellowship is one of the significant advantages and assets of the peer self-help movement, providing desperately needed positive relationships both for social isolates and individuals caught up in a negative social network (Glasser, 1998).

Recreational and leisure skills are closely tied to social networks, and the *recreational leisure environment* of many individuals with substance abuse problems is tied solely to drug and alcohol acquisition and consumption. They do not have hobbies or recreation lives, or if they do, alcohol and drugs are involved. Harvey's situation is a good example of this phenomenon. He had positive recreational and leisure outlets, but alcohol was always involved. Indeed, in one counseling session he lamented that he would never be able to bowl again because he could not conceive of bowling without beer drinking. Other clients have no leisure skills other than passive solitary activities such as television or reading and may become bored during recovery, a significant precursor to relapse (Lewis, Dana, & Blevins, 1994). This may be an especially difficult problem for individuals in recovery from illegal stimulant dependence, who have a high need for stimulation and excitement and low tolerance for boredom.

A *history of institutionalization* can create an adverse environmental situation for individuals with drug and alcohol problems, some of which can be related to treatment itself. Institutional environments nearly always have firm strictures against drug and alcohol use, and any use of drugs or alcohol is considered abusive use in a de facto sense. While these strictures are logical and appropriate in correctional or treatment settings, they may have limited validity in other settings, such as physical disability rehabilitation settings. As Shipley, Taylor, and Falvo (1990) and Helwig and Holicky (1994) noted, some institutions (i.e., hospitals and independent living centers, respectively) may completely ignore the presence of alcohol or drug problems, influencing the availability and appropriateness of treatment and the ultimate recovery of the individual. Having a history of institutionalization for drug and alcohol treatment or as result of an abuse- or dependence-related legal offense can adversely affect employment and educational opportunities as well as add a life-enduring stigma. Therapeutic communities have a long and positive tradition of service to individuals with drug dependence problems, but their philosophy of total allegiance to and involvement in the community presents difficulties for some individuals who have been unable to leave the therapeutic community environment and function in the real world. Secondary gain and disincentive for recovery are obstacles presented by some treatment systems. For many years, individuals who were dependent on drugs and alcohol were eligible for Social Security disability benefits. Although they were technically required to be drug or alcohol free, most were not, and they had little incentive to become abstinent. In the mid-nineties, the SSDI system removed more than 200,000 individuals with a primary disability of drug or alcohol dependence from their roles. However, many immediately reapplied for benefits on the basis of other coexisting disabilities, and many were reinstated. For some individuals, institutionalization may confer status: Some gangs may reward prison sentences by awarding higher ranking in the gang; participation in treatment, conversely, may be seen as a sign of weakness.

Finally, *environmental isolation* may catalyze or exacerbate drug or alcohol problems. The emerging recognition of drug and alcohol problems among individuals with disabilities, the elderly, and other groups may be traced to their relative isolation from the environment.

Discussion Question: Discuss groups for whom environmental isolation poses a high risk for drug and alcohol problems.

Issues of Choice

In his latest work, *Choice Theory: A New Psychology of Personal Freedom,* reality therapy theorist William Glasser writes ". . . for all practical purposes, we choose *everything* we do, including the misery we feel" (1998, p. 3). In this newest evolution of his work, Glasser suggests people have the ability to choose to be in control of their lives, instead of relinquishing that control to other people or to a dependency. Accordingly, for all people, the decision to begin using and to continue using drugs and alcohol is based on choice. This choice is not the dichotomous choice of the moral model that suggests that dependence is bad, and therefore, choosing to drink or use drugs is bad. Rather than this simplistic black or white dichotomy, choice implies the freedom, ability, and responsibility to choose between at least two options and to modify or expand those options as needed. It is a cognitive process affected by both personal development and the environment, and consequently, substance abuse or dependence severely limit options or impair the ability to choose.

Most people are relatively good at making choices, even though most of the time they do not have a complete understanding of the repertoire of choice options available to them. They understand that consequences follow choices and that most of the time, good choices lead to positive consequences, and poor choices lead to negative consequences. Moreover, people learn from their choices.

While people choose to begin to use drugs and alcohol, nobody chooses to become a substance abuser. Substance abuse and dependence result from constrained choice options limited by personal and environmental factors beyond the cognitive control of the individual. In some situations, that constraint is vividly seen. Individuals who are physically addicted to drugs or alcohol have nearly all cognitive choice options overridden by the physical demands of the body. They may want to quit using, but that choice falters quickly in the pain of withdrawal. The power and seductiveness of crack dependence is so strong, and the reward for smoking is so great, that other, more rational choices are discarded. How else can you explain mothers abandoning babies? Once detoxification occurs and the pain and craving begin to subside, more subtle constraint mechanisms take over. For everyone, and especially for people in recovery, choosing to drink or use drugs is a very highly complex choice, despite the simple slogans and rhetoric. Intricate decision-making skills are required, including judgment, analysis, and an understanding of consequences. However, when powerful development is impaired, or when the environment is fraught with problems, good choices may not ensue. As counselors we need to understand that becoming dependent and maintaining dependence is *not* a rational choice option. Rather, it is an option dictated by powerful internal and external forces, reacted to by poor choices. In the same vein, recovery *is* a choice option only if individuals have a full range of choices available to them and the freedom, ability, and responsibility to exercise those choices. Treatment and rehabilitation must go beyond abstinence, therefore, and include the remediation of developmental deficits and the evolution of skills to meet the demands and assaults of the environment.

SUMMARY

Based on the disease concept popularized by E. M. Jellinek and Alcoholics Anonymous in the 1930s and 1940s, treatment for alcoholism and drug addiction as a medical intervention grew markedly in the 1960s and 1970s. The "traditional treatment model" involved confronting denial, education about the disease concept, inpatient counseling based on AA's 12-Step model, and then discharge follow-up by a support group such as AA or NA. The field of rehabilitation counseling traces its roots back to the early 1900s and federal legislation designed to help people with disabilities obtain employment. Although substance abuse and dependence were recognized as disabling conditions, rehabilitation counselors usually deferred to the chemical dependency field to work with clients who had alcohol or drug problems. Aside from referral, the substance abuse treatment and rehabilitation counseling fields had little organized or coordinated contact with one another.

A systematic examination of the literature demonstrates that alcoholism/ addiction is a bona fide disabling condition, meeting rehabilitation's three disability criteria (it is a medically diagnosable condition, results in functional limitations, and there is a reasonable expectation that the person having this condition can benefit from services). Additionally, alcoholism and addiction were found to be disabling conditions under the Americans with Disabilities Act. Clearly, all types of drug addictions should be directly addressed by rehabilitation counselors in their work with clients. Rather than emphasizing the medical model and its diagnostic criteria of disease, rehabilitation counselors should focus on the functional limitations that result from the disability. The advantages of a functional limitations emphasis include consideration for variability among people with the same diagnosis; the logical link between functional limitations and rehabilitation goals and planning; reduction of stereotyping clients based on diagnosis or disability; and consideration of the person's assets and the developmental, sociocultural, or environmental conditions that impede or enhance rehabilitation.

Substance abuse and dependence disabilities experience both personal development and environmental problems and therefore are classified under the developmental-environmental realm of disability (Livneh & Male, 1993). Developmental or environmental problems do not cause substance abuse or addiction, but they can markedly increase the potential for such problems. Developmental issues for the substance abuser often occur at adolescence where three patterns of risk emerge: Normal experimentation with alcohol or drugs escalates to severe abuse or dependency; alcohol or drugs are selected as a maladaptive coping strategy to deal with stress and peer pressure (e.g., gangs); and there is concurrent emphasis on alcohol or drug lifestyles. Environmental issues affecting substance abusers typically include vocational, educational, community, and institutional/caregiving organizations. Rehabilitation of clients' substance abuse problems must be holistic and address not only the psychological developmental issues of the person but his or her environmental challenges as well.

4

Drugs and the Central Nervous System

The study of drugs affecting the cognitive and emotional states of the user is known as psychopharmacology. Although there has been research in this area for many years, the "psychopharmacology revolution" began in the 1950s with the development of antipsychotic drugs. Ray and Ksir (1996) stated that, at this time, "We came to accept the notion that drugs could have powerful and selective effects on our mind, our emotions, and our perceptions" (p. 7), largely because newly discovered antipsychotic drugs had freed thousands of patients from mental hospitals. More recently, the increased understanding of neurotransmitters, brain structure, and their functioning continues this revolution and promises to increase our understanding of just how psychoactive drugs work and why some people become addicted to them.

A basic understanding of the workings of the brain is essential to understanding substance abuse and addiction. This chapter will present an overview of the structure and function of the nervous system; discuss brain chemistry, neurotransmitters and message conduction; and finally review what is currently known about the neurochemical basis of alcohol and drug addiction.

THE HUMAN NERVOUS SYSTEM

The nervous system is divided into two subsystems: the *peripheral nervous system* (PNS) and the *central nervous system* (CNS). The PNS consists of the neurons (nerve cells) that exist outside of the brain and spinal cord. It is subdivided into the somatic and autonomic systems. The somatic system regulates or controls sensory and motor functions that are typically under conscious control of the individual. The somatic system allows one to be aware of touch, smell, sight, and sound, and to contract and relax voluntary muscle groups (e.g., arms and legs) in order to move about the external environment. The autonomic system controls or regulates the internal environment of the body (e.g., heart rate, blood pressure, hormone levels) and is usually not under the conscious control of the individual. The PNS nerves transmit information from the internal and external environments to the CNS and from the CNS to peripheral areas of the body. The entire nervous system is a very complex network of specialized cells that serves as a pathway for communication that enables the body to perform its functions. A closer examination of nerve cell structure and function will be helpful before discussing the CNS.

Neuron Structure

Specialized cells, called neurons, are the most basic unit of the nervous system. Neurons generate and transmit neural impulses. Each neuron consists of a number of components:

Cell body	The largest portion of the cell containing the nucleus
Axon	A singular process that conveys messages away from the cell body to other, adjoining neurons in the system. Axons are usually covered with a fatty sheath, called *myelin,* which acts as

insulation around the "nerve wire" that sends messages to adjoining neurons.

Terminal   The end of the axon may divide into multiple branches. At
branches   the endings of each are stored chemicals; these storage areas are
          called *vesicles.*

Dendrites   Multiple processes or projections from the cell body that receive incoming messages and convey these messages inward, toward the cell body

Receptors   Subcellular structures that are part of the cell membrane (usually the dendrites). Receptors are able to detect the presence of chemical substances called *neurotransmitters* that are released from adjoining nerve cells' vesicles and transmit the signal.

The neuron is specially designed to transmit messages within the larger nervous system. Communication takes place via an electrical and chemical chain of events. The billions of neurons comprising the nervous system, although part of the same system, do not come into direct contact with one another. Each neuron is separated by a very small space (about 1/10,000 of an inch across) that is referred to as a synaptic gap or simply the *synapse.* In order to communicate with other cells, each neuron must bridge the synaptic gap with its message. The neuron terminal that is releasing the neurotransmitter is referred to as the presynaptic terminal, while the receiving dendrite is referred to as the postsynaptic terminal (see Figure 4.1).

The communication process begins when there is a change in the electrical state of the neuron, which may be caused by external (e.g., touching a hot stove) or internal (e.g., having a thought) stimuli. The process of conducting messages across the nervous system is complex; however, a simplified version of it may be divided into a number of steps, shown in Figure 4.2. First, a neuron generates an

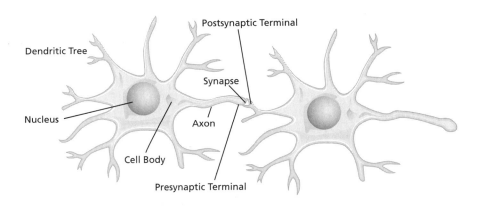

FIGURE 4.1 Components of neuronal structure

Source: from "Alcohol and the Brain," by M. E. Charness, in *Alcohol Health and Research World, 1990, 14(2),* 85–89. Reprinted by permission of the author.

electrical pulse that travels down its axon. Second, the electrical pulse reaches the end of the axon or terminal where chemicals called neurotransmitters are stored in vesicles. Third, the electrical pulse causes the neurotransmitters to be released into the synapse. Fourth, the neurotransmitter molecules saturate the synapse, and some attach or slot into receptor sites in adjacent (postsynaptic) cells. Fifth, after attaching to the receptor site, the neurotransmitter induces a change in the membrane structure that alters the chemical composition of the cell, which allows the message to be transmitted to the adjoining cell. Sixth, the electrical state of the adjoining cell is altered, and it initiates an electrical pulse that travels down the axon to release its own neurotransmitters.

The alteration that occurs in the target neuron may entail the transmission of secondary messengers that intervene between the original message and its ultimate effect on the nerve cell. The secondary messenger interprets the neurotransmitter attaching to the receptor site and uses this information to alter the firing rate and general metabolic activity of the neuron (Snyder, 1986). Hence, the electrical and chemical activity within and between neurons may be compared to a domino-like sequence, with one cell firing off, causing adjoining cells to change their internal state and to fire, which in turn causes other adjoining cells to fire, and so on. The process is very fast because of the speed of electrical conduction and the small gaps between neurons. It takes only microseconds for the neurotransmitters to cross the synapse and attach to its receptor sites. Synaptic transmission is quite brief; as soon as the neurotransmitter interacts its receptor sites, it is cleared away, preparing the neuron for the next release of neurotransmitter activity. The process of clearing the synapse takes less

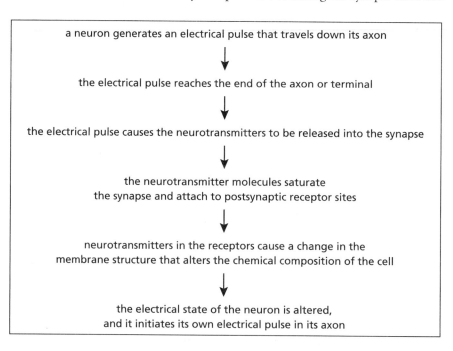

FIGURE 4.2 Sequence of message transmission within and between neurons

than $\frac{1}{100}$ of a second and is done in a number of ways. Enzymes may be used to destroy the neurotransmitter molecules that haven't attached to receptor sites, surrounding glia (specialized cells found throughout the CNS) may pump it away, or the neurotransmitter will be pumped back into the axon that released it in a process called *reuptake*. The reuptake mechanism is important because it conserves the supply of the cell's neurotransmitters.

The Central Nervous System

All human behavior, whether it is observable or not, requires CNS activity. The CNS is comprised of two interactive units: the spinal cord and the brain (Figure 4.3). The spinal cord is protected by the vertebrae of the spinal column. Openings along both sides of the vertebral column allow motor and sensor

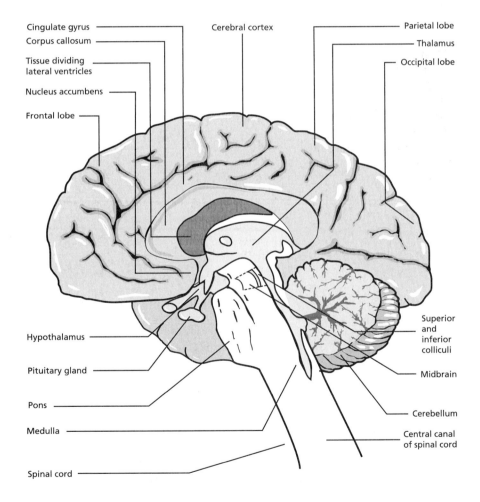

FIGURE 4.3 A sagittal section through the human brain

Source: Kalat (1991) *Biological psychology*, 6th ed., (Brooks/Cole Pub.)

spinal nerve roots to exit and communicate with the peripheral nervous system. The spinal cord is responsible for transmitting messages both to and from the brain. The nerves in the CNS do not regenerate as they do in the PNS; once CNS nerve cells are destroyed by injury or disease, they cannot typically be regenerated.

The second part of the CNS—the brain—interprets, coordinates, and directs impulses in response to internal and external stimuli. It organizes and directs motor activity and is the seat of cognitive processes such as learning, memory, and thinking; it is also the source of emotional responses. The brain, along with the autonomic nervous system, coordinates and regulates the function of internal organs so that the body functions as a unit. The myelinated fibers that conduct nerve messages and make up the inner part of the brain are referred to as white matter. Gray matter is the nonmyelinated nerve fibers that make up the outer portion of the brain that receives, sorts, and processes messages. The brain is the primary center for the integration, coordination, initiation, and interpretation of neural messages.

There are a number of structures in the brain that are divided into regions, but it should be noted here that the brain is quite probably the most complex structure in the known universe, and these divisions and their functions are not always completely understood. Proceeding inward, the brain is roughly divided into three major functional areas: *cerebral cortex, limbic system,* and *brain stem.* The cortex is the outmost part of the brain, with the limbic system and brain stem located deeper within the brain. It has been theorized that the brain has evolved throughout human history, with the brain stem being the most ancient and the cortex the most recent development. According to Beaumont (1983) the brain's evolution consisted of a series of layers wrapped around a central core consisting of the top of the spinal cord and the brain stem, with each successive layer adding a more sophisticated level of function that progressively extended the functional capacity of the system. Other important areas in the brain include the basal ganglia, hypothalamus, and the reticular activating system.

In humans, the *cortex* is the most developed part of the brain and comprises about two-thirds of its mass. The gray matter that makes up the cortex has three areas of function: motor, sensory, and associational. Motor functions allow us to move about the environment; sensory functions allow us to perceive the environment through vision, hearing, smell, and so forth; and the associational functions consist of higher cognitive information processing that includes memory, reasoning, judgment, abstract thinking, and consciousness. Certain regions of the cortex are connected with the reward systems located in the limbic system and allow for drive-motivated behavior (e.g., eating behavior to relieve hunger). These connections between the limbic system and the cortex are thought to be at the root of compulsive psychoactive drug use. This topic will be discussed more fully later in this chapter.

The brain is separated into right and left hemispheres, which in turn are divided into four major areas or lobes. The rational portion of the mind is located in the left hemisphere of the brain; it performs verbal, analytical, and sequential thinking. The right hemisphere is the intuitive and creative half of the brain; it is also responsible for spatial abilities. The major lobes of the brain are referred to as the frontal, parietal, temporal, and occipital lobes.

The frontal lobe controls voluntary and skilled movement. It is also involved with higher intellectual functions of foresight, analytical thinking, and judgment. The parietal lobe is considered to be the sensory area; it is responsible for integrating and interpreting sensation (light touch, pressure, pain, temperature). Some memory functions, especially those that are associated with sensations such as smell, reside in the parietal lobe. The temporal lobe interprets and distinguishes incoming auditory messages; it is responsible for hearing and understanding sounds. The occipital lobe controls the reception and interpretation of visual stimuli and is responsible for sight. Several parts of the cortex are involved in language; Wernicke's Area is responsible for receptive languages (it overlaps temporal, occipital, and parietal lobes), and Broca's Area is responsible for expressive language (it is found in the frontal lobe area).

The *limbic system*, found in the inner portion of the brain, consists of a number of structures such as the hippocampus (meaning "seahorse"), fornix (meaning "vaulted chamber"), and cigulate (beltlike) gyrus. There are significant linkages between the limbic system and the basal ganglia (which are bits of gray matter embedded in the inner white matter of the brain and are centers of activity). The limbic system, sometimes referred to as the visceral brain, is the center for emotions such as anger, aggression, and mood. It also regulates many behaviors responsible for survival, including hunger, thirst, and reproduction/sexual behavior. There appears to be overlap between the functions controlled by the limbic system and the hypothalamus, the distinction being that the limbic system organizes behaviors centered around these emotions and needs, whereas the hypothalamus is more concerned with the initiation of behavior in light of the current level of need motivation (Beaumont, 1983). The hypothalamus is also an important link between the brain and the pituitary gland, which controls many of the endocrine glands to regulate hormonal production. Several structures within the limbic system are critical to the rewarding effects of drugs because the sensation of pleasure or euphoria originates here.

The *brain stem* is located at the base of the brain and is formed by three primary structures: the medulla oblongata (oblong marrow), the pons (bridge), and the midbrain. The cerebellum sits astride the brain stem and forms massive connections with it as well. The brain stem controls our most basic bodily functions, including breathing, heartbeat, salivation, blood pressure, and the retching reflex. The cerebellum controls the coordination and integration of voluntary movement and equilibrium and balance of the body. Clearly, these very basic functions are the minimal requirements for human life, supporting the notion that this part of the brain evolved first. The reticular formation, including the ascending reticular activating system, is a netlike structure that runs throughout the brain stem. The neurons in this structure receive inputs from sensory pathways on their upward path (toward the cortex) and result in a generalized arousal of the whole forebrain and is important in maintaining arousal or wakefulness or attention. The 12 pairs of cranial nerves enter the brain at the brain stem level; the cranial nerves are unique because they are the only nerves that enter the brain directly without being routed through the spinal cord. The cranial nerves contain both motor and sensory nerve functions and are important for olfactory (smell), optic (vision), auditory (hearing and equilibrium), and vagus (taste) functions.

BRAIN CHEMISTRY AND NEUROTRANSMITTERS

The brain depends on chemicals to function. It may be viewed as a master pharmacist, dispensing the proper types and amounts of neurochemical (drugs), based on the body's particular needs at the time (e.g., sleep, attention, memory, movement). The brain is, in fact, unique among the organs in terms of the ability of chemicals, such as psychoactive drugs, to move through it to sites of action. However, not all chemicals that enter the body are allowed to enter the brain. A "blood-brain barrier" acts to keep certain chemicals in the blood out of the brain's neurons and glial cells. Glia are the cells that surround and give support to neurons; glia cells comprise about 85 percent of all cells in the brain. The blood-brain barrier is found in the capillaries surrounding the brain's neurons. The barrier is essentially a tightly packed lining in the capillaries that is selective in terms of what substances are allowed in and what substances are kept out, based on molecular size and solubility in the membrane. Overall, water soluble substances are kept out, and fat soluble substances are allowed in. Certain kinds of drugs only act on the peripheral nervous system because of the blood-brain barrier (e.g., antitumor agents). Partially fat-soluble drugs (e.g., morphine) must enter the brain slowly, wheras fat-soluble drugs (e.g., heroin) enter the brain very quickly. Hence, the blood-brain barrier can affect the rapidity of action of certain drugs and thereby influences the drug's potency. For instance, crack cocaine is more fat soluble than cocaine hydrochloride (the powdered kind), so it is able to cross the blood-brain barrier more quickly and give a faster, more powerful effect. Drugs that are readily dissolved in fat or oils are referred to as lipophilic, or "fat loving." Other drugs are water soluble and are referred to as hydrophilic, or "water loving."

As mentioned earlier, the brain depends on chemicals known as neurotransmitters to bridge synaptic gaps and conduct messages. Neurotransmitters are not the only neurochemicals that affect brain functioning. Hormones are chemicals secreted from specialized cells (i.e., endocrine glands) that enter the bloodstream and impact on organ and body functioning. An important distinction between hormones and neurotransmitters is that hormonal influences tend to be broad, impacting various parts of the body, whereas neurotransmitters are focused on the nervous system.

Acetylcholine was the first neurotransmitter to be discovered (in 1921) by the German pharmacologist Otto Loewi. Interestingly, Loewi isolated acetylcholine in the heart, not the brain, via an experiment on the vagus nerve (a nerve extending down from the brain stem that regulates heart function). Currently, there have been close to 100 neurotransmitters identified, 45 of which were identified after the mid-1970s (Snyder, 1986). Because of the recency of research on neurotransmitters, no one yet knows how many neurotransmitters may be discovered in the future.

Neurotransmitters may be either excitatory or inhibitory. Excitatory neurotransmitters will cause a neuron to "fire," or pass along, a message; inhibitory neurotransmitters will prevent a neuron from firing a message. Neurotransmitters attach, or "slot into," receptor sites the same way a key (the neurotransmitter) may fit into a lock (the receptor). Neurotransmitters may be very specific, only attaching to specific sites, or they may function like a passkey, attaching to several different receptors. Similarly, some drugs may act on all receptor subtypes for a particular neurotransmitter, while others act on specific receptor subtypes. This accounts for the fact that two different drugs can affect the same neurotransmitter system (e.g., LSD and Prozac both act on the serotonin system) but have markedly different effects on cognition, emotions, and behaviors.

Neurotransmitters may be classified in a number of different ways. One scheme employs categories based on chemical makeup and separates them into *amino acids, neuropeptides,* and *aminergic* (including catecholnergic). The first category, amino acids, are very simple organic compounds that are the building blocks of proteins. It has been estimated that about 90 percent of all neurotransmitters are amino acids. Examples of amino acid–based neurotransmitters are Glutamate, GABA, and Substance P. The second group is the neuropeptides; these neurotransmitters are a synthesis from amino acids. A peptide containing a sequence of over 100 amino acids is a protein, so peptides are an intermediate step between amino acids and proteins. Neuropeptides comprise about 8 percent of all neurotransmitters, for example, beta-endorphins and eutephilus. The third category, the aminergic neurotransmitters, are nitrogen-based organic compounds. Aminergic neurotransmitters comprise about 2 percent of all neurotransmitters and include serotonin and acetylcholine; catecholamine neurotransmitters are part of this group and include dopamine and norepinephrine. Table 4.1 identifies the primary neurotransmitters affected by psychoactive drugs, their action, and the major drugs that affect their action.

Acetylcholine is a neurotransmitter involved in muscle movement, memory, motivation, and arousal. Receptor sites for it are located in the nucleus basalis in the lower part of the basal ganglia and project into much of the cerebral cortex. Acetylcholine, its receptor sites, and an enzyme that catalyzes its creation have all been found to be greatly reduced in patients with Alzheimer's disease; this is understandable given acetylcholine's role in memory and the functional memory loss experienced by Alzheimer's patients.

Catecholamines are a group of neurotransmitters that have a chemical structure based on the catechol nucleus and have been linked to emotional states. The major neurotransmitters in this category are dopamine, epinephrine, and norepinephrine. *Dopamine* was discovered in 1958 in the corpus striatum, a part of the brain regulating motor behavior. This basal ganglia dopamine pathway is damaged in patients with Parkinson's disease, and these

Table 4.1 Neurotransmitters Affected by Psychoactive Drugs

Neurotransmitter and Function	Drugs That Impact the Neurotransmitter System
Acetylcholine	
Memory, muscle movement, motivation, heart rate, sexual behavior, sleep	PCP, marijuana, LSD, nicotine, cocaine
Dopamine	
Muscle movement, pleasure, energy	Virtually every drug that induces feelings of pleasure, including cocaine, amphetamine, opiates, marijuana, heroin, PCP
Endorphins	
Analgesia (pain relief), reward mechanisms	All opiates, such as heroin or morphine, alcohol, solvent inhalants
GABA	
Sleep, inhibition, anxiety or tension	Alcohol, marijuana, barbiturates, benzodiazepines
Norepinephrine	
Arousal and alertness, energy, pleasure	Most stimulants, including cocaine, amphetamine, nicotine
Serotonin	
Aggression, depression, sleep, appetite, dominance	LSD, alcohol, cocaine, amphetamines, MDA, and certain antidepressants
Substance P	
Pain	Analgesics, such as opiates and opioids, cocaine when applied locally to a mucus membrane

people experience tremors, rigidity, and other muscular control problems. Another dopamine pathway that leads from the midbrain is the mesolimbic. It projects into the frontal cortex and is part of the medial forebrain bundle. The Dopamine Theory of Reward holds that all addictive drugs stimulate this particular dopamine pathway, which is responsible for the motivating properties of virtually all positively reinforcing stimuli. In other words, when dopamine is triggered in the mesolimbic area of the brain, it has a reward function that signals to the rest of the brain to continue whatever it was doing to receive that stimulation. Hence, dopamine has sometimes been referred to as the "pleasure neurotransmitter." People with depression experience anhedonia, a loss of interest or pleasure in activities. Scientists believe that this symptom may result from lowered dopamine levels in the brain.

Epinephrine, also known as adrenalin, is primarily found in the bloodstream, while *norepinephrine,* or noradrenalin, discovered in the 1930s, is found extensively in the nervous system. These neurotransmitters may be understood as "energy chemicals"; they are released in greater amounts during the day and decrease at night during inactivity. Norepinephrine, especially, influences the level of arousal and alertness and may be important for regulating waking and REM sleep. These two neurotransmitters also mediate the body's emergency responses, such as increased heart rate, bronchi dilation, and elevation of blood pressure. This response has been termed the "fight or flight" response.

Another class of neurotransmitters is referred to as opioid. This name was chosen because scientists were aware of the opioid drug class before they discovered opioidlike chemicals in the brain. The binding site for opiate drugs was discovered in 1974 by three different laboratories (Winger, Hofmann, & Woods, 1992). This led to the speculation that there were morphinelike drugs that existed naturally in the brain and were involved in regulating pain. Two molecules were isolated and named leu-enkephalin and met-enkephalin; both acted like morphine but were much more potent. Shortly thereafter, a group of morphine-like chemicals named *endorphins* were isolated; the word *endorphin* literally means "morphine within" (endogenous + morphine = endorphin). Endorphins have an important pain-relief function. Beta-endorphin is found in relatively small quantities in long-axon neurons connecting the hypothalamus, forebrain limbic structures, the medial thalamus, and the locus ceruleus; it is specifically associated with the brain's opiate receptors. Enkephalins are more ubiquitous in short-axon neurons in the basal ganglia, hypothalamus, amygdala, and the substantia nigra. Endorphins are also released from the pituitary gland, and enkephalins may be released from the adrenal gland under conditions of stress (Akil, Madden, Patrick, & Barchas, 1976). When released from glands, these neurotransmitters function like hormones. How they affect the body is not well understood; some research into the "runner's high" has focused on endorphin release in response to the stress placed on the body by marathon runners.

Gamma-aminobutyric acid (GABA) is one of the amino acid transmitters in the brain, as indicated earlier. It is found almost exclusively in the brain and has an important inhibitory effect, reducing the firing of neurons. It is not organized into discrete pathways the way dopamine or some other neurotransmitters are. GABA may be responsible for regulating anxiety or tension. When the functioning of GABA is increased, the perception of anxiety may be reduced because of GABA's inhibitory action. Glutamic acid is another amino acid transmitter, but it has an excitatory function. People who experience a reaction to monosodium glutamate (MSG) have jaw pain and a flushing sensation because it triggers the release of this neurotransmitter. Glutamic acid may also be involved with memory.

Serotonin is found in a group of cell bodies located in the raphe nuclei of the brain stem. It is generally considered to be an inhibitory neurotransmitter and may slow the firing of neurons that alert the brain to incoming stimuli. Serotonin-containing neurons are thought to regulate many behaviors, including aggression, anxiety, depression, and sleep. Some of the relatively new antidepressants, such as Prozac, Zoloft, and Paxil, affect the serotonin system almost exclusively. The basic structure of the serotonin is the indole nucleus; drugs such as LSD and psilocybin have the same chemical structure as indolin, and drugs in this class are referred to as indoles.

Substance P is a neuropeptide found in the brain and throughout the body, especially the skin, that acts on neurons carrying pain messages. Any substance or event that causes an increase of substance P in a synaptic gap would result in the sensation of pain. For instance, foods that are considered "hot," such as red chili peppers, contain capsaicin, a chemical that releases substance P into various synapses and causes pain, which we interpret as heat. Opiates that relieve pain do so, in part, by blocking the release of substance P.

Discussion   Human behavior has a biological/neurological basis. How will
Question: our increased understanding of what goes on in the brain affect
                   how we treat people with alcohol or drug problems?

PSYCHOACTIVE DRUGS
AND BODY FUNCTIONING

A drug is any substance, natural or artificial, other than food, that by its chemical nature alters structure or function in the living organism. Psychoactive drugs are those that affect the cognitive and/or emotional state of the user. The effects of psychoactive drugs vary enormously, depending on a number of factors, including (1) the drug's chemical makeup (this factor is complicated for illicit or street drugs because so many other substances may be mixed with the drug); (2) the level of dose (this is also affected by method of ingestion); (3) the presence of other drugs in the person's system (a synergistic effect may occur when more than one drug is present in the bloodstream, thereby compounding the drug's potency, making overdose more likely); and (4) the particular characteristics of the individual user, including body chemistry, personality, and circumstances of use (mind set and setting during use).

Psychoactive drugs can influence neurotransmitter functioning in several ways. In general, there are two types of drugs, based on their effects on neurotransmitters (Kalat, 1998). An agonist is any drug that mimics or increases the effects of a neurotransmitter, whereas an antagonist is any drug that blocks or reduces the neurotransmitter effects. Neurotransmitters are manufactured or synthesized by neurons using enzymes that transform the "precursor molecules" into neurotransmitters. For example, the amino acid protein tyrosine is used to synthesize neurotransmitter dopamine; d,l–phenylalanine is used to make adrenaline and noradrenaline. Some drugs act as antagonists and inhibit the formative enzymes and therefore impede the production of neurotransmitters. For instance, blood pressure medication can block the formation of norepinephrine, which is responsible for elevating blood pressure. Other drugs interfere with the storage and release of neurotransmitters. If a drug causes neurotransmitters to leak out of the vesicles, the neurotransmitter may be broken down by enzymes, thus causing a depletion of the store of that neurotransmitter, also an antagonist function. Other drugs may act as agonists and infiltrate the vesicles, literally pushing the neurotransmitter into the synaptic gap and causing the neurons to fire or be inhibited (depending on the neurotransmitter's function). Still other agonist drugs inhibit enzymes that degrade neurotransmitters, thus increasing the amount of the neurotransmitter, while other drugs block the reuptake mechanism. Finally, some drugs bear a chemical resemblance to neurotransmitters (an agonist function) and slot directly into receptor sites; these drugs may mimic the

Table 4.2 The Actions of Psychoactive Drugs on Neurotransmitter Functioning

Agonist Actions That Tend to Stimulate or Increase Neurotransmitter Function

1. Crowding out neurotransmitters from their storage vesicles and forcing them into the synaptic gaps
2. Blocking the reuptake of the neurotransmitters after their release into the synaptic gap
3. Blocking enzymes responsible for degrading the neurotransmitters after their release into the synaptic gap
4. Binding to the receptor sites and mimicking the actions of the neurotransmitters
5. Facilitating the transmission of secondary messages that are triggered by the neurotransmitters

Antagonist Actions That Tend to Inhibit or Reduce Neurotransmitter Function

1. Disruption of the neurotransmitter storage system, causing them to leak out and be broken down
2. Blocking the release of neurotransmitters into the synaptic gap
3. Inhibiting the precursor enzymes that are necessary for the production of neurotransmitters
4. Binding to the receptor sites and blocking the neurotransmitters
5. Inhibiting the transmission of secondary messengers that are triggered by the neurotransmitters

neurotransmitter and be treated as such by the receptor, while others may block the receptor site without causing the message response to be transmitted (an antagonist function). Table 4.2 depicts the inhibiting and stimulating actions of psychoactive drugs on neurotransmitters.

The biochemical functioning of the brain may be altered when repeatedly exposed to psychoactive drugs. Several concepts are important to the understanding to the disruption of normal brain functioning by drugs; these concepts are metabolism, homeostasis, tolerance, physical dependence, and withdrawal.

The process of *metabolism* refers to the body processing, transforming, and eliminating foreign materials such as food and drugs. In the metabolism of food, matter is changed into energy (usually referred to as calories) and waste. The body reacts to drugs as though they were toxins and attempts to eliminate the drugs by metabolizing and eventually neutralizing them. Metabolism of drugs is performed primarily via the liver, but the blood, lymph, kidneys, or other body tissue that recognizes the drug as a foreign substance may assist in absorption and elimination. The liver metabolizes drugs by changing their chemical structure. With alcohol, for instance, the body is able to eliminate it at a rate of one-quarter to one-half ounce of absolute alcohol in one hour (equivalent to about one drink per hour). The liver, using enzymes that it produces, metabolized about 90 percent of all the alcohol that enters the body by converting it to acetaldehyde (a toxin), which is then converted to acetic acid and then water, oxygen, and carbon dioxide. The remaining 10 percent of alcohol is removed via excretion by the urinary tract, lungs, and skin.

Metabolism generally decreases the effects of drugs over time, but some drugs, such as valium, are transformed by the liver's enzymes into three or four compounds that have greater, rather than lesser, effects on the user. The speed at which a drug is metabolized and eliminated from the body varies from drug to drug and is referred to as the drug's "half-life." Half-life is the amount of time it takes to remove half of the drug from the system and is expressed in units of time, for example, hours (e.g., the half-life of a long-acting drug such as dalmane is 90–200 hours, while the half-life of a short-acting drug such as halcion is 2–6 hours). Half-life is the major factor in determining how long a drug will affect the user and how long it can be detected in the body. A number of factors, such as age, gender, race, the presence of other drugs in the system, and certain types of disabilities can all influence the metabolism of drugs. Drugs may be consumed at such a rate that they build up in the user's system, forcing the body to find a new chemical balance and adjust to a state where drugs are continually present.

Homeostasis refers to the body's ability to regulate and hold its internal environment in balance. There are a number of bodily functions that must function within certain limits or parameters. Body temperature is probably the most familiar. When the body deviates from the normal 98.6 degrees, it will either raise (e.g., by shivering) or lower (e.g., by perspiring) its temperature to try to maintain its thermal balance. Other body levels held in balance are blood sugar, heart rate, blood pressure, water content, acidity, and sodium content. Interestingly, the body will adapt to variations in the environment, compensating for such things as reduced oxygen found at higher elevations. Similarly, when the body is repeatedly exposed to psychoactive drugs, is will change its homeostatic functioning to accommodate the ubiquitous presence of the drug in its system. This process results in tolerance to the drug and is understood to be physical dependence.

The body adapts to the repeated exposure to psychoactive drugs in a number of ways, and increased *tolerance* to the drugs being used is one of these adaptations. There are a variety of types of drug tolerance. Focusing on the brain, *pharmacodynamic tolerance* relates to a reduction in the sensitivity of neurons to the drug. For example, if the brain is repeatedly exposed to a depressant, such as alcohol, it compensates by reducing the amount of GABA (an inhibitory neurotransmitter) that is produced or by reducing the number of GABA receptor sites (literally changing the structure of the brain). This adjustment occurs when the brain is repeatedly exposed to a drug over time and compensates for the drug saturation in the brain. Literally, the brain has learned to produce less GABA because of the presence of another inhibitor, alcohol. Similarly, research has shown that when the brain is repeatedly exposed to opiates, it will generate more opiate receptor sites or even produce opiate antagonists that counteract the effects of opiates. The end result in either case is the drug user requiring greater amounts of the drug to experience its euphoric effects. *Acute tolerance* refers to a single episode of drug use that results in an increased tolerance. In other words, subsequent doses of a drug, during a single episode or binge, seem to have less effect than the initial dose of the drug (e.g., the first hit of cocaine will produce a greater feeling of euphoria than the second hit taken an hour later). *Drug disposition tolerance* occurs when the use of a drug causes an increase in the rate of its metabolism or excretion. For instance, the liver will produce more enzymes to metabolize barbiturates or alcohol when repeatedly exposed to these drugs. Essentially, with practice, the liver becomes more efficient at eliminating a particular drug. The increased metabolism of the drug reduces the effect of later dosages, leading to an increase in the size of the dose by the user, which will in turn again raise the activity of enzymes to metabolize the drug. *Cross-tolerance* refers to a drug user's increased tolerance to different drugs that are in the same classification. For instance, alcoholics have an increased tolerance for barbiturates, another depressant. This implies that the body makes similar physiological changes when responding to similar psychoactive drugs. *Behavioral tolerance* refers to the process of learning to adapt to the effects of drugs from a behavioral standpoint. The drug user learns strategies to compensate for being under the influence. For instance, most people would be unable to walk a straight line or speak clearly when their blood alcohol levels are above .10 (the legal level of alcohol intoxication); however, people with high alcohol tolerance can frequently pass behavioral tests of sobriety because they've learned to compensate for drug-induced impairments. That is one reason why law enforcement must ultimately use blood tests to determine blood alcohol levels. In summary, tolerance results in small dosages having no effect; large dosages having limited euphoric effects; and dosages that would be fatal to nontolerant people taken without causing death. However, tolerance isn't always a never-ending escalation. *Reverse tolerance* occurs when someone experiences a marked reduction in his or her tolerance to the effects of a drug. For instance, alcoholics destroy liver cells through their repeated and increasing use of alcohol. Since the liver is responsible for metabolizing alcohol, its damage results in its reduced efficiency at removing the drug from the user's system. Hence, alcoholics with cirrhosis of the liver may stay drunk all day on a few beers because the alcohol isn't being removed from their blood, and it passes through the body time and again without being changed or metabolized.

Physical, or tissue, dependence is a concept closely related to tolerance; it is the adaption of the brain to the drug, and when the drug becomes absent, the user experiences "abnormal" neuron functioning that results in withdrawal symptoms because of the changes in the homeostasis of the brain. One might develop tolerance to a drug but not be dependent on it. For instance, many social drinkers have a somewhat increased tolerance to alcohol, but they are not dependent on it for normal functioning. Up until recently, the concept of physical dependence, along with tolerance, was relied on to diagnose addiction. In order for a drug to be addictive, it had to cause changes in brain cells (alter its homeostasis) after prolonged use. As a result, more of the drug must be taken to achieve the initial effect or euphoria (tolerance). When the drug is absent from the system, the brain responds by producing withdrawal symptoms because it is out of balance. Essentially, there are three characteristics of *withdrawal:* (1) the development of symptoms, such as sweating, chills, diarrhea, or pain, that result directly from the cessation or reduction of the drug by the user; (2) the symptoms cause distress or impairment in social, occupational, or other areas of functioning; and (3) the symptoms are not due to other medical conditions or a mental disorder (DSM–IV, 1994). Different drugs have differing patterns of withdrawal symptoms. Heroin and other opiate withdrawal produces diarrhea, chills, fever, runny nose. Alcohol withdrawal produces tremors, sweating, rapid heart rate, and hallucinations. Valium withdrawal produces seizures, and caffeine withdrawal produces frontal headaches (caffeine withdrawal can occur with as little as two cups of coffee use daily).

Inaba and Cohen (1997) identified three types of withdrawal. First, *nonpurposive withdrawal* refers to the objective, physical signs of withdrawal, such as tremors, vomiting, seizures, and so on. The locus ceruleus is a structure in the brain that seems to be important in withdrawal symptoms. Withdrawal symptoms from alcohol, opioids, and benzodiazepines are treated with clonidine, a drug that suppresses locus ceruleus hyperactivity. Second, *purposive withdrawal* refers to an active manipulation by the user who will exaggerate withdrawal symptoms or complain of withdrawal symptoms when none exist in an effort to obtain the drug. This manipulation may or may not be conscious; when it is unconscious, it is understood to be a conversion reaction from the expectation of the withdrawal process (i.e., the anticipation of withdrawal symptoms result in a self-fulfilling prophecy or placebo effect). Third, *protracted withdrawal* refers to a recurrence of withdrawal symptoms long after one has detoxified. The user experiences a symptom "flashback," frequently due to some stimulus or trigger in the environment. Withdrawal symptoms and hence craving for the drug heroin may be triggered by the smell of burnt matches; for alcoholics it may be the sight of a magazine ad for whiskey; for cocaine users it may be the sight of powdered sugar. These environmental stimuli have become paired with drug use and their effects; the addict becomes conditioned to these secondary stimuli or cues much in the same way that Pavlov's dogs learned to salivate at the sound of a bell. Protracted withdrawal may cause the recovered addict to relapse and begin using drugs again. This is potentially dangerous since the former user's tolerance has been lowered by abstinence, and overdose can occur if he or she attempts to resume a former level of consumption.

Discussion Questions: Have you ever developed a habit? If so, can you draw some parallels of the concepts of tolerance, homeostasis, and withdrawal to understanding your own behavior in relationship to that habit? How would you feel if you were forced to give up a habit?

THE NEUROCHEMISTRY OF ADDICTION

We know today that there is a clear and compelling neurochemical basis for alcohol and other drug addictions, rather than attributing it to a weak will or moral failings. Miller and Gold (1993) argued that there were four major factors that demonstrate that alcohol and drug addictions share the same neurochemical etiology:

1. Addiction to alcohol and other drugs typically occur in combination; that is, there is a strong tendency toward multiple addictions.

2. Family and other genetic studies appear to demonstrate an inherited vulnerability or predisposition for the acquisition of addiction.

3. Multiple addictions can be reliably diagnosed as independent or separate disorders in alcohol and drug users.

4. Recent animal and human studies have consistently found neurochemical, neurophysiological, neuropharmacological, and psychopharmacological mechanisms common to both alcohol and other drug addictions.

It appears that we are now in a position to formulate a theory for a common neurochemistry of addiction, comparable to that which has been done for schizophrenia and manic–depressive illness.

Addiction traditionally has been defined as consisting of two diagnosable conditions: physical tolerance to the drug (increasing amounts of the drug are need to achieve an effect) and physical dependence (the drug is required to function "normally"; if the drug is removed withdrawal occurs). Using only these two criteria cocaine may be viewed as only moderately addictive because its withdrawal symptoms are relatively brief and mild—most of which may be psychological rather than physiological in nature. A broader, and more complete definition of addiction should also take into account the cognitive and behavioral components of addiction. Someone is considered addicted if there is a strong craving or need for the drug, which is concomitant to drug-seeking behavior, even in the absence of withdrawal symptoms. This definition would confirm cocaine as a highly addictive drug because users, even after detoxification, report very strong craving and high rates of relapse. Goldstein (1989) defined addiction as the behavioral pattern of drug use, including an overwhelming involvement or compulsive use, excessive time and energy spent obtaining the drug, and a high tendency to relapse, even after withdrawal symptoms have ceased. Miller and Gold (1993) argued that addiction is "a primary disorder manifested by predictable and consistent characteristics not dependent on other conditions. A neurochemical basis underlies the loss of control inherent in the addictive drive to use alcohol and other drugs" (p. 122).

The DSM-IV provides the following definition of psychoactive substance dependence (addiction) and is relied on by psychiatrists, psychologists, and other professionals for diagnosing addiction. In order for a person to be considered addicted, he or she must demonstrate at least three of the following characteristics or behaviors:

1. The substance is often taken in larger amounts or over a longer period than the person intended.

2. There is a persistent desire (or one or more unsuccessful attempts) to cut down or control substance use.

3. A great deal of time is spent in activities necessary to get the substance (e.g., theft), taking the substance (e.g., chain smoking), or recovering from its effects (e.g., hangovers).

4. Frequent intoxication or withdrawal symptoms occur when the user is otherwise expected to fulfill major role obligations at work, school, or home (e.g., does not go to work because of a hangover, goes to school intoxicated, under-the-influence while taking care of children) or when substance use is physically hazardous (e.g., drives when intoxicated).

5. Important social, occupational, or recreational activities are given up or reduced because of substance use.

6. Substance use is continued despite the user's knowledge of having a persistent or recurrent social, psychological, or physical problem that is caused or exacerbated by the use of the substance (e.g., keeps using heroin despite family arguments about it, cocaine-induced depression, or an ulcer is irritated by drinking).

7. Marked tolerance to the drug or a need for markedly increased amounts of the substance (e.g., a 50 percent increase) in order to achieve intoxication or desired effect, or markedly diminished effect with continued use of the same amount.

8. Characteristic withdrawal symptoms are present when drug use is discontinued.

9. The substance is often taken to relieve or avoid withdrawal symptoms.

(*Note:* The last two criteria may not apply to cannabis, hallucinogens, or phencyclidine (PCP) because these drugs do not result in appreciable physical dependence or withdrawal.)

Discussion Questions: Is it meaningful to talk about addictions outside of the realm of alcohol and drug use? What is meant by gambling, food, or sex addictions?

From a neurochemical perspective, what takes place in the brain that causes someone to develop an addiction to a psychoactive drug? There is no clear explanation for why some people become addicted to psychoactive drugs while others do not. Research centering on biological factors examines the brain functioning of animals that have somewhat similar brain structures as humans (e.g., rats, cats, primates). Researchers in this area have attempted to identify the locations of reward in the brain, attempting to identify the neurochemistry of both euphoria and craving. What is known today is that drugs with reinforcing properties (i.e., those that result in drug-seeking behavior in the user) act by "hijacking" the reward pathways in the brain that are responsible for the survival of the species (Abbot, 1992). Behaviors necessary for immediate survival include eating and drinking, while long-term survival of the species depends on such behaviors as sex and mothering. These behaviors, in humans, are perceived as being intrinsically pleasurable. The drive to repeat these behaviors is located in the "reward pathways" of the brain. Three major brain systems have been identified as being responsible for the intrinsic reward or hedonic effects of drugs. These systems are heavily populated with receptor sites for dopamine, opioid, and GABA. The primary location of these systems is in the midbrain-forebrain-extrapyramidal circuit, including the medial forebrain bundle, ventral tegmental area, and the nucleus accumbens. In fact, the nucleus accumbens has been referred to as the "pleasure center" of the brain. Generally, the rewarding properties of drugs affect the brain's reward system. This reward system has a multidetermined neuropharmacological basis that seems to involve the same neuroanatomical elements or structures (Koob, 1992); the dopamine, opioid and GABA systems play key roles in the reward (and therefore the addiction) process.

There are two major dopamine systems in the ventral midbrain, with the mesocorticolimbic dopamine system being implicated in drug reinforcement. The cell bodies in this system connect the ventral tegmental area and the nucleus accumbens, essentially an interface between the midbrain and forebrain. The mesocorticolimbic dopamine system seems to act as a filtering and gatekeeping mechanism for signals from the limbic regions of the brain that mediate basic biological drives and motivation that are ultimately translated into motor activity by the extrapyramidal motor system (Koob, 1992).

The opioid peptides are found throughout the brain and form three major systems that are defined by their precursor molecules: Beta-endorphins from proopiomelanocortin, enkephalins from proenkephalin, and dynorphin from prodynorphin. These systems modulate the nociceptive response to pain (decrease pain sensations), reward, and homeostatic functions that relate to eating, drinking, and temperature regulation (DiChiara & North, 1992).

Finally, GABA is the most widely distributed inhibitory neurotransmitter in the CNS. A major function of the GABA system is anxiolytic or tension reducing. GABA's receptor sites are readily acted on by alcohol, barbiturates, and benzodiazepines. All of these drugs have classic sedative/hypnotic actions that include euphoria, disinhibition, anxiety reduction, sedation, and hypnosis. GABA function in the limbic and extrapyramidal regions of the brain, including the ventral forebrain and nucleus accumbens, appears to influence and contribute to drug reward because it is responsible for lowering endogenous stress or tension. In summary, the reward system in the brain is very ancient and very powerful. Its primitive origins were necessary to continue the species because behavior that resulted in survival had to be reinforced. Research with rats has demonstrated that when these regions of the brain are exposed to certain psychoactive drugs, some rats will continue to take the drug to the exclusion of all other survival behaviors.

An important problem in understanding the neural basis for drug addiction is "Why will drug addicts continue to use drugs, despite increased tolerance and the negative consequences of drug use?" It seems paradoxical that addicts continue to use drugs despite the reduction in pleasure that they receive from the drug (due to the many forms of tolerance they develop) and the negative or harmful consequences of their continued use (such as going through withdrawal symptoms or being fired from a job due to drug-related absenteeism). Robinson and Berridge (1993) developed the Incentive-Sensitization Theory of Addiction in an attempt to explain why addicts continue to crave drugs (drug wanting) despite the reduction in the subjective pleasure that they receive from drugs (drug liking). There are four main points to the Incentive-Sensitization Theory. First, all addictive drugs are capable of enhancing the function of dopamine transmission (specifically mesotelencephalic dopamine). This implies that all addictions tend to act on the same brain systems and have a similar etiology. Second, *incentive salience* is an important psychological component in the development of addiction. Incentive salience is the ability to transform the perception of stimuli (e.g., the sight of white powder, the smell of alcohol) into a salient conception, making the stimuli desirable or wanted. This psychological function is accomplished when mesotelencephalic dopamine transmission is activated. Third, in some individuals, especially those who are prone to addiction, the repeated use of an addictive drug creates incremental neuroadaptations in this neural system, which results in an increasing and perhaps permanent hypersensitization to the drug and other stimuli that have become paired with drug use (e.g., the sight of a needle becomes paired with the high experienced from heroin use). These stimuli become powerful triggers or cues for drug-taking behavior. The dopamine system is involved with associative learning; hence, drug use and drug-related stimuli easily become paired with feelings of anticipation and result in learned behavior that is repeated. This process results in excessive incentive salience being given to drug-taking and drug-related stimuli; normal wanting becomes excessive drug craving, which in turn results in compulsive drug use. In short, there is a qualitative difference in the brain function of drug addicts and alcoholics because of the neuroadaptions caused by the brain's prolonged exposure to the drug. Fourth, the sensitization of the neural systems that result in drug wanting or craving (i.e., incentive salience) can operate independently from neural system changes that are responsible for either the euphoria produced by drugs (drug liking) or from drug withdrawal (negative reinforcement). In other words, repeated drug use only sensitizes the neural system responsible for "wanting" alone, not the neural systems that induce feelings of pleasure (euphoria) or discomfort (withdrawal).

This theory explains why an addictive drug can be wanted more and more (craving) despite the fact that the drug may be liked less and less (diminished euphoria because of drug tolerance). It also accounts for the persistence of drug craving and drug use relapse, even long after the discontinuation of drug use, because the changes in the dopamine system are theorized to be long-standing if not permanent.

Currently there are no research data identifying the exact nature of neuroadaptions in the brain's nerve pathways that may result because of prolonged drug use as described in the Incentive-Salience Theory of Addiction. On the other hand, there does appear to be substantial evidence, based on animal models and clinical studies with humans, supporting a neurochemical basis of drug addiction. The mechanisms of addiction relate, at least initially, to the intrinsic feelings of pleasure or euphoria that addictive drugs induce (i.e., positive reinforcement) and subsequently to the negative reinforcement that occurs when one takes a drug to relieve the aversive symptoms of withdrawal. In addition, the learned behavior of drug use, when engaged in repeatedly, may sensitize certain regions of the brain responsible for reward. This sensitization is long-standing or even permanent and results in unrelenting drug craving in some people. Because addictive drugs act on those areas of the brain that are associated with basic drive states (hunger, thirst, sex), mood, and other instinctual behaviors, addiction may be conceptualized as an acquired drive, one that arises spontaneously, repeatedly, and persistently (Miller & Gold, 1993). The addiction drive is then manifest in behaviors related to the preoccupation with drug seeking, impulsive and compulsive use, and frequent relapse. In summary, research tends to indicate that there is a specific brain chemistry disorder that is the primary cause of the complex array of physical, emotional, and behavioral symptoms known as addiction. The mapping and understanding of the "neurochemical gateway" of addiction is still in its infancy, however, and future research and discovery will determine its exact nature.

Discussion   Why is it important to uncover a neurochemical basis for
Questions: alcohol or drug addictions? What are the ramifications for
funding for substance abuse research or treatment?

SUMMARY

This chapter presented some of the biological information necessary to understanding how drugs act on the user. The neuron is the basic unit of the nervous system, including the brain. The major divisions of the brain were briefly described. The cerebral cortex is the largest and most complex part of the brain and is responsible for motor, sensory, and associational functions. Associational functions include judgment, abstract reasoning, and consciousness. The cortex has significant connections with the limbic system, or the emotional center of the brain. This inner part of the brain regulates many behaviors responsible for the survival of the species, including behaviors related to hunger, thirst, and reproduction. In order for these behaviors to be repeated, they must be reinforced by feelings of pleasure, and the limbic system is home to the pleasure centers of the brain that are always targeted by psychoactive drugs. The brain stem is the most ancient part of the brain, and it regulates such basic functions as respiration, heart rate, blood pressure, and the retching reflex.

Neuron structures (such as axons, dendrites, synapses, and receptors) were identified and described in terms of their role in the transmission of neural messages. Neurotransmitters were characterized as the chemical messengers within the brain and were classified as either excitatory (tending to cause the neurons to send a message, or fire off) or inhibitory (preventing the neuron from sending a message). Several neurotransmitters directly affected by psychoactive drugs were presented, including acetylcholine, dopamine, endorphins, GABA, norepinephrine, and serotonin.

Concepts related to drug addiction and the disruption of normal brain functioning were presented. Metabolism is the process of transforming, processing, and eliminating drugs. Homeostasis is the body's ability to regulate and hold its internal environment in balance. Tolerance occurs when, after repeated use, the user needs larger and larger dosages of the drug to achieve the desired effect. Several types of tolerance occur, including pharmacodynamic, acute, drug disposition, cross, and behavioral tolerances. Physical dependence is the body's adaption to the drug-saturated state of the habitual user. When the level of the drug in the body is reduced, the habitual user experiences abnormal neuron functioning that results in drug withdrawal symptoms.

Finally, newly emerging information regarding the neurochemistry of addiction was discussed. There seems to be clear and compelling evidence that addictions have a biological rather than a purely psychological basis. Miller and Gold (1993) pointed to supporting research that has found (1) addiction to alcohol and other drugs typically occur in combination; that is there is a strong tendency toward multiple addictions; (2) family and other genetic studies appear to demonstrate an inherited vulnerability or predisposition for the acquisition of addiction; (3) multiple addictions can be reliably diagnosed as independent, or separate disorders, in alcohol and drug users; and (4) recent animal and human studies have consistently found neurochemical, neurophysiological, neuropharmacological, and psychopharmacological mechanisms common to both alcohol and other drug addictions. Abbot (1992) believes that the reinforcing properties of psychoactive drugs work by "hijacking" the reward pathways in the brain that are responsible for the survival of the species; hence, addiction may be conceptualized as an acquired drive. The Incentive-Salience Theory of Addiction was presented as a way to understand the distinctions between the reinforcing properties of drugs (i.e., feelings of euphoria) and the overpowering urges to use drugs (i.e., craving) despite the negative consequences that occur with addictive use.

5

Drugs of Abuse

CHAPTER 5 OUTLINE

I. Stimulants

    A. Amphetamines and Cocaine

    B. Caffeine and Nicotine

    C. Other Recreational Stimulants

II. Depressants

    A. Alcohol

    B. Opiates and Opioids

    C. Sedative-Hypnotics

    D. Inhalants

III. Hallucinogens

    A. Indoles

    B. Catechols

    C. Marijuana and Hashish

    D. Other Hallucinogens

IV. Summary

There are many ways to categorize drugs. The Controlled Substances Act (1970) created five drug categories or schedules that classify drugs based on their pharmacologic properties, patterns of potential abuse, and dependence-producing liability. Still another strategy for classifying drugs relies primarily on the user. Snyder (1986) placed psychoactive drugs in the following categories: opiates (e.g., morphine, heroin), neuroleptics (e.g., antischizophrenic drugs such as chlorpromazine), stimulants (e.g., amphetamines, cocaine), antianxiety agents (e.g., diazepam, chlordiazepoxide), antidepressants (e.g., amitriptyline, imipramine), psychedelics (e.g., LSD, mescaline), and sedative-hypnotics (e.g., phenobarbital, chloral hydrate). For the purposes of this chapter, however, we will focus on three broad drug categories that tend to be widely used recreationally and are most often drugs of abuse. These categories of drugs are stimulants, depressants, and hallucinogens. Stimulants include, but aren't limited to, amphetamines, cocaine, caffeine, nicotine, and other recreational stimulants (e.g., khat). Depressant drugs include alcohol, opiates and opioids (narcotics), sedative–hypnotics, and inhalants. The hallucinogenic drug class includes indoles (e.g., lysergic acid diethylamide, or LSD), catechols (e.g., peyote/mescaline) tetrahydrocannabinol (e.g., marijuana/hashish), and other hallucinogens (e.g., belladonna, amphetamine derivatives such as MDA).

STIMULANTS

Throughout our history, mankind has known about naturally occurring stimulants such as coffee beans, coca leaves, tobacco, and khat leaves. As a class, stimulants are those drugs that act directly on the central nervous system to create an increased state of electrical activity and accelerated mental processes. Their effects on other systems include increased blood pressure, faster heart rate, higher body temperature, and constriction of peripheral blood vessels. Generally, the subjective intoxicating effects of stimulants consist of mood elevation, feelings of pleasure or euphoria, increased energy and alertness, increased sense of well-being and self-confidence, and decreased fatigue and appetite. Stimulants have been used medically for treating depression, sleeping disorders (e.g., narcolepsy), and hyperactivity. Using a stimulant to treat hyperactivity in children may seem counterintuitive, but stimulants such as Ritalin have been very effective at calming hyperactive children. It has been theorized that hyperactive children are understimulated, and they act out as a way of self-stimulation. Giving these children small amounts of a stimulant obviates their need for self-stimulation, and the children are able to remain quiet and focus their attention.

Amphetamines and Cocaine

Amphetamines, along with cocaine, are probably the most powerful and widely abused stimulants. Amphetamines are synthetic drugs and include d,l amphetamine, methamphetamine, dextroamphetamine, and dextromethamphetamine. Common street names for this drug class are speed, meth, crank, crystal, and ice (these latter two names refer to the crystalline form of dextromethamphet-amine). The pharmacological properties of amphetamines, along with cocaine, make them highly effective CNS stimulants. The effects of amphetamines and cocaine are similar, but amphetamines are cheaper to make, easier to use, and have a greater half-life, giving them a longer-lasting effect. Amphetamines produce their stimulating effects by causing dopamine and norepinephrine to be released into the synapses in parts of the brain associated with pleasure, especially the nucleus accumbens. Also, the drug's molecules occupy the reuptake mechanism so that the neurotransmitters, having been released into the synapse, are not taken back up as readily and therefore stay active in the synapse longer (Kalat, 1998).

For centuries, Chinese used a medicinal tea having an active ingredient of ephedrine. Amphetamine was isolated from ephedrine and patented in 1932, and its first medical application was as a bronchial dilator for treating asthma and to counter low blood pressure (Ray & Ksir, 1996). A Benzedrine inhaler was sold over the counter as early as 1932. Later, amphetamines were widely used as "pep pills" and diet aids because of their appetite suppression effects. Rather than being a panacea for the overweight, users would develop tolerance that reduced the appetite suppression characteristics, requiring users to take ever-increasing amounts of the drug after only four to six months. During the 1960s amphetamines became a widely popular and profitable recreational drug, resulting in the emergence of illegal laboratories that manufactured amphetamines. In 1970 amphetamines began to be regulated by the federal government (Controlled Substance Act, 1970). "Speed," the most desired drug on the streets in the 1960s, has reemerged in the 1990s in the form of methamphetamine (Ray & Ksir, 1996). Methamphetamine is sold in liquid ampule form for injection and is sometimes referred to as "meth" or "crank." It is a derivative of amphetamine with a more potent effect on the CNS. "Ice" (dextromethamphetamine) is also a very potent and long-lasting derivative of amphetamines; it gets its name because of its smokeable, crystalline form.

Typically, amphetamines are taken orally in pill form, but injecting (shooting), inhaling (snorting), and smoking have been increasingly used. The peak effects of the amphetamines take place about 2 to 3 hours after oral ingestion. The duration of effect, or the "high," lasts about 4 to 6 hours; the half-life of most amphetamines is about 10 to 12 hours. Amphetamines are completely eliminated from the body about two days after last use (Ray & Ksir, 1996). In moderate dosages, amphetamines cause an increase in heart rate, blood pressure, and respiration. Appetite is reduced, and the user's mood becomes elevated with a mild euphoria. The feeling of fatigue is reduced, and the user maintains wakefulness. High doses disrupt neurotransmitter balance, and prolonged use can result in sleep deprivation, hallucinations, malnutrition, and extreme paranoia that is associated with violence. It is even possible for cardiovascular problems to develop. The disruption of the brain's chemistry essentially consists of a depletion of the brain's supplies of norepinephrine and dopamine, and returning to a normal balance can take weeks or months. The user, having depleted the supplies of these two important neurotransmitters, suffers from severe physical and mental depression during the recovery period. Like borrowing money from a loan shark, payback is often a painful process.

Cocaine is a naturally produced drug; a grave in Peru dating from about A.D. 500 contains the first record of coca leaf use. Coca leaves contain about 2 percent cocaine, and cocaine hydrochloride (a stable salt in powder form) was isolated from the coca leaf in about 1860. Because extraction produces pure cocaine, powder cocaine is much more potent than just chewing the leaf the way South American peasants do. Cocaine is made by mixing leaves with a solvent such as gasoline and soaking the mixture to create a mash. When the excess liquid is filtered out, a coca paste remains. In South America, paste is often smoked with tobacco, another CNS stimulant. The paste may then be made into cocaine hydrochloride, a stable salt that may be snorted or mixed with water and injected; freebasing requires mixing cocaine with a solvent such as ether to allow smoking. Crack cocaine became popular in 1980s when it was discovered that mixing coke with water and baking soda, then drying it, could make coke into a stable, smokeable form. The cocaine "rocks" could then be "cracked" into smaller pieces that produce a rapid, short-term high for about $10 to $20.

Cocaine has a very complex chemical structure that doesn't resemble, chemically, any known neurotransmitter. Its mechanism of action is to interfere with the reuptake of several neurotransmitters such as norepinephrine, dopamine, and serotonin. Its euphoric effects probably come from blocking the reuptake of dopamine and serotonin within the brain's limbic system; PET scan data show that cocaine works in large part by occupying or blocking dopamine transporter sites, preventing the reuptake of dopamine. It is this abnormally long presence of dopamine in the brain that is believed to cause the effects associated with cocaine. The absorption of cocaine is very slow when ingested by chewing the coca leaf, and the psychoactive effects are more moderate in nature. Snorting cocaine hydrochloride (the stable salt-based powder) results in quick absorption through nasal mucosa, and its proximity to the brain gives it a more potent effect. Intravenous injection allows cocaine to reach the brain in about 15 to 30 seconds, and when freebased or smoked, such as with crack cocaine, it reaches the brain in about 5 to 8 seconds (the lungs provide a very large mucous membrane surface area for absorption and rapid blood circulation to the brain). Cocaine molecules are metabolized by enzymes in the blood and liver and have a half-life of about an hour; the drug can be found in the urine for about 8 hours after ingestion.

Cocaine is not entirely without legal applications; physicians have used the drug for a number of purposes. Historically, it was also used for the treatment of depression and, interestingly, for morphine addiction. Its addictive properties were soon discovered, and cocaine was no longer used for this purpose. As noted in Chapter 2, cocaine was the active ingredient in a number of popular patent medicines sold in the United States during the turn of the century. Cocaine's effectiveness as a local anesthetic was discovered in 1860 and was used for eye surgery and dentistry. Today, medicine has discovered other local anesthetics that don't cause CNS stimulation; however, cocaine is still prescribed for nasal, laryngeal, and esophageal procedures because it is absorbed so well by mucous membranes.

Like amphetamines, cocaine produces an increased sense of well-being, euphoria, increased energy, and decreased fatigue. There is no evidence that occasional use of small amounts is a threat to the user's health; however, because of its powerful rewarding effects, it is very easy to develop a tolerance and increase dosage levels to the point of toxicity. Acute cocaine poisoning causes profound CNS stimulation, convulsions, and respiratory and cardiac arrest—similar to amphetamine overdose. Also, rare and severe toxic reactions do occur that cause cardiac failure. Cocaine, when used with alcohol, can produce a new chemical within the body called cocaethylene, which may be several times more toxic than cocaine itself. Cocaethylene was discovered in the early 1990s and has a longer duration of action, is more selective in blocking dopamine but not serotonin reuptake, and may be more lethal, given the high rate of drug-related deaths involving the mix of cocaine and alcohol; still scientists are not certain of all of its effects as of yet (see Randall, 1992).

The negative effects of stimulants such as cocaine include tremors, increased muscle tension, irritability, and anger (memory and orientation are not affected except with high dosages). Overdose or toxicity effects include bruxism (clenched jaw), paranoia, compulsive behavior, obsessive thoughts, auditory and visual hallucinations, coma, and even death. Chronic use can lead to nasal septum inflammation due to snorting and malnourishment because of neglected eating habits. Binging, a common problem with cocaine, leads to paranoia and hallucinations. If used by pregnant women, it can be very dangerous to fetuses—the "crack baby" phenomenon began in the 1980s and entails premature delivery, smaller head circumference, below average body weight, and increased susceptibility to infant diseases.

Withdrawal symptoms that occur with cocaine addiction are also common to amphetamine addiction. The major symptoms tend to be more psychological rather than physical in nature; they include anhedonia (the lack of ability to feel pleasure), anergia (lack of energy, motivation, or initiative), and an intense craving for the drug. There are, however, no life-threatening or physically painful symptoms of withdrawal. The treatment for amphetamine and cocaine abuse or addiction requires abstinence from all stimulating chemicals (including nicotine or caffeine). Nutritional approaches aimed at enhancing the depleted supply of neurotransmitters are also an important part of treatment.

Caffeine and Nicotine

The most widely used stimulants in the world tend to be of milder stimulating effect. Caffeine, which is found in the drug class of xanthines, is probably the most widely used stimulant in the world. It has been estimated that up to 92 percent of the U.S. population consumes caffeine on a regular basis (Winger, Hofmann, & Woods, 1992). Coffee was first discovered in the Middle East (there are in fact Arabian legends of its discovery by a goatherd named Kaldi whose sheep were acting excitedly after eating red berries) and spread to Europe by the 13th century. In low dosages, the caffeine in coffee causes increased alertness, heart rate, and blood pressure, and decreased fatigue. The absorption of caffeine, taken orally, peaks in about a half-hour, with the maximum CNS impact taking place in about 2 hours. The half-life of caffeine is about 3 hours, with about 90 percent of the drug being metabolized or absorbed and 10 percent being excreted, primarily through the urine. Caffeine works by blocking the brain's receptors for a neurotransmitter/neuromodulator known as adenosine (Ray & Ksir, 1996). Adenosine acts as an inhibitor, producing sedation; caffeine blocks the receptors for adenosine and results in a mild stimulating effect on the CNS.

With excessive use, caffeine can irritate the lining of the stomach and cause nervousness, irritability, muscle tension, and insomnia. At extreme doses, such as 10 grams or the equivalent to 100 cups of coffee, it will cause convulsions that produce respiratory arrest and possibly death. Dependence on the caffeine in coffee takes place at about 500 mg (5 cups of coffee) per day, and may be accompanied by some of the toxic effects, such as anxiety, and insomnia. Withdrawal from the caffeine in coffee has been well documented. People who drink as little as 2 cups per day may experience frontal headaches about 18 hours after they discontinue their coffee consumption. Fortunately, the level of dependence is rather mild, and withdrawal symptoms dissipate after a few days. Of course, coffee isn't the only source of caffeine; it is found in lesser amounts in tea, soft drinks, cocoa/chocolate, headache medicines, and over-the-counter stimulants. Table 5.1 depicts the amount of caffeine, in milligrams, contained in commonly used drinks, foods, and medicines.

Discussion Questions: Do any of the consumer products you use on a regular basis contain caffeine? Were you aware of it, and, if not, how do you feel about it?

Table 5.1 Caffeine Levels from Various Sources

Caffeine Source	Average Amount of Caffeine (in milligrams)
1 Cup Espresso	200 mg
1 Dose of Vivarin	200 mg
1 Cup Brewed Drip Coffee	115 mg
1 No-Doz Tablet	100 mg
1 Cup Percolated Coffee	80 mg
1 Can of Coca-Cola	80 mg
2 oz serving of Chocolate	40 mg
2 Anacin Tablets	32 mg
1 Cup Chocolate Milk	5 mg
1 Cup Decaffeinated Coffee	3 mg

Note: Dosages identified were selected based on typical serving size.

Nicotine, a relatively mild stimulant, is probably the most deadly, giving smokers a 70 percent greater mortality ratio than nonsmokers (Winger et al., 1992). Cigarette smoking can cause heart disease and lung cancer. The Surgeon General's Report (1979) stated that cigarette smoking was the single most important environmental factor in premature death in the United States. Premature mortality in the United States directly attributed to smoking is about 400,000 deaths per year, or about 20 percent of all deaths (Bartecchi et al., 1994).

Nicotine is the psychoactive ingredient found in Nicotiana tabacum, or the tobacco plant. Native Americans have known about tobacco for centuries; documented use by the Mayan culture dates back over 2000 years. The methods of tobacco use vary and include cigarettes, cigars, pipe smoking, and smokeless tobacco or chew. The patterns of use also vary widely, from the occasional cigar smoker to the cigarette chain-smoker. An intermediate pattern of use can be characterized as spaced use, with the first smoke taken upon waking and smoking at intervals varying from every 15 minutes to every 2 hours (Winger et al., 1992). Nicotine blood levels will rise and fall according to this pattern of use, with nicotine entering the bloodstream immediately as it is absorbed by the lungs (after inhalation, it takes about seven seconds for nicotine to reach the brain). The effects of nicotine on nervous system functioning has been extensively studied and found to be complex. Effects are dose related and center on the nicotine receptors in the brain. In small dosages, nicotine mimics the effect of acetylcholine and causes the release of acetylcholine and norepinephrine. In addition, blood and brain levels of serotonin, endogenous opioid peptides, and dopamine are found to be elevated after smoking. The effects on the user include constricted blood vessels, increased heart rate and blood pressure, decreased appetite, and slight mood elevation. Cigarette smoking has toxic effects from the irritation caused by tar and smoke; nicotine is itself considered to be a toxin and is commercially used as a pesticide. Nicotine poisoning can cause nausea, vomiting, weakness, convulsions, coma, and even death. Contact with tobacco leaves by tobacco workers handling the leaves can lead to nicotine poisoning, especially in nonsmokers who have no tolerance to the effects of nicotine (Surgeon General's Report, 1988). Tolerance to the drug takes place quickly, even faster than with cocaine. Because of nicotine's strength and speed of action (e.g., the rapid onset of light-headedness and nausea), the body will rapidly attempt to protect itself by adapting its neurochemistry almost immediately to the effects of smoking. In fact, some have argued that nicotine is the most addictive drug in existence, resulting in a craving that may last a lifetime after withdrawal (Inaba & Cohen, 1997). Despite its highly addictive properties and lethal consequences of long-term use, nicotine continues to be a legal drug. Political pressure from tobacco companies, tobacco-growing states, and the 54 million smokers in the United States have caused tobacco products to be exempt from laws that make it illegal to sell cancer-causing agents for human consumption. Recent changes in the political landscape and legal arena have resulted in tobacco companies being sued by various states for the health-related costs caused by smoking. This has resulted in liability settlements that have cost the tobacco companies billions of dollars, a cost sure to be passed on to smokers. These changes will likely affect how tobacco use is regulated in the future.

Other Recreational Stimulants

There are a variety of other stimulants that are used and abused throughout the world. Amphetamine congeners such as Ritalin, Preludin, and Fastin result in stimulating effects similar to amphetamines. Ritalin (methylphenidate) is probably the most widely prescribed of these drugs and is used to treat hyperactivity or attention deficit disorder in children (Ray & Ksir, 1996). Ephedrine, a nonprescription antiasthmatic drug, has been sold as a legal stimulant that is sometimes referred to as a "look-alike" because it is made to look identical to prescription stimulants. Ephedrine is an extract of the ephedra bush, found growing in desert regions throughout the world. It may also be brewed as a stimulating tea, a practice that has continued in China for over 4000 years; the dried plant is still sold in herbalist shops today.

Methylenedioxymethamphetamine (MDMA) is a stimulant referred to as "ecstasy" that gained popularity in California in the 1970s and 1980s. It was a legal drug, used to treat depression, that soon gained popularity on the streets. It was being manufactured by illegal designer-drug laboratories that were circumventing the Drug Schedules. Because of its widespread abuse, MDMA was placed in the Schedule I category under the Controlled Substance Act, classifying it as an addictive drug with no medical applications. Although MDMA produces stimulating effects similar to amphetamines (e.g., increased heart rate and blood pressure), it will also result in some perceptual changes such as increased sensitivity to light and blurred vision. Other effects include jaw clenching, sweating, and ataxia. Its method of action seems to be the release of serotonin (a neurotransmitter involved with the senses) and dopamine, which is involved with pleasure. Some research has shown that long-term use of MDMA results in permanent degeneration of the serotonin system and up to a 50 percent decrease in serotonin levels in the brain (De Souza, Battaglia, & Insel, 1990).

A plant known as khat (*Catha edulis*) is a widely used and abused drug in the Middle East. Like the coca leaf, the khat leaf may be chewed to achieve a stimulating effect from its active ingredient, cathinone. Cathinone is a natural methamphetaminelike chemical that produces increased sociability, energy, alertness, and decreased fatigue and appetite. The spread of khat has been limited, partly because its potency begins to decrease about 48 hours after the khat leaves are harvested. Chronic or abusive khat use results in physical exhaustion, depression, and irritable, even violent, behavior.

Another stimulant widely used in the East and Middle East is the betel nut. Although not common in the U.S., more than 200 million people use it as a recreational drug and medicine (Inaba & Cohen, 1997). Like khat, the betel nut is chewed and slowly absorbed into the bloodstream via the digestive tract. Its effects, similar to espresso or cigarettes, result in mild euphoria, increased energy, and elevation of mood. Chronic use of the betel nut has been linked to mouth and esophageal cancer.

DEPRESSANTS

Depressants are those drugs that cause disinhibition and reduced anxiety at low dosages, sedation and ataxia with intermediate-sized dosages, and anesthesia and coma with large dosages. As the category's name implies, these drugs depress the overall functioning of the central nervous system. Some mimic the actions of the body's natural chemicals, while others work directly on the brain and enhance the action of GABA on receptors that regulate anxiety in the brain; still others act in ways yet unknown. The primary types of drugs found in this classification are alcohol, opiates/opioids, sedative-hypnotics (barbiturates and benzodiazepines), and inhalants. Beverage alcohol is the most widely used and abused depressant in the world. Opiates and opioids include heroin and methadone. Sedative-hypnotics are a wide range of synthetic drugs that tranquilize and produce sleep. Inhalants include substances that give off fumes, including organic solvents, volatile nitrites, and nitrous oxide.

According to Winger et al. (1992), the epidemiology of abuse of the alcohol, barbiturates, and benzodiazepines may vary. There are, however, similar pharmacologic sequelae:

1. Chronic use results in physiologic dependence and withdrawal syndromes having similar characteristics.

2. There is cross-dependence among these drugs, and withdrawal from one depressant can be lessened by administration of one of the other depressants.

3. The withdrawal symptoms of alcohol and many of the barbiturates can be fatal, progressively moving from tremor, to convulsions, to delirium, to cardiovascular collapse.

4. Although moderate cross-tolerance from depressants occurs with many of these drugs (a tolerance for one depressant results in a tolerance for another), tolerance does not prevent a fatal overdose from CNS depressants.

Alcohol

There are a number of variations on the basic alcohol molecule, including ethyl alcohol, ethanol, and grain alcohol. Alcohol is widely used as a solvent in industry, where it is denatured by adding a toxin that makes it unpalatable or poisonous. Alcohol is also an excellent medium for chemical reactions. Methanol, which goes into gasoline, is denatured ethanol, and other chemicals are added to it for purposes of combustion. Methyl alcohol is wood alcohol and causes blindness among other disorders when consumed. Ethanol or beverage alcohol is produced by a process known as *fermentation;* this is the basis for all alcoholic beverages. Fermentation is the process where yeasts act on sugar in the presence of water. In other words, $C_6H_{12}O_6$ (glucose) + H_2O (water) is transformed into C_2H_6O (ethyl alcohol) + CO_2 (carbon dioxide). This is how beer and wine are produced, using the sugars in grains and hops to create beer, and grapes or other fruit-based sugars to make wine. *Distillation* increases the potency of the fermented beverage; the solution containing the alcohol is heated, and the vapors are collected and condensed into liquid form again. Distilled alcohol can be produced to make a variety of liquors: brandy from grapes; vodka from potatoes; scotch, whiskey, and bourbon from a variety of grains; gin from juniper berries; and tequila from cactus. The flavor of the alcoholic beverage comes from substances used to produce the alcohol or from other ingredients that may be added.

Absorption of alcohol begins in the mouth through the epithelium. About 20 percent of consumed alcohol enters the bloodstream through the stomach, and most (80 percent) enters the bloodstream through the small intestine. Alcohol is spread throughout the body via passive diffusion, where its concentration is distributed relatively evenly throughout the body. Because it is water soluble, the greatest concentration of alcohol occurs in those parts of the body that are less dense and contain the most water; the blood and body organs will have the highest concentrations.

The human body eliminates alcohol at a rate of one-quarter to one-half ounce (.25 to .50 oz) of absolute alcohol per hour. One-half ounce of absolute alcohol is generally contained in a 12-ounce can of beer, a 4-ounce glass of wine, a 2-ounce glass of sherry, or a 1-ounce shot of whiskey. Although differing in serving size, each of these drinks is equivalent in terms of its intoxicating effects because they each contain about the same amount of alcohol. Alcoholic content of liquor is measured by "proof," which is expressed as a number reflecting twice the percentage of alcohol found in the beverage (e.g., a bottle of 80 proof whiskey contains about 40 percent alcohol). Absolute alcohol cannot be produced economically, and some of it evaporates quickly. Hence, the "pure alcohol" in grain alcohol is really about 95 pecent, or 190 proof.

The only way to eliminate alcohol from the body is through the passage of time (giving a drunk a cup of coffee to sober him or her up will only result in a more wide awake drunk). Elimination occurs through both metabolism and excretion. Metabolism of alcohol is performed primarily by the liver, which eliminates about 90 percent of the alcohol that has been consumed. The liver converts alcohol into acetaldehyde by removing 2 hydrogen molecules. Acetaldehyde (CH_3CHO) is a highly toxic substance that is quickly converted to acetic acid and then water, oxygen, and carbon dioxide. As indicated earlier, a healthy liver is capable of eliminating about one-half ounce of absolute alcohol per hour. The remaining amount of alcohol not metabolized is excreted by the urinary tract, perspiration through the skin, and by exhalation from the lungs.

BAC and Intoxication The amount or level of alcohol contained in the body after its consumption is measured by blood alcohol concentration (BAC). BAC is an expression of the percentage of alcohol in the blood by weight. The body of an average-sized person contains about 6 to 8 quarts of blood; additionally, much of the rest of the body contains varying amounts of water as well. The larger the person, the more water content in which the alcohol is dispersed. BAC reflects the milligrams of alcohol per 100 milliliters of blood and is expressed in decimal form. For instance, 100 mg of alcohol per 100 ml of blood is expressed as a BAC of .10 percent, which is generally recognized to be legally intoxicated. There are a number of factors that influence BAC for any individual; size and weight are probably the most important. Larger people have more blood and water in their bodies. Therefore, alcohol becomes more diluted within their bodies. Hence, the large person who drinks the same amount of alcohol as a small person will have a comparatively lower BAC level. Gender is another factor affecting BAC because, when compared to males, females (1) are smaller; (2) have more fatty tissue that alcohol does not easily penetrate; and (3) have hormones that affect BAC levels during the menstrual cycle (higher premenstrually but lower on the first day of the cycle). Coupling these factors to the fact that women tend to have lower metabolism rates than men means that women, as a group, will have higher BAC levels than men even though they've consumed the same amount of alcohol over the same time period.

Another factor affecting the rate of alcohol absorption is the presence or absence of food in the stomach; a full stomach slows alcohol's passage to the small intestine, thus slowing its entry into the bloodstream. Finally, the presence of other drugs in the user's system can act to speed up alcohol's absorption, a phenomenon referred to as a "synergistic effect." Drug synergism can occur with all of the depressants and results in inadvertent overdoses and about 4000 deaths per year (Inaba & Cohen, 1997). The primary reason for drug interactions relates to the liver being overburdened in metabolizing more than one drug at a time, resulting in higher concentrations of depressants entering the bloodstream. Physical dependence and tolerance to the drug does not markedly effect BAC until the liver has been damaged and tolerance drops— then alcoholics have an increase in BAC/drinks-per-hour ratio.

Alcohol will depress CNS functioning, but it also has a disinhibiting effect. Before the 20th century, it was thought that alcohol had a stimulant effect at low levels and acted as a depressant at higher levels (Winger, et al., 1992). The "stimulating" features of low dosages of alcohol were increased talkativeness, self-confidence, exaggerated behavior, and euphoria. Today, alcohol is considered to be a depressant, and its stimulating effects are understood to result from the depression of those parts of the brain responsible for controlling inhibition. Under the influence of alcohol, people are more likely to act out on impulses and less likely to keep in check stimulating behavior that is suppressed by anxiety or thoughts of punishment. Research by De Wit, Pierri, and Johanson (1989) indicated that most people choose to consume alcohol for its disinhibiting effects than for its depressing effects.

The observable behaviors displayed by people under the influence of alcohol vary markedly. Harney and Harger (1965) found that about 10 percent of the population of drinkers appears to be intoxicated (i.e., slurred speech, obvious loss of inhibitions, and motor problems) with a BAC of .05. At BAC

Table 5.2 BAC, Subjective Effects, and the Number of Drinks per Hour

BAC	Number Drinks per Hour	Effects on the Drinker
.02–.05	1–2 drinks/hr	Feelings of congeniality, mild euphoria, lowered alertness
.05–.08	3–4 drinks/hr	Reduction of normal inhibitions, feelings of excitement, decrease in motor coordination, possible increase in aggressive behavior
.09–.15	5–6 drinks/hr	Impaired concentration and motor coordination, slowed reaction times, confusion, reduced judgment, legal intoxication in most states
.15–.30	7–9 drinks/hr	Stupor or extreme grogginess, extreme incoordination and staggering, loss of consciousness or passing out
.30–.40	10–12 drinks/hr	Coma, surgical anesthesia, reduction of oxygen to the brain and destruction of brain cells, resulting in potential brain damage
.40–.50	12–15 drinks/hr	Death in the nontolerant individual

levels of .10 to .15 (legally drunk), 64 percent appeared intoxicated; only at BAC levels of .20 or more do all drinkers appear visibly intoxicated. It is even more difficult to detect, from observation alone, who and who is not intoxicated among alcoholics. Because of physical dependence and tolerance, alcoholics with BACs as high as .30 (a level that would put a normal person in a stupor) may only appear mildly intoxicated (Mendelson & Mello, 1966). As a benchmark describing the effects of alcohol on behavior, Table 5.2 depicts various BAC levels, number of drinks consumed per hour by an average-sized adult, and alcohol's concomitant behavioral effects. As a rule of thumb, people are able to metabolize about one-half to one drink per hour; any more than that and the alcohol begins to build up in the system, and the person's BAC level rises. The more drinks over a given time period, the faster the BAC level rises.

The precise effects of alcohol on neurotransmitter functioning is currently being researched. Alcohol easily crosses the blood–brain barrier due to its simple chemical structure. Generally, it interferes with neurotransmitters by competing with them for neurotransmitter receptor sites. The primary neurotransmitter systems affected by alcohol are GABA, serotonin, and acetylcholine. GABA is responsible for regulating anxiety; receptors for GABA are found in high concentrations in the cerebellum (controlling motor coordination), the hippocampus (involved in information retrieval), and the cerebral cortex (responsible for general cognitive processing). Serotonin is involved in sleep and sensory experiences, including euphoria. Acetylcholine is involved in muscle movement, memory, motivation, and arousal. Alcohol also appears to have an impact on the reticular activating system, which controls sensory input and output. Blood alcohol levels at the .4 to .5 level suppress the medulla oblongata (part of the brain stem), causing death from respiratory failure. An alcohol antagonist has been discovered that will counteract the intoxicating effects of alcohol. Kolata (1986) reported that a drug (RO 15-4513) allowed rats that were so intoxicated that they couldn't roll over to stand up, walk normally, and appear sober within two minutes of an injection. This drug will probably never be marketed for public use because it acts as a convulsant and does not lower the user's BAC level. Lithium, a drug used to treat bipolar disorder (manic-depression) has also been found to be useful in countering the intoxicating effects of alcohol and reducing the urge to continue drinking.

Negative Consequences of Alcohol Abuse   Hangovers are a well-known consequence of overdrinking. Symptoms include thirst, upset stomach, fatigue, headache, depression, and anxiety. There are many theories about the cause or causes of hangovers. They may be symptoms of withdrawal of a short-term exposure to alcohol—hence, "the hair of the dog that bit you" temporarily relieves symptoms. Other theories center on congeners; these are natural products of fermentation such as maltose, organic acids, acacia, and salts. Congeners affect the taste, smell, and color of alcohol, but some congeners are very toxic. Therefore, some types of alcoholic drinks are more likely to result in a hangover and will produce stronger hangovers. Most beers have only .01 percent congeners, while some wines (a drink that tends to produce stronger hangovers) have about .04 percent congeners. The only real treatment for a hanger is time to sleep it off and non–stomach-irritating analgesic for headache or other pain.

Alcohol abuse has a significant negative impact on several body systems, most notably the liver. The liver is responsible of eliminating about 90 percent of the alcohol consumed, and liver disease frequently occurs in alcoholics because alcohol disturbs the metabolic machinery of the liver. Three diseases may result from alcohol abuse: fatty liver, alcoholic hepatitis, and cirrhosis, sometimes referred to as Stages I, II, and III of liver disease, respectively. Fatty liver may be acute, caused by an episode of binge drinking, or chronic, occurring in alcoholics who drink heavily and steadily. Fatty liver may be asymptomatic and develops when the liver becomes infiltrated with fat while it is otherwise occupied with metabolizing alcohol. When alcohol is consumed in excess, it acts as a nonspecific stressor that causes a release of fatty acids from adipose tissue and results in an increase in free fatty acids and triglycerides that infiltrate the liver. Fatty liver is a reversible disease characterized by liver enlargement and tenderness; liver function test results vary, but fatty liver is rarely fatal.

Alcoholic hepatitis, a sometimes fatal disease, is characterized by inflammation and death of liver cells; the inflammation is caused by a virus or a toxin. For alcoholics, symptoms usually begin just after a heavy episode of drinking. Symptoms include an enlarged liver, abdominal pain, vomiting, and weakness. Ascites, which is edema or a buildup of fluid in the abdominal cavity, may also result from long-term drinking. Hence, an alcoholic who eats very little may still have a swollen belly. Alcoholic hepatitis may also cause an enlargement of the spleen and gastrointestinal bleeding. It is diagnosed by elevated liver enzyme signs and jaundice or buildup of bile in the blood. As indicated earlier, hepatitis is an inflammation of the liver. Alcoholic hepatitis is distinguished from viral hepatitis by a history of heavy drinking. Fortunately, it is usually reversible; successfully treatment involves removing the toxin from the system and allowing the liver time to heal.

Cirrhosis of the liver results from typically 10 or more years of alcohol abuse and occurs in about 10 percent of all people who have been diagnosed as alcoholics. It is the seventh leading cause of death in the United States (Ray & Ksir, 1996). Cirrhosis results when dead liver cells are replaced with fibrous (scar) tissue, leaving some healthy liver cells to survive as islands surrounded by fibrotic tissue. Cirrhosis is caused by poor nutrition and prolonged alcohol consumption. Initially the liver is enlarged and tender; later it becomes small, hard, and nontender because of the buildup of scar tissue. The clinical signs and symptoms of cirrhosis are similar to those of alcoholic hepatitis. Major complications include ascites and esophageal varices or varicose veins in the lower esophagus and stomach due to back pressure from blood unable to enter the liver (frequently, retching may burst these swollen veins, causing the patient to vomit blood). Hepatic encephalopathy may also occur, causing mental functioning to be progressively impaired, leading to coma. The mechanisms are unclear, but it may result from biochemical triggers in the brain related to impaired liver functioning. Cirrhosis may be accompanied by portal hypertension, resulting from the backflow of blood from the liver to the heart via the inferior vena cava due to compressed vessels in the liver. About 50 percent of alcoholics with cirrhosis die of it five years after diagnosis. Its treatment requires abstention from alcohol, correction of malnutrition, infection control, and management of complications that may have occurred.

Chronic alcohol abuse can also lead to brain dysfunction. One of the major manifestations of damage to brain functioning is Wernicke-Korsakoff syndrome. Wernicke's disease symptoms consist of confusion, apprehension, ataxia (incoordination of voluntary muscle movement), and nystagmus (jerky movements of the eye muscles). Wernicke's disease is thought to be related to thiamine (vitamin B_1) deficiency, resulting from a poor diet, poor absorption in the intestine, and inability of the body to metabolize thiamine. Wernicke's, by itself, is usually reversible, often dramatically so with administration of thiamine. Unfortunately, about 80 percent of those with Wernicke's disease will develop Korsakoff's psychosis (Reuler, Girard, & Cooney, 1985). Korsakoff's psychosis may appear without the vitamin deficiency, but some believe that they are linked, with Wernicke's being the acute and Korsakoff's the chronic form of the same disease (Thomson, Jeyasingham, & Pratt, 1987). Korsakoff's is characterized by short-term memory loss, confabulation, polyneuritis (inflammation of nerves), disorientation, muttering, delirium, insomnia, and hallucinations. The general disorientation and mental impairment seem to be due to widespread brain damage. Recovery from Korsakoff's psychosis is unlikely, with many patients ending up in nursing homes or VA hospitals.

It is unclear how much alcohol exposure is needed before brain damage occurs. Most studies on moderate drinking levels find no consistent evidence of brain damage. Most alcoholics, however, show some signs of brain damage: "From 50 to 75 percent of detoxified, long-term alcohol-dependent individuals show significant impairments in tests of problem solving, perception, and memory. Many of these alcohol-dependent individuals have demonstrable brain abnormalities. . . ." (Alcohol and Health, 1990, p, 124). Because CNS tissue tends not to regenerate after it has been damaged, recovery from alcohol-related brain damage is limited. Abstinence from alcohol may result in the recovery of some cognitive functions and partial recovery of brain atrophy (shrinking of brain tissues), and significant reversal of other brain abnormalities that show up on computerized tomography (CT) scans, with the prognosis being somewhat better for those abstaining alcoholics who are under age 40 (Alcohol and Health, 1990).

The effects of alcohol on the heart include cardiomyopathy, coronary artery disease, high blood pressure, and dysrhythmia. These disorders may be caused by the direct toxic effects on muscle and/or nerve fibers and the reduction in thiamine. Cardiomyopathy is a disease of heart muscle characterized by edema, fatigue, palpitations, and cyanosis in individuals under 50. The prognosis is good with abstinence from alcohol. Hypertension is more prevalent in alcoholics than in the general population, as is coronary artery disease—the narrowing of the arteries supplying the heart with blood. Dysrhythmias, such as speeding, slowing, and irregular heart beat, are caused by alcohol's disruption of the electrodynamics that govern heart rate. Not all alcohol use is harmful, however. Moderate use of one or two drinks per day has been found to have beneficial effects on the heart. When compared to alcohol abstainers, regular moderate drinkers have a lower risk of coronary artery disease. One reason for this benefit may be alcohol's ability to increase high-density lipoprotein blood levels and lower the more harmful low-density lipoproteins. Alcohol also decreases blood platelet aggregation and coagulation and has an anxiolytic effect that reduces the moderate drinker's levels of stress. These health benefits do not, however, outweigh the risks of any alcohol consumption for recovering alcoholics, people who are at risk for developing alcoholism (e.g., having a family history), and pregnant women (Winger et al., 1992).

There are a number of gastrointestinal tract problems caused by alcohol abuse, most notably involving the esophagus, stomach, and pancreas. The esophagus, having been directly exposed to alcohol, has a greater risk of developing cancer in alcoholics than nonalcoholics. Alcohol will reduce the speed in which the stomach empties; it interferes with gastroesophageal sphincters, stimulates gastric secretion, and damages the lining of the stomach. Heavy alcohol consumption is a leading cause of acute pancreatitis, which is manifest by intense abdominal pain, nausea, vomiting, fever, and tachycardia. More than 75 percent of patients with chronic pancreatitis have a history of heavy drinking (Van Thiel et al., 1981). Pancreatitis usually occurs after 5 to 10 years of heavy drinking, and by the time symptoms appear, chronic changes have already occurred in the pancreas. Regulation of the metabolism of sugar is disrupted within the pancreas, and the risk of developing diabetes is increased. Although there are large individual variations, a study of people who developed pancreatitis showed that, as a group, they were having about 12 drinks per day (Alcohol and Health, 1990).

The peripheral nervous system is also adversely affected by chronic alcohol abuse. Peripheral neuropathy is manifest by tingling and burning, especially in the feet and sometimes in the hands; toothachelike pain and muscle weakness may also be present. The cause may be related to nutritional intake and/or the direct toxic effect of alcohol on nerve endings. Fortunately, the symptoms abate with abstinence from alcohol and proper nutrition.

Discussion Questions: On what basis does society decide which drugs are legal (socially acceptable) and which are illegal (socially unacceptable)? What kinds of societal attitude changes toward psychoactive drugs do you anticipate in the future?

Opiates and Opioids

Traditionally referred to as narcotics, opiates/opioids is one of the oldest and most researched drug classifications. Opiates are naturally occurring chemicals that are derivatives from *Papaver somniferum,* or the opium poppy, while opioids are similar synthetic drugs. People have known about and used opiates throughout history; the Sumerians used them 5000 years ago; the ancient Egyptians called them a cure and a killer. More recently, opium use was introduced to the United States by Chinese immigrants who came to work on railroad construction at the turn of the century. One of the principal effects of opium is pain reduction. On experiencing damage to its tissues, the body releases a neurotransmitter (Substance P) is to protect itself from further damage. Substance P is experienced as pain. If the pain is intense, the body responds by releasing endorphins to inhibit the transmission of the pain messages. If the pain is still too intense, physicians use opiates or opioids to supplement endorphins by preventing the release of pain neurotransmitters and by blocking these receptor sites. The patient, once given the drug, experiences pain relief and sedation but rarely euphoria. When taken by pain-free individuals, however, this class of drugs causes sensation and feelings of pleasure or euphoria. Opiates/opioids attach to the neurotransmitter receptor sites in the limbic system, resulting in artificially induced euphoria. In addition to the feelings of pleasure, opiates/opioids produce physical effects that include muscle relaxation, head nodding, drooping eyelids, constipation, reduced hormone production, dry skin, and cough suppression. Some of the negative side effects of narcotics include shallow breathing, clammy skin, nausea, vomiting, slowed speech, difficulty concentrating, and depression. Overdose or toxicity effects include tachycardia, convulsions, coma, and death.

Opiates and opioids cross the placental barrier in pregnant women; consequently babies born to addicted mothers are also addicted. They also have low birth weights and are in danger from potentially fatal withdrawal symptoms. Additionally, stillbirth and a variety of other neonatal problems are common.

The major types of opiates are opium, morphine, codeine, heroin, dilaudid, percodan, and vicodin (some of these drugs, such as heroin, are actually semisynthetic drugs but are considered to be opiates). Opium is the direct extract of the poppy. It may be consumed by smoking or ingested orally, which was common at the turn of the century in the form of laudanum and patent medicines. Morphine is an extract from opium and is about ten times more potent. Morphine is widely used in medicine as a painkiller that can be administered orally or by injection. Morphine gets its name from Morpheus, the Greek god of dreams. Codeine is a morphine extract and probably the most widely used opiate; it is also one of the most widely abused prescription drugs. It is commonly prescribed for coughs but also for pain, such as in Tylenol with codeine. Codeine may be abused when taken with Doriden, a sleeping pill, to produce a heroinlike euphoria.

Heroin is an extract from morphine and is about 2.5 times more potent (hence, it's about 25 times more potent than opium). Heroin was first isolated in 1874 and was named after Heros, the Greek god of heroes. Ironically, heroin was hoped to have the heroic ability to treat pain without the addictive properties of opium and morphine, it was even used to treat opium and morphine addiction. Heroin may be smoked or snorted, but injection is the preferred Western method of ingestion, where the heroin powder is "cooked" with water. The street purity of heroin varies greatly, and it is frequently cut with a wide variety of chemicals. Overdose occurs when the nervous system shuts down due to the drug overload, the user has a slowed heart rate, blood pressure drops, respiration slows, and lungs fill with fluid. Heroin overdose can happen so quickly that the user is often found with the needle still in his or her arm.

Other opiates include percodan, dilaudid, and vicodin. Percodan is most often taken orally and acts after about 30 minutes and will last about four to six hours. Its painkilling properties are weaker than morphine but stronger than codeine. Dilaudid, an extract of morphine, is another short-acting painkiller that is stronger than morphine and may be taken either orally or injected. Vicodin is an opiate that is commonly prescribed for acute, short-term pain. These drugs are used as pain medication and are commonly found in rehabilitation populations who are affected by either acute and chronic pain.

Opioids are synthetically manufactured opiates; all are prescription drugs with known medical applications. Fentanyl is a widely used analgesic used for sedation and pain control in surgical procedures. It is relatively short-acting with a duration of about two hours. Demerol is most often injected and is a relatively strong analgesic; it has become the drug of choice among the drug-abusing medical community. Talwin is used to treat chronic or longstanding pain; it may be taken orally or injected. Darvon is prescribed to treat relatively mild to moderate pain and is often used by dentists; it is a short-acting painkiller that lasts for about four to six hours.

Methadone is probably the widest-known opioid. It is a fentanyl derivative that is used in federally licensed "methadone clinics" to block withdrawal symptoms and reduce cravings for heroin and other opiates/opioids. It is addictive and euphoric for nonaddicts, but its euphoric effects are much less than heroin's, and it will block withdrawal and drug craving for up to 72 hours. Much controversy exists over whether it is appropriate to use an opioid (that is addictive) to combat an opiate addiction. The metabolic deficiency theory of Dole and Nyswander (1967) suggested that addicts suffer from a biochemical disease or deficit that requires opiates for relief; this theory played a crucial role in justifying methadone programming. Today, there are about 100,000 heroin addicts receiving methadone treatment programming, which has been expanded to include a variety of psychological and vocational services. Naloxone and Naltrexone are two other drugs that have been used to treat heroin addiction. They are short-acting opiate antagonists that block the neurochemical and euphoric effects of opiates/opioids. In addition to blocking the high, these drugs are important in treating acute overdose. Recently, Naltrexone has been used effectively to treat the craving for alcohol; an NIAAA press release stated, "Separate NIAAA-supported, three-month trials [found] that Naltrexone helped to prevent early return to heavy drinking in a significant proportion of treated patients. In addition, patients who received Naltrexone reported less alcohol craving and fewer drinking days than patients given a placebo" (National Institute on Alcoholism and Alcohol Abuse, 1995, online).

The addictive characteristics of opiates and opioids have been well documented. Opiates and opioids cause euphoria because they bind into endorphin receptor sites located in the pleasure centers of the brain, most notably the nucleus accumbens and the ventral tegmental areas (Watson, Trujillo, Herman, & Akil, 1989). As discussed in Chapter 4, opiates and opioids are chemically similar to endorphins and hence are very effective pain relievers. The body is extremely efficient in tolerating the effects of opiates, so that the drugs appear to weaken with each successive dose. Cross-tolerance also readily occurs; for example, tolerance to heroin causes tolerance to morphine and the synthetic opioids. Tolerance to opiates and opioids results from a number of sources; the body will become more efficient and speed up its metabolism of the opiate substance, nerve cells become desensitized to the drug's effects, and brain chemistry is altered in other ways to compensate for the drug effects. Tissue dependence occurs quickly; after only two to three weeks of use, the body needs the drug to function at its new balance, or homeostasis. Short-acting opiates (e.g., heroin, morphine) have intense but brief withdrawal, whereas the longer-acting drugs have milder but more long-term withdrawal symptoms. Withdrawal symptoms typically consist of flulike symptoms of diarrhea, chills, nausea, cramps, watery eyes, and loss of appetite. Compulsion or drug craving may begin with experimentation or euphoria seeking, and continuation of use is based on blockage of pain from withdrawal, dependence on the drug to stay normal, or at the biochemical level to overcome endorphin deficiency. Consequently, we see both physical and psychological dependence playing important parts in the addiction to opiates and opioids.

Sedative-Hypnotics

In the United States, over 150 million prescriptions for sedative-hypnotics are written each year, almost all of which are in pill form and taken orally (Inaba & Cohen, 1997). These drugs are used to reduce anxiety, tranquilize, induce sleep, control high blood pressure, and reduce or eliminate seizures. Generally, sedatives are used for calming or lowering anxiety, while hypnotics are used for inducing sleep; however, some sedatives are used to induce sleep, and some hypnotics are used as sedatives—hence, the distinction is often blurred. There are three classifications of sedative-hypnotics: barbiturates, benzodiazepines, and nonbarbiturate sedative-hypnotics.

Barbiturates were first synthesized in 1868, and today there are about 2400 different known compounds. After alcohol, barbiturates are the most frequently abused CNS depressants in the United States (Winger et al., 1992). Barbiturates, as a class, are an effective hypnotic that induce sleep and depress breathing and motor coordination; their site of action is localized to the brain stem. The intoxication produced by barbiturates is very similar to alcohol, including the reduction in inhibitions, but they differ in that they don't suppress appetite, so malnutrition is less of a problem for sedative-hypnotic abusers. Barbiturates may be slow acting (12 to 24 hours), such as phenobarbital used to treat the seizures caused by epilepsy, or fast acting (4 to 6 hours), such as seconal, which is used to induce sleep. The barbiturate Pentothal is used as an anesthetic in surgery. One of the dangers of barbiturate prescriptions is that they have a relatively low safety index, meaning that their treatment dose is relatively close to a toxic dose. Tolerance to barbiturates develops due to physiologic changes in the liver, allowing it to more rapidly metabolize the drugs. Withdrawal from barbiturates is dangerous, possibly resulting in convulsions, hallucinations, nausea and vomiting, delirium, tremors, and other physical signs of hyperexcitability.

Benzodiazepines include such widely prescribed drugs as Valium, Librium, Ativan, Halcion, and Xanax. This class of drugs was developed in the 1950s and came into wide use in the 1960s as an alternative to barbiturates used to treat anxiety. The primary advantage of benzodiazepines over barbiturates is that they have a very safe chemical index; the therapeutic dose is far below the toxic dose. Also, benzodiazepines are able to reduce anxiety over a wider dosage range, making it easier for physicians to find a therapeutic dose for anxiety without producing unwanted sedation. Other applications include the treatment of panic attack (Xanax), insomnia (Halcion), and as a sedative during surgery (Valium). Some potential problems of benzodiazepine use are their relatively long half-life in the body, which can result in addiction occurring at relatively low levels, and an unpredictable pattern of withdrawal symptoms having the potential for seizures. More people have died from Valium withdrawal than from Valium overdose. Generally, withdrawal occurs after a few months of high dosage use or a year of lower dose use. Other withdrawal symptoms include anxiety; hypersensitivity to light and noise; and disturbances to sleep, memory, and concentration. One of the most dangerous patterns of use is to combine a benzodiazepine with another CNS depressant such as alcohol to create a synergistic effect that can easily lead to drug overdose.

Tolerance to benzodiazepines is related to increased liver efficiency, and age-related tolerance occurs with younger people tolerating higher doses than older individuals. The effect on a senior citizen may be up to ten times stronger than the same level dose with an adolescent. Neurochemically, benzodiazepines

Table 5.3 Commonly Prescribed Benzodiazepines

Long-Acting (usually taken 1 to 2 times per day or every other day)
  Valium (diazepam)
  Clonopin (clonazepam)
  Librium (chlordiazepoxide)
  Dalame (flurazepam)
  Centrax (prazepam)
  Tranxene (clorazepate)

Intermediate/Short-Acting (usually taken 3 to 4 times per day or at night)
  Restoril (temazepam)
  Xanax (alprazolam)
  Serax (oxazepam)
  Ativan (lorazepam)
  Halcion (triazolam)

affect the brain by interacting with or acting like gamma aminobutyric acid (GABA), the brain's most effective inhibitory neurotransmitter. In addition, the neurotransmitters of serotonin and dopamine have been found to be affected by Valium. Table 5.3 presents a list of the most commonly prescribed long-acting and intermediate/short-acting benzodiazepines.

Nonbarbiturate sedative–hypnotics include such drugs as Quaalude, Doriden, Placidyl, Miltown (meprobamate), and buspirone. Quaaludes, a once popular drug, are hard to obtain in the United States because of its history of heavy abuse and overdose when used with other drugs. Doriden is a short-acting hypnotic used to treat insomnia; it is combined with codeine by drug abusers to produce extended periods of euphoria and relaxation. Placidyl is about as potent as Doriden but is shorter-acting. Miltown was very popular in the 1950s and led to the modern recognition of addiction caused by a legally prescribed drug. Buspirone does not produce CNS depression or synergize with alcohol and has very limited abuse or dependence potential. It has been used in Europe as an anxiolytic, but it may be most effective on only mild cases of anxiety.

Negative effects of sedatives include slurred speech, poor concentration, memory loss (blackouts), poor judgment, and limited attention span. Overdose or toxicity effects include strabismus, vertigo, shock, coma, and death (death occurs because brain stem respiratory centers are repressed to the degree of cessation). The synergistic effect of combining alcohol with another depressant accounts for high fatality rates associated with this drug class.

Inhalants

Inhalants are a group of volatile chemicals, meaning that they easily evaporate, making inhalation the easiest route of ingestion. These chemicals may be inhaled directly from the container (sniffing), by soaking a rag and placing it in the mouth or next to the nose ("huffing"), or by spraying it into a plastic bag that is then placed over the nose and mouth (bagging). Inhalants are a diverse group of products—many of which are sold over the counter with no restrictions—that can produce psychoactive effects. The products are used commercially for a number of legitimate purposes and include paint solvents, glues, motor fuels, cleaning agents, aerosol sprays (e.g., hair sprays) and aerosolized food products (e.g., whipped cream), anesthetic gases (nitrous oxide), and nitrates (e.g., butyl nitrite). Because many of these substances are widely available and found in homes, offices, garages, and retail stores, they are often the first psychoactive substances used by adolescents who are experimenting with drug use. Because of their ease of use, wide availability, low cost, and legality, inhalants have been referred to as a gateway drug that will lead to illicit drug use.

After alcohol and tobacco, inhalants are probably the most widely abused drug by adolescents, with 12- to 17-year-olds making up the largest group of current users (Substance Abuse and Mental Health Services Administration, 1993). The intoxication produced by most inhalants is comparable to that produced by alcohol. Inhalants act as a CNS depressant and tend to slow down the function of the brain and spinal cord. At low-level dosages, users experience relaxation, lightheadedness, giddiness, and reduced inhibitions. At high-level doses, the senses are numbed, hallucinations may occur, and the user may lose consciousness or lapse into a coma. Some of the side effects of use include inflamed nasal tissue, headaches, nausea/vomiting, dizziness, slurred speech, reduced muscle coordination, vision problems, and seizure. The length of action may vary from several seconds up to one hour, depending on the inhalant and level of dose. Tolerance to inhalants can develop with use over time, however, and physical dependence does not seem to develop. Because most inhalants are not intended for consumption, they pose a number of dangers to the user. Fatal accidents resulting from suffocation can occur from inhaling vapors inside plastic bags. Lead poisoning may develop from the vapors of lead-based paints, transmission fluids, and other petroleum products. Oily sprays, when inhaled, can coat the lungs and reduce the amount of oxygen available to the brain and induce asphyxiation. Some inhalants are quite toxic, including carbon tetrachloride, leaded gasoline, and toluene (the chemical found in glues, solvents, and thinners).

HALLUCINOGENS

Most hallucinogens disrupt serotonin functioning, the neurotransmitter responsible for controlling the senses. The subjective effects of hallucinogenic drugs make them somewhat unique among psychoactive drugs. Like stimulants, they cause the elevation of some bodily functions, such as heart rate, blood pressure, and body temperature. The user's pupils will be dilated, and salivation will increase. The subjective effects of hallucinogens are quite remarkable, however, causing an altered sense of reality. Perception is modified or distorted, colors appear brighter than normal, moving objects may be followed by afterimages or tracers, and multiple images or overlapping images may be seen. A mixing of the senses, called synesthesia, may occur, where sounds appear as visual images, or a visual picture may be changed with the rhythm of music. In addition to the distortion of the senses, hallucinogen users experience an enhanced emotionality—they may perceive exceptionally beautiful or awe-inspiring images, or intense sadness or fear may accompany objects breaking apart or moving away.

Indoles

Hallucinogenic plants have been used for many centuries as medicines and for religious or spiritual purposes. The basic structure of the neurotransmitter serotonin is the *indole nucleus*. Serotonin is a neurotransmitter that is involved in sleep and sensory experiences, including euphoria. LSD and psilocybin have the same chemical structure as indolin and are called indoles. LSD or "acid" is d-lysergic acid diethylamide (discovered accidentally when absorbed through the fingers of a German researcher investigating a fungus alkaloid that infects grain). LSD is very potent; it takes very little to produce effects. LSD is generally taken orally and has a half-life of three hours after being metabolized in the liver. Tolerance develops quickly; initial dose levels become ineffective after only three to four days of repeated use. Cross-tolerance has been shown between LSD, psilocybin, and mescaline; interestingly, users tend not to develop physical dependence or withdrawal from LSD.

The high induced by LSD varies with each episode of use; nonetheless, the experiences tend to be similar, following a sequential pattern. The "trip" will last six to nine hours, with initial effects (dizzy, hot or cold, dry mouth) being noticed in 20 minutes. Then, diminished and altered levels of mood and perception occur after about 30 to 40 minutes. One hour after ingestion, full-blown intoxication occurs; changes in perceptions of self, usually depersonalization or an "out-of-body feeling," occur after about two hours. Trips may be placed into two broad categories, either expansive or constrictive. Expansive highs are perceived as a good trip, accompanied by feelings of insight, creativity, and pleasure. Constrictive trips, however, are characterized by the user showing little movement, feelings of being threatened, and paranoia. Panic reactions may be an averse consequence of use, where the user has a feeling of impending doom or death, with an accompanying fight or flight reaction. Constrictive experiences are more likely to occur when the drug is taken in unfamiliar or uncontrolled environments or when the user's initial mood is negative. As the drug's effect diminishes, normal psychological controls, perceptions, and mood return.

"Flashbacks," the unexpected memory of or reexperience of a trip, occur in regular users of LSD after a period of abstention from the drug. Flashbacks entail many of the drug's effects, such as hallucinations, distortion of the senses, and other psychoticlike symptoms. The experiences of flashbacks may be mild or so strong as to convince the person that they have actually ingested LSD. Flashbacks are more common in those who have bad trips and are also more likely to occur under situations of stress or anxiety. Overdose or toxicity effects are relatively nonexistent. LSD is not generally toxic and has never been linked to even one death.

Other indole hallucinogens include morning glory, psilocybin, DMT, and cohoba. Morning glory seeds have a psychoactive hallucinogenic effect because they contain several alkaloids and d–lysergic acid amide, which is about one-tenth as potent as LSD but still affects serotonin functioning. Psilocybin is the active ingredient in several different mushrooms of Mexico, often referred to as "magic mushrooms." The most potent of the mushrooms is *psilocybe mexicana*. When dried these mushrooms contain about 0.2 percent to 0.5 percent psilocybin. Dimethyltryptamine was synthesized in the 1930s; on the streets it is commonly referred to as DMT. Additionally, DMT is the active agent in cohoba snuff widely used in South America; cohoba is snorted, smoked or injected because it produces no effect if swallowed. The psychoactive effects last about an hour, and tolerance is rapidly established, making repeated use of cohoba less and less effective.

Catechols

Catechol hallucinogens have a chemical structure based on the catechol nucleus, but their hallucinogenic effects are similar to the indoles. The catechol nucleus is the basic molecular structure of catecholamine neurotransmitters, dopamine, and norepinephrine. Catechol hallucinogens include peyote/mescaline; amphetamine derivatives that have little stimulating effect but produce hallucinations, such as DOM (or STP) and MDA; and phencyclidine (PCP). Mescaline is the active ingredient of the peyote cactus button. Mescaline is taken orally, but it doesn't pass through the blood-brain barrier well, so larger doses are required for effect. The maximum effect after ingestion is experienced in about ½ to 2 hours. The half-life of mescaline is about 6 hours, but it may persist in the brain for up to 10 hours. DOM or STP refers to 2,5-dimethoxy-4-methylamphetamine. It is about 100 times more potent than mescaline, yet still only ⅓th as potent as LSD. DOM also tends to produce more acute and chronic toxic reactions than any of the other hallucinogens.

PCP, sometimes referred to as angel dust, was originally developed as an analgesic and today is used legally as an animal anesthetic. When taken by humans, however, PCP induces hallucinogenic effects. PCP can be smoked in a joint, snorted, taken orally, or injected. It tends to distort sensory messages, acts as a disinhibitor, and produces a sense of depersonalization or a separation of the mind from the body. Adverse reactions to PCP include elevated blood pressure, violent or combative behavior, tremors, agitation, and paranoia. High dosages may result in seizure, coma, cardiovascular instability, and kidney failure. Effects of a small dose last about 2 hours, and bigger dosages can remain in effect for up to 48 hours. PCP is stored in the body's fat cells, and traces of it can be detected for months after its use. PCP use is dangerous because users, if they become violent, are anesthetized and may injure themselves without realizing it.

Marijuana and Hashish

The active ingredient in marijuana is tetrahydrocannabinol or THC, the amount of which varies greatly depending on the variety of the plant and how it was grown. Hashish is the more potent resin of the marijuana plant; it is made by boiling the plants in alcohol, filtering out the solids, and reducing the liquid to a thick, sticky oil. Hashish has a very high THC content, ranging from 7 percent to 14 percent. Ganja consists of dried marijuana plant material but only from the tops of the plants having flowers (female plants); its THC is around 4 percent to 8 percent. Sinsemilla is a form of marijuana that literally means "without seeds." It has an average THC content of about 4 percent to 5 percent. Low-grade marijuana, sometimes referred to as "ditch weed," is about 1 percent THC.

After caffeine, nicotine, and alcohol, marijuana and its variations are probably the most widely used psychoactive drugs in the United States. Marijuana has been classified here as a hallucinogen because it distorts perceptions of time and space, although it has also been incorrectly classified as a narcotic and is currently a Schedule I drug on the Controlled Substances Act schedules. Like other hallucinogens, there tends to be little physical dependence or physical withdrawal from the drug. Unlike many of the other hallucinogens, marijuana acts like a depressant, causing sedation, decreased motor activity, and reduced reaction to pain. It raises the seizure threshold and blocks convulsions. When used in combination with depressants such as alcohol, THC will have a synergisticlike result and heighten their effects. Unlike depressants, however, marijuana use will elevate blood pressure and heart rate. Blood vessels will dilate, especially in the whites of the eyes, giving the user bloodshot eyes. Because THC lowers blood glucose levels, the appetite of the user is increased. This effect has led to marijuana being used combat nausea and weight loss in people receiving chemotherapy for cancer and in AIDS patients. Nonetheless, marijuana is currently a Schedule I drug, meaning that the government considers it to be a highly addictive and abuse-prone drug with no medical applications— in the same classifications as heroin.

Generally the leaves from the marijuana plant are dried and smoked, but they may also be taken orally. Marijuana's intoxicating effects include euphoria, relaxed inhibitions, disoriented behavior, distorted perceptions of space and time, and impairment in the process of transferring short-term into long-term memory. Some of the negative side effects of marijuana include nausea, dizziness, vomiting, panic reactions, paranoid states, fatigue, and reduced motivation. Like the other hallucinogens, there is no physical tolerance or withdrawal clearly documented with marijuana use. However, discontinuing use may result in psychological symptoms such as insomnia, anxiety, hyperactivity, and drug craving.

The neurochemical action of THC on the brain is not well known. Since variations of the THC molecule produce differing effects, it appears that the drug is selective in its action on receptor sites. THC will stimulate the release of dopamine (which regulates pleasure) and serotonin (which regulates sensory experiences) from their presynaptic storage in the vesicles; it also influences the function of acetylcholine (regulating memory) and GABA (regulating anxiety). Herkenham et al. (1990) identified specific receptor sites for marijuana, the exact functions of these "cannabinoid receptors" are not currently known. It has been theorized that the brain has naturally occurring substances that resemble the molecular structure of THC that may be involved with the regulation of pain, learning, memory, and other behaviors affected by marijuana (Fishbein & Pease, 1996). The limbic system is especially affected by THC, and the hippocampus, amygdala, and medial forebrain bundle have many THC binding sites. This probably accounts for marijuana's euphoric, sedation, and anxiolytic effects. THC binding sites are also found in the basal ganglia, cerebral cortex, and cerebellum, regions of the brain regulating higher thought processes, perception, and memory. Very few binding THC sites are located in the brain stem, so even very high dosages of THC do not impair breathing or heart function, and overdose is not fatal. Very high dosages will, however, induce hallucinations and panic states described as a toxic psychosis. There is no known THC antagonist, meaning no drug appears to interfere with its effects.

After marijuana is smoked, the THC is absorbed by the lungs; the longer the smoke is held in the lungs, the higher the dose. THC, being fat soluble, is quickly spread throughout the body, and its physical and psychological effects are soon felt. THC blood levels peak in about 30 minutes after use, and its physical and psychological effects last for up to 3 hours. The half-life of THC is about 19 hours; its metabolized by-products (about 45 metabolites from marijuana have been identified) may be found in the blood for up to 50 hours. It may take up to 1 month to completely eliminate THC and its metabolites from the body; being fat soluble, THC is readily stored in the body's fat cells and body organs—most notably in the brain, adrenal gland, liver, lungs, ovaries, and testes. Three days after discontinuing use, about 50 percent of the total THC ingested will be found in the organs and fatty tissues (Fishbein & Pease, 1996). It will be slowly released into the bloodstream and eliminated by the feces, urine, and plasma. Because of its ease of storage and slow release, THC detected in urine or blood samples may be unrelated psychological or behavioral functioning, which makes it difficult to prove impairment from standard drug testing.

Other Hallucinogens

Belladonna is a plant whose name means "beautiful woman"; it was indeed used by ancient Greeks and Egyptians to dilate the pupils to enhance their beauty. Belladonna is a poisonous plant that also contains an active hallucinogenic alkaloid, atropine. This drug blocks the acetylcholine receptor site in the parasympathetic system. The psychoactive effects of this drug cause delirium, sensations of flight or falling, and impaired attention. Mandrake is another ancient hallucinogen that contains atropine. Amanita mushrooms, specifically fly agaric and panther, have been known to create hallucinations, delirium, and hypnotic or dreamlike states that may last up to eight hours. Bufotonin is a toxin excreted by the bufo toad, and morning glory seeds contains ololiuqui. Both are naturally occurring hallucinogens that cause initial excitement, pupil dilation, elevated blood pressure, distortions in the perceptions of time and space, changes in body perceptions, and other distortions of the senses. All tend to act on the neurotransmitter serotonin. Two other naturally occurring hallucinogens are myristicin and elemicin, the active chemicals in the spices of nutmeg and mace, respectively. Neurochemically similar to mescaline, these hallucinogens produce similar effects. One to two teaspoons of these spices will cause feelings of euphoria, sensory changes, excitation, and depersonalization. The onset of action is slow, taking from two to five hours, and they tend to produce anxiety, vomiting, nausea, headaches, vertigo, and tremors, making repeated use of large dosages of these spices less likely.

SUMMARY

This chapter grouped drugs into three major categories: stimulants, depressants, and hallucinogens. Stimulants are those drugs that act directly on the central nervous system to create an increased state of electrical activity and accelerated mental processes, increase heart rate, blood pressure, body temperature and respiration, while decreasing the feelings of fatigue and appetite. Many stimulants occur naturally, such as coffee beans, cocoa leaves, tobacco, and khat leaves, and have been with us since the earliest days of recorded history. These more mild stimulants continue to be the most widely used stimulants in the world today. More powerful stimulants such as amphetamines (d,l amphetamine, methamphetamine, dextroamphetamine, and dextromethamphetamine), cocaine hydrochloride, and crack cocaine are probably the most widely abused illegal stimulants in the United States. The pharmacological properties of amphetamines, along with cocaine, make them the most effective CNS stimulants because they act on the neurotransmitters norepinephrine and dopamine.

Depressant drugs are on the other end of the psychoactive continuum, tending to reduce respiration, heart rate, and blood pressure and induce relaxation and decrease inhibitions in the user; large dosages result in anesthesia and coma. Alcohol is a widely used, readily available depressant. Used in moderation there are no negative, and even some positive, health-related consequences. However, alcohol abuse leads to very clear and dangerous health problems and damage to key organs (liver, heart, and brain). The level of alcohol dose is expressed in the amount of alcohol in the bloodstream, or blood alcohol concentration (BAC). The opiates are direct extracts from the opium poppy and include opium, morphine, codeine, and heroin. Opioids are synthetically manufactured opiates. All are prescription drugs with known medical applications. Fentanyl, demerol, talwin, and darvon are widely perscribed opiates used in the treatment of pain. Methadone is probably the best-known synthetic opioid and is used to block withdrawal symptoms and reduce craving for heroin and other opiates/opioids.

Sedative-hypnotic drugs are used to reduce anxiety, tranquilize, induce sleep, control high blood pressure, and reduce or eliminate seizures. There are three classifications of sedative-hypnotics: barbiturates, benzodiazepines, and nonbarbiturate sedative-hypnotics. Barbiturates were first synthesized in 1868, and today there are about 2400 different known compounds. Barbiturates may be slow acting, such as phenobarbital, or fast acting, such as seconal. Some like pentothal are used as an anesthetic in surgery. Benzodiazepines include such widely prescribed drugs as Valium, Librium, Ativan, Halcion, and Xanax. Applications of these drugs include the treatment of panic attack, insomnia, and as a sedative during surgery. Nonbarbiturate sedative-hypnotics include such drugs as Quaalude, Doriden, Placidyl, Miltown (meprobamate), and buspirone.

Inhalants are a diverse group of products often sold over the counter with no restrictions, such as glues, motor fuels, cleaning agents, and aerosol sprays. When inhaled, these products produce psychoactive effects similar to depressant drugs. At low dosages, users experience relaxation, lightheadedness, giddiness, and reduced inhibitions. At high-level doses, the senses are numbed, hallucinations may occur, and the user may lose consciousness or lapse into a coma. Some of the side effects of use include inflamed nasal tissue, headaches, nausea/vomiting, dizziness, slurred speech, reduced muscle coordination, vision problems, and seizure.

Hallucinogens include indoles, catechols, marijuana, and other hallucinogens. These drugs tend to disrupt serotonin functioning and distort sensory perception. The subjective effects are remarkable, causing an altered sense of reality and enhanced emotionality, where exceptional beauty, awe-inspiring images, or intense sadness or fear may be induced from ordinary objects. Indoles are those hallucinogens that have a molecular structure based on the indole nucleus, the same structure as the neurotransmitter serotonin. LSD, psilocybin, morning glory, and DMT fall into the indole classification.

Catechols are drugs with a catechol nuclear structure, which is similar to the neurotransmitters of dopamine and norepinephrine. Peyote and mescaline and amphetamine derivatives such as DOM, MDA, and PCP fall into this category. Tetrahydrocannibinol (THC) 1 is the active ingredient in marijuana and its resin, hashish. After caffeine, nicotine, and alcohol, marijuana is probably the most widely used psychoactive drug in the United States. Marijuana relaxes inhibitions and distorts the perception of time and space, and it impairs short-term memory. THC seems to affect dopamine and GABA; recently, "cannabinoid" receptor sites have been found in the brain, suggesting that the brain produces chemicals similar in structure to THC. Other drugs falling into the hallucinogenic classification include belladonna, mandrake, amanita mushrooms, myristicin (found in nutmeg), and elemicin (found in mace). All of these act on serotonin, and, in addition to their hallucinogenic effects, produce symptoms of nausea, headaches, and vertigo in the user.

6

Group Counseling

CHAPTER 6 OUTLINE

A PRIMARY TREATMENT MODALITY

Group counseling has achieved a position of considerable stature in the reper-toire of treatment approaches used in both inpatient and outpatient chemical dependency treatment programs (Doweiko, 1996). This acceptance of group counseling as a primary treatment modality is linked to a number of factors. First, the popularity and perceived success of Alcoholics Anonymous and simi-lar peer self-help groups has undoubtedly served as the impetus for the domi-nance of the group model in treatment programs. Group counseling was the undergirding of the therapeutic community model of treatment in this coun-try as well (Bratter, Collabolletta, Fossbender, Pennacchia, & Rubel, 1985). Second, administrators regard group counseling as a cost-efficient and staff-efficient way to provide professional services simultaneously to a large number of clients (Zastrow, 1989), an important consideration when caseload sizes continue to grow and staffing complements remain the same or shrink. From a clinical perspective, the insight and experience of both the group leader and the group members are available to participants in groups (Matuschka, 1985). Ultimately, however, group counseling has been popular because groups serve as a microcosm of society for group members (Yalom, 1970). Group has proven to be a safe place to (1) explore risks, (2) learn about and try out new behaviors, (3) observe and model the behaviors and actions of others, (4) ex-plore relationships and relationship styles, and (5) to learn more effective cop-ing and living strategies.

While group counseling has valuable uses and has become widespread, questions have been raised about its efficacy with individuals who have psy-choactive dependence problems. Doweiko (1996) asserts that the effectiveness of group counseling with individuals who have dependence problems has not been supported in the literature. Lewis, Dana, and Blevins (1994) have sug-gested that group counseling in psychoactive substance dependence treatment has primarily been limited to two forms, a verbal confrontational model aimed at combating client denial and resistance, or a didactic model focused on pro-viding information about drug, alcohol, or the recovery process to a passive and often cognitively impaired or cognitively-depressed audience. "These methods are inconsistent with what is known about human behavior change and may lack the very characteristics that make group work effective" (p. 127). Group activities that focus on denial, resistence, repression, and similar defense mechanisms ignore a basic premise. Defense mechanisms are unconscious ef-forts of the mind to protect the individual from psychological assault. Attempts to batter down defense mechanisms through verbal confrontation may only strengthen them, leaving both the group and the individual frustrated, con-fused, and unsuccessful.

Providing instructions about the effects of drugs and alcohol to a group of passive learners who may be suffering the residual impact of their dependence violates basic principles of adult education. All individuals in recovery have learned firsthand—and very actively—about the effects of drug and alcohol. They do not need to learn effect issues; they need to be able to observe, learn, model, and practice recovery behaviors that will allow them to be successful. Finally, many treatment agencies have a set array of didactic groups in which all clients participate, irrespective of their diagnosis, previous treatment history, current treatment needs, or status in recovery. As Miller (1992) points out, standardized treatment, no matter how comprehensive, has much less impact than treatment that is individualized. Counselors with little or no group leadership training or experience are required to lead groups because of schedule demands and the agency plan of operation, with often disastrous results for both clients and counselor.

Perhaps, however, the problem is not that group counseling approaches are ineffective in treating psychoactive substance dependency. Rather it is that substance abuse counselors have an insufficient understanding of the dynamics of group formation, group activities, and group process, and limited knowledge of the personal and professional characteristics necessary to conduct successful group counseling. This chapter examines types of groups offered in dependency treatment programs, reviews strategies for successful group counseling, and examines important and necessary counselor skills, abilities, and characteristics for conducting group counseling.

TYPES OF GROUPS

Psychoactive dependence treatment programs have traditionally offered four types of treatment groups: counseling groups, didactic groups, peer self-help groups, and self-improvement groups. *Counseling groups* focus on creating intrapsychic change within the individual. They highlight personal growth and development and often center on rededication of inappropriate behaviors and the acquisition of new, optimally functional skills (Corey, 1995). Recovery from any disabling condition is difficult; recovery from psychoactive chemical dependency is affected by and affects interpersonal relationships, the social world, the vocational environment, and often the physical environment (Lewis, Dana, & Blevins, 1994; Monti, Rohsenow, Colby, & Abrams, 1995). Coping with the many changes inherent in recovery can be an emotionally trying experience. Moreover, the chemical changes occurring in the body, including continued cravings for drugs and alcohol, can heighten the emotionality of recovery, and group can be a significant asset to help individuals deal with these powerful emotions. Recovery is a lonely experience for many dependent people, who typically feel insecure, inadequate, inferior, and are in poor emotional health as a result of the dependency process (Taricone, Bordieri, & Scalia, 1989). They are often forced to give up old friends, companions, acquaintances, and all former socialization experiences, and they often become alienated from family members. For these individuals, counseling groups serve as a format to deal with their losses, begin to reconstruct their lives, and rebuild their relational skills. Finally, recovery is a confrontational life experience. Individuals in recovery are forced to confront the reality of the past, often for the first time, along with confronting the reality of the need for change. Zastrow

(1989) asserts that individuals in dependency treatment are giving up a multitude of relationships centered around drugs or alcohol and that they experience a grieving process akin to that described by Elizabeth Kubler-Ross. Most people require the support, guidance, and encouragement of group counseling as they deal with their losses and face the challenges of recovery.

Didactic groups have the specific goal of imparting information, often through a specific teaching-learning process. These are the groups conducted in treatment facilities to acquaint clients with the 12 Steps or the effects of drugs and alcohol. Didactic groups that employ active participation strategies, are well designed, and are tailored to the needs of the individual clients can serve a valuable educational purpose. However, too often didactic groups are passive experiences in which somnambulant clients dutifully watch old videos or listen to boring, poorly developed, and poorly presented lectures.

Discussion   Discuss strategies that might be used to improve the way
Question: didactic information is delivered in groups.

Peer self-help groups are voluntary groups for people who have common problems. They include Alcoholics Anonymous, Narcotics Anonymous, Cocaine Anonymous, and similar groups. These groups are discussed at length in Chapter 8. Many treatment centers conduct a variant of the peer self-help model, called *support groups.* Support groups differ from pure peer self-help groups in two important ways: They are led by a staff member of the treatment facility who is often a person in recovery (Kirstein, 1987), and attendance is usually a mandatory part of treatment. In most other ways, these groups are similar in content and style to traditional peer self-help groups.

Discussion   Bring in a listing of local peer self-help groups. Discuss the
Question: availability of peer self-help groups of various types in the
                 community.

Self-improvement groups are often referred to as activity or task groups. These groups combine the basic elements of counseling and didactic groups to the extent that they focus on behavioral and psychological change by teaching new skills. Decreased social isolation, relationship development or rebuilding, life transitions management, relapse prevention skills, and similar activities are often the goals of self-improvement groups. Assertiveness training groups, attitudinal awareness groups, drink refusal training groups, and quality recovery groups are but a few of the group types falling under the broad rubric of self-improvement groups. Self-improvement groups that focus on self-esteem and self-worth issues, such as those described by Enns (1992), are especially important for women recovering from dependency problems.

Discussion   Discuss some of the self-improvement groups available in the
Question: community and in treatments. Why are these groups an impor-
                 tant part of dependency treatment and rehabilitation?

NECESSARY ELEMENTS FOR
EFFECTIVE GROUP COUNSELING

A number of authors have identified the elements required for effective group counseling. The first is creating within the group a sense of *safety and security* for group members. The members must be able to trust that the group experience will be positive, productive, and supportive (Corey, 1995). Unlike other parts of their lives, the group is a place where members can abandon facades and discuss their problems and emotions honestly and openly. In turn, group members have a chance to hear the problems and solutions of other group members and to react and act in a genuine manner. No matter what the type of group, in the early stages of group development it is the leader's task to create a sense of safety and security by demonstrating a positive attitude toward the group process, by defining the rules and norms of the group so that group members will know what to expect, and by demonstrating trust and trustworthiness. Later in the group process, safety and security will become a function of the group dynamics as cohesion among group members emerges. Groups with individuals recovering tend to be highly volatile, and it is very common for sensitive issues such as incest, spouse abuse, and child abuse to come up spontaneously and abruptly. Creating a sense of trust, safety, and security facilitates the cathartic release of the strong emotional feelings attached to these volatile issues and frees the group members to further explore additional sensitive concerns.

Yalom, in his classic text *The Theory and Practice of Group Psychotherapy,* writes that the "instillation of hope" is crucial to all forms of group counseling (1970). He argues that "not only is hope required to keep the patient (*sic*) in therapy so that other curative factors may take effect, but faith in a treatment mode can in itself be highly therapeutic" (p. 9). Many individuals entering recovery are bereft of hope and beset with feelings of low self-esteem, depression, and being lost and alone. Group can provide a sense of purpose, a feeling of progress, and a sense of optimism as individuals observe and feel personal change and as they see change in others. A tremendous ability to infuse and instill hope is one of the reasons Alcoholics Anonymous is perceived as so successful (Yalom, 1970). The faith and hope in AA that guides many people through recovery has at the same time established the perception of universal effectiveness of peer self-help models (McCrady & Delaney, 1995). Early in the group process the leader sends a significant message about hope. If group members perceive the leader to be upbeat, positive, and a firm believer in the efficacy of the group process, the group members are likely to derive a strong sense of hope from the group dynamics.

Discussion Question: What are some strategies to instill a sense of hope into the group process?

Closely tied to hope, and indeed deriving from it, is the force of altruism within groups. *Altruism* refers to the ability to be of help to others in the group setting. Yalom (1970) notes that significant breakthroughs can occur for clients with low self-esteem when they discover that their experiences and insights help fellow group members.

Cohesion describes the sense of belonging, feeling of closeness and solidarity, and feeling of understanding felt by group members. It is a necessary element of the group process to promote self-disclosure and mutual support and to promote the continued activities of the group (Corey, 1995; Yalom, 1970). Without the unifying force of cohesion, the group will be little more than a discussion forum, with few if any therapeutic gains accomplished by group members. However, Corey (1995) cautions that too much cohesion can be too much of a good thing. Groups that are not challenged to move forward by the group leader may settle into a self-perpetuating state. "The group enjoys the comfort and security of the unity it has earned, but no progress is made" (p. 111).

Discussion   What can the group leader do to build cohesion in the group?
Questions: What can group members do?

Many clients enter group believing that their problems are unique and unusual, but through the group process they quickly learn that there are common threads running through the lives of fellow group members. Yalom (1970) refers to this as "universality." Usually a great feeling of relief comes over group members when they discover that they are not alone on the journey to recovery. Other people have made the same mistakes, had the same struggles, experienced the same losses and frustrations, and have the same feelings.

Discussion   Ask students to write on a slip of paper a feeling they had
Question: when they first entered college or graduate school. Collect the
slips of paper and read aloud the problems looking for themes
in content and feeling (I was excited; I was anxious; I thought
everyone else was smarter than I was; I missed my family; etc.),
thus demonstrating the principle of universality.

The opportunity for vicarious learning is another powerful element of group counseling. *Vicarious learning* is a learning process that occurs indirectly as a result of observing the behavior or actions of other group members or the group leader and includes imitative behaviors such as modeling and mirroring (Corey, 1995). Indeed, one of the earliest and continuing tasks of the group leader is to model appropriate group behavior for the members. By observing and following the leader's style and mannerisms, group members conform to the expectations of the group norms. Mirroring is a form of vicarious learning in which group members see parts of themselves reflected in the actions and behaviors of other group members, and it is a significant contributor to positive change within the group (Riorden, 1992).

Discussion   Describe some ways a group leader or group members might
Question: model appropriate behavior for group members.

Group counseling affords an opportunity for interpersonal learning not easily found in individual counseling. *Interpersonal learning* deals with comprehending the effect of the self on other individuals and the impact of others on the self. Yalom (1970) suggests interpersonal learning is a function of three issues: the importance of interpersonal relationships, the corrective emotional experience, and the role of the group as a microcosm of society. Interpersonal relationships and the microcosmic aspect of group are closely bound. Individuals in group are forced to deal with, to interact with, and to react to other people from all spectrums of society. The corrective emotional experience is an intense, risky expression of emotion that happens because the group is cohesive enough and supportive enough to allow members to risk. Following the emotional expression there is a time to review the content and process of the expression, along with a chance to analyze the appropriateness or inappropriateness of the emotional response. Consequently, the group member, according to Yalom develops a more profound "ability to interact with others more deeply and honestly" (p.23), which is not as likely to eventuate in individual counseling. The evidence suggests that these cathartic experiences often signal a turning point for individuals in group therapy. Ultimately as group members increase their comprehension of events and relationships within the group, they grow more aware of their comprehension of events and responsibilities in the outside world.

Discussion Question: Often singular events change and shape our lives. What are some of the corrective emotional events that have occurred in the lives of class members to change their lives?

THE STAGES OF GROUP DEVELOPMENT

All groups progress through a series of stages of group development. A number of theorists (Corey, 1995; Yalom, 1970; Zastrow, 1989) have identified four or five stage patterns that typically begin with a formation, or definitive stage, followed in order by transition, action, working, and termination stages.

Definitive Stage During the definitive stage—the earliest meeting of the group—individuals strive to achieve an understanding of where and how they fit in the group and the roles they have in the group. This is the time, also, when individual members look for acceptance and approval, and they look for structure in the group process. They want to know what will be happening and may be anxious and dependent. The group leader's tasks in the definitive stage are to set the rules and guidelines for the group to allay anxieties and to provide support and encouragement for participation. As the group progresses through this stage, it gradually defines the structure and meaning of the group, the goals and functions required to meet those goals, and the boundaries within which the group will operate.

One of the earliest tasks of the definitive stage is to decide if the group is to have an open or closed membership. In some settings this decision may be preordained by agency policy. Open membership groups are very common in dependency treatment centers and are open to new members throughout the life (often indefinite) of the group. Closed groups are closed to new members once the group has begun. Corey (1995) points out that open membership groups have the advantage of continuous new stimulation as new members join the group and old members leave. In addition, the wisdom and insight of long-term group members is available to new members as they join. Of course, the major disadvantage of open groups is that they may never reach a level of cohesion. Furthermore, new members must always play catch-up. Closed groups are more likely to reach greater levels of stability and cohesion, but group dynamics will suffer if group members drop out or if the energy level of the group diminishes.

In a variant of the open–closed dichotomy, Alcoholics Anonymous and other peer self-help groups conduct open and closed meetings that are somewhat different from open and closed groups. Open meetings are open to anyone who wishes to attend; closed meetings are limited to individuals who identify themselves as members of the AA fellowship. Typically these meetings have a set of discussion topics (Step meetings; Big Book meetings), but they do not have a strictly closed membership. Any AA member can come and go at any time.

Discussion Question: What are some of the advantages and disadvantages (administrative, clinical, counselor-centered, client-centered) of open and closed groups?

Transition Stage   The transition stage is a time of heightened anxiety, defensiveness conflict, and struggles for control (Corey, 1995). Individuals test their power and position within the group, often challenging their peers and the group leader. By this stage of the group, they have a sense of the group norms; now they must determine the safety of the group process and the level of trust they give and feel. It is a time of action, reaction, interaction, and transaction. The transition stage is a time of resistance. For some members that resistance may take the form of behavioral or verbal acting out, while others may withdraw into limited participation or even silence. It is important to remember that resistance at this stage is a normal and expected part of the group process. Counselors need to guard against categorizing members according to the behaviors and verbalizations seen during this stage (Corey, 1995). To do so may cast a member into a role from which there is no escape and, ultimately, no positive outcome from counseling.

Action Stage   In the action stage, the group moves from a period of personal involvement to a time of group involvement. Independence becomes replaced by interdependence on each other. Cohesion begins to develop, group members begin to make greater personal commitments toward group participation and take more risks, and group processes become more important than individual needs and self-involvement.

Working Stage The action stage segues into the working stage of group dynamics when group involvement and productivity are at their peak. This stage is distinguished from the action stage by the activities of the members. In the action stage, members are still responding to personal needs and working on personal issues. Throughout the working stage there is a greater emphasis on group issues. Honesty and openness have become natural and vital parts of the group process, and there is greater opportunity for in-depth problem exploration and resolution.

Termination Stage Most groups naturally reach a termination point, and that termination is typically seen as a positive event. The termination stage can be a time of intense productivity and emotionality as group members develop a sense of urgency to complete unfinished personal or group business (Zastrow, 1989). Group cohesion is at a peak, and the willingness to work on group issues in an efficient, productive manner is apparent. For many, termination is a time of anticipated loss and anxiety, as natural feelings of separation and doubt begin to surface. Indeed, a test of the success of the group may be the comfort felt by members and the willingness to leave the group. On an individual level, a member who is feeling insecure about future success may actually regress in behaviors and actions in order to stay in the safety of the group. During this stage, the group leader has the often difficult task of helping group members work through their anxieties and feelings about separation and moving forward. Ultimately the goal of any group is independence and improved functioning—points that the leader should stress throughout the group process.

The Case of Ronnie

Ron was a 16-year-old adolescent finishing a course of inpatient treatment for his inhalant and crack cocaine dependencies. The product of a single-parent, female-led family, he had experienced a number of difficulties with male role models in his life. He made excellent progress in counseling group, quickly becoming committed and involved in the goals of the group, and showed a dedication to developing an insightful understanding of the issues affecting his life. He described his group leader, a 40-year-old male counselor as being "the most important person in [his] life." During his tenth group session, the group leader suggested that Ronnie seemed ready to move on to the next phase in his treatment. That night Ronnie broke curfew at the facility and set fire to a small shed on the grounds.

Discussion Questions: What occurred with Ronnie? How might these problems have been prevented?

Termination of participation in chemical dependency groups is especially a time of high anxiety and emotionality. For many clients, leaving the safety and support of the group engenders very high levels of stress and tension. Natural doubts surface about the ability to put into practice new behaviors and new skills as they enter a new life phase and face new expectations. To decrease stress and boost levels of self-confidence, many facilities conduct formal group departure rituals that frequently include giving a symbolic token of "graduation" to the terminating members. Usually these symbols are coin-sized metal disks inscribed with AA or NA slogans or similar motivational phrases. Hence, these rituals became known as "coining out." The symbols serve a dual purpose: They serve as very real evidence of the completion of group and of the client's readiness to move on, and they provide a daily reminder of the knowledge, insight, and skill learned in group. Coining out ceremonies are memorable events, and many individuals carry their coins with them throughout life until the coins have been worn smooth of all engraving and art.

Discussion Question: What are some other termination rituals that might be used in ending group?

GETTING STARTED: GUIDELINES FOR FORMING AND LEADING A GROUP

As is the case with many activities, the key to successful group leadership rests with careful advance preparation. Four elements of the group process must be considered prior to implementing group activities, regardless of whether the group is a single-event activity group or a multisession counseling group: the goals of the group, the participants in the group, the logistics of the group, and the format of group activities.

Defining the *goals and objectives* of the group is imperative. Group members typically enter group with at best a vague idea of what they want to get out of the group process. If the leader is unwilling or unable to add structure to the group process, the group will invariably flounder. This is not to imply that goal setting is a unilateral task of the group leader, although it may be in some situations. Didactic groups that focus on teaching a specific skill (writing a resume, for example) are typically conceptualized by the leader with little input from group members about the goals of the group. Discussion and input from all of the group members is essential in specifying the goals of counseling group. Selecting goals that *can* be achieved by the group members is also vital. Often groups in dependency treatment centers are structured in their topics and format. Unfortunately what may seem to be a reasonable goal for one group of clients may not be reasonable or appropriate for another group.

Each group is composed of different individuals with unique and specific characteristics. While it may be tempting to assume all individuals with dependency problems are alike, this is simply not the case. The leader's task, to the extent that it is possible, is to determine the unique and specific *characteristics* of group members and to appropriately tailor group activities to meet their needs and skill levels. It is absolutely essential to identify group needs, expectations, and skills as precisely as possible. Often, for example, group activities may involve tasks that require a relatively high level of reading skill, analysis, and comprehension (e.g., when reading and discussing a section from one of the many self-help texts). In this situation the leader should determine if the group members are literate or if any of the group members have a learning disability that may preclude full participation in the reading and comprehension activities. The gender composition of the group is also important. Historically women have been in the minority in treatment, often representing only 10 percent to 20 percent of the treatment population. The possibility that some activities may be gender specific or gender exclusionary must be considered. Finally, the size of the group is important. Most group practitioners recommend a group size ranging from 8 to 12 members. A group with too many members challenges the ability of the leader to attend to the needs of all of the members, and important issues may get lost in the shuffle. One solution for an overly large group is to work with a cotherapist. Groups that are too small may be lacking in stimulation and interaction.

Group logistics include issues such as the meeting time and place, resources (i.e., video monitors, flip charts, writing materials, etc.) required for group activities and room and seating arrangements for the participants. Nothing is more embarrassing or frustrating to both the group and the leader than not having the needed resources or being forced to work in a room or setting that is uncomfortable in size or structure.

Carefully planning the *format of group activities* is essential. For new groups an ice-breaking activity may be needed to stimulate group interaction. Sessions for more mature groups should include relevant content that is logical in presentation, illustrated by examples if needed and paced to meet the needs of the group. However, flexibility is an important format characteristic because, despite the best-conceived intentions, group activities rarely go exactly as planned. Finally the group leader should take time to relax and reflect upon the group session before it begins to get into the right mind-set. Some individuals are born group leaders, but most are made—through training, practice, hard work, and experience.

A MODEL FOR CONDUCTING
ACTIVITIES IN A GROUP

One of the most difficult tasks, and one for which counselors are the least well prepared, is the task of conducting informative and interesting didactic or self-improvement groups in treatment facilities. Counseling groups are self-generating and self-perpetuating through the actions and interactions of all of the group members. However, the success and stimulation of didactic and self-improvement groups rest with the group leader's thoughtful choice of an appropriate activity to foster the desired insight and learning. Cole (1993) suggests a "7-Step Model for Group Dynamics" for group leaders who are conducting activity-oriented groups.

The first step of Cole's model is *introduction,* in which it is the leader's initial task to make a self-introduction that includes the leader's credentials for conducting the group. The leader should ask all group members to introduce themselves and make an effort to learn the names of all of the group members as quickly as possible. Following these introductions, the group leader clarifies the goals and objectives of the group session and sets the agenda for the group, including stating the specific purpose of the group. Often rehabilitation professionals assume that clients know and understand the reason for treatment activities. This is not always the case, and it is important to be explicit in setting the agenda to achieve maximum benefit for participants. Corey (1995) notes that groups may flounder or be aimless when the leader has done an inadequate job of preparation, direction, and guidance.

The second phase is to conduct the *activity,* which may be preselected by the group leader or may be selected by the group members. Cole asserts that timing and appropriateness are important for activities to be successful. It must be possible to accomplish the activity in the allotted time. In addition it must be appropriate to the skill level of the group, consistent with the therapeutic needs of the group, and within the physical and mental capacities of the group. Counselors are often called upon to facilitate exercise or recreation groups in treatment centers, for example. Therapeutic recreation activities for a group of adolescents would be different from activities selected for a group of middle-aged adults. Care must be taken to conduct activities that can be performed safely by clients whose health may be jeopardized by long-term alcohol or drug abuse. Finally, the activity must be consistent with the knowledge and skill level of the group leader. In didactic and self-improvement groups, members expect the leader to have a high degree of knowledge and expertise. The road to group failure is not paved by good intentions on the part of the leader but by poor preparation.

Following completion of the group activity, group members are invited to *share* their experience, thoughts, or actual work products with the rest of the group. If the activity has been watching a video, group members can share their individual learning experiences. If the activity involved a concrete task—for example, creating a resume—group members are invited to share their actual completed work. During this sharing phase, the emphasis is on the actual content of the participants' work or experience, concentrating on the cognitive, factual, and observable outcomes of the group activity. It is the leader's duty to encourage and support participation and discussion and to model appropriate levels of involvement. This step is a good time for the leader to evaluate the objective success of the activity.

The sharing phase leads directly to and is intricately linked with the *processing* step, during which group members express their subjective feelings about the activity, their participation, and the participation of other group members and the leader. Rutan and Stone (1993) argue that the content or overt meaning of any given comment or group event cannot be separated from the process or covert meaning of the comment or event. The linkage may be direct, or the content message may be a symbolic representation of hidden or underlying dynamics. In either case it falls to the leader to attend to the underlying currents flowing between content and process issues. Unless overt and covert power struggles, avoidance and withdrawal reactions, domination issues, and other concerns are addressed, the risk of ignoring or missing important group dynamics is very real (Rutan & Stone, 1993).

According to Cole's model, the leader has three final challenges: *generalizing* the outcome of the activity to other settings; reviewing the *application* of the activity to other life situations; and *summarizing* the events of the group to highlight the important points. Both the generalizing and application tasks address the issue of transfer of learning. The critics of group activities in treatment centers suggest that the activities lack a real-world orientation or that the teaching methods and objectives utilized in activities are inconsistent with real-life needs and demands. These are valid criticisms in many cases and are best addressed in the planning stages of an activity. Alternatively, even if appropriate activities and teaching methods are selected, clients may be unable to make the connection between the treatment environment and the outside world. By generalizing and reviewing the application of the learned principles, the group leader assists clients in making connections between treatment efforts and real-world functioning. Finally, the leader summarizes the group activities, reiterating the important points and setting the stage for future group sessions. Cole notes that it is especially important to end group on time to allow clients to move on to the next segment in their rehabilitation programs.

GROUP LEADERSHIP

The success or failure of a group is dependent on several factors: the characteristics of and contributions of the group members; the activities and techniques used to foster group growth and development; and the personal and professional attributes of the group leader (Corey, 1995). It is important to be clear about one thing. Leadership of a group does not rest solely with the designated leader. Indeed, leadership occurs when one member of the group influences other members to move the group toward reaching its goals. Consequently, because all members have the ability to sway the group, all members have both the capacity and responsibility for leadership. However, there is a distinction between leadership behavior and being in the position of being the designated group leader and being directly responsible for the scheduling logistics, activities, and ultimate outcome of the group (Zastrow, 1989).

Trait approach theories of leadership postulate that leaders have inherent characteristics that distinguish them from followers. However, the research seeking to explain or define those inherent characteristics has been inconclusive and at times contradictory (Zastrow, 1989). The differing types of leadership required for different groups suggest the importance of training for leadership over genetic traits. For example, leading a very focused activity group requires skills different from those needed to lead a support group or a counseling group. In contrast to the trait approach, *position* approach theories of leadership examine leadership abilities by focusing on the behavior of individuals who are in leadership positions. This line of research has yielded mixed results, too, largely because there is little consistency in how individuals acquire leadership positions. Some inherit their positions; others study for years to acquire theirs; some become leaders through merit; and some become leaders by default. Since group counseling is such a dominant force in dependency treatment, nearly every counselor will be expected to assume a group leadership role at some point. Undoubtedly some counselors are intuitively talented group leaders, yet every counselor has the potential to be a competent group leader with sufficient training, practice, and diligence.

Discussion Questions: Think about some of the leaders you know. Did they get their leadership role because of their traits? What are some of the traits you find valuable in a leader? Think of some of the traits possessed by leaders you know. How do you think these traits were acquired? What kind of traits would be important for leading a counseling group in a dependency treatment setting?

Leadership Styles

Several distinct leadership styles have been identified. *Authoritarian* leaders tend to make all of the decisions and assume all responsibility for the group. An authoritarian leader remains aloof from the group membership, fosters dependence, and generally tries to act in an efficient and decisive manner. Group members are likely to respond to authoritarian leadership out of a sense of compliance and not necessarily from a commitment to the goals of the group. Individuals who are conducting didactic groups that focus on the accomplishment of a specific task need authoritarian skills. Authoritarian leaders who are unsuccessful in carrying out their leadership role often generate factionalism within the group as members jockey for positions of favor with a resultant decline in group morale.

Discussion Question: Discuss other group situations in which authoritarian skills would be helpful.

Democratic leaders seek the maximum involvement and participation of all group members in every decision while at the same time maintaining an objective approach. Policies and procedures are discussed with the group, and responsibility is spread across group members rather than concentrated in the group leader. As a by-product of this democratic style, all issues of dissatisfaction and concern become public issues, and conflicts are confronted and dealt with openly. If conflict resolution occurs, group members develop strong personal commitments to the success of the group. However, if conflicts are not resolved, the leader may be seen as weak and ineffective. Decision making in democratically led groups may be slow and confusing, as input is solicited from all sides and parties.

Discussion Questions: When is a democratic style most useful? Least useful?

Zastrow (1989) writes that *laissez-faire* leaders demonstrate minimal participation in the group activities, delineate few guidelines, and impose little structure, leaving group members to their own resources. "Group members seldom function well under a laissez-faire style, which may be effective *only* when the members are committed to a course of action, have the resources to implement it, and need minimal leadership to reach their goals" (p. 41). Unfortunately many counselors who are ill-prepared to do group work tend to operate under the guise of this style. Probably the reality is that they do not have a defined sense of personal, professional group leadership style.

While not well researched or theoretically driven, two other styles are commonly seen in dependency group counseling. *Confrontive* leaders are very oriented to the here and now, have charismatic qualities, and may not be oriented to the needs of group members. Lewis, Dana, and Blevins (1994), in their criticism of group counseling in dependency treatment, argue that confrontation strategies frequently result in group member compliance with the confrontations of the leader or other group members without truly internalizing the underlying values. Long-lasting, sustained behavior change is not implemented by the group member, and former, destructive behaviors are quickly renewed. Confrontation is a valuable counseling strategy if it goes beyond demanding compliance and incorporates the characteristics of caring and concern and specific, descriptive, and well-timed feedback (Hutchins & Cole, 1992). Indeed, confrontation is a necessary part of the group counseling process to maintain the movement of the group and to train group members to be self-confrontive of problems needing resolution (Corey, 1995).

Discussion Question: When is confrontation appropriate in group counseling? Demonstrate ineffective and effective use of confrontation.

Charismatic leaders set themselves up as the ideal. This has been a common, although often unacknowledged, model in chemical dependency treatment. These group leaders believe in a particular style of recovery—often one that they went through themselves—and they refuse to recognize the validity or viability of other recovery options. "I got sober this way, and you should get sober this way" is the explicit message delivered to anyone who will listen. Charisma is very seductive for both the counselor and the clients. However, reliance on this style works only as long as no mistakes are made, no failures are evident, and unswerving loyalty is present—usually impossible criteria to meet. Client perceptions, attitudes, and loyalties change rapidly if the charismatic leader fails in any fashion.

Discussion Question: List some charismatic leaders. What are the characteristics that make them charismatic?

BASIC ROLES AND FUNCTIONS
OF THE GROUP LEADER

The fundamental concern of any group leader in any group type is to shape the group culture into one that will be conducive to and supportive of positive change. This concern is met through performing specific tasks aimed at accomplishing the goals and objectives of the group and by performing specific maintenance activities promoting the emotional and social stability of the group (Johnson & Johnson, 1975). In accomplishing these activities, the leader may assume the role of technical, teaching expert or of model-setting participant as ways to shape the culture of the group.

Direction is a basic leadership function. At the initiation of group activities, the leader provides structure for the members by setting forth the behavioral and ethical guidelines for group behavior, including confidentiality policies and procedures. With the increasing utilization of group work in outpatient settings, confidentiality directives should go beyond iterations of state and federal regulation to include guidelines about respecting the rights of fellow group members in the local community. As the group process continues, the leader has the responsibility to guide and stimulate, but not dominate, the group activities. Using appropriate levels of self-disclosure, modeling desired behaviors, and maintaining a strict sense of personal honesty and commitment to the goals of the group are vitally important. If the leader does not demonstrate a belief in the efficacy of the group, neither will the members.

In dependency treatment, tolerance is a necessary leader function, especially early in the group process. Individuals in recovery are facing significant issues of loss, abandonment, rejection, separation, guilt, and anger. Emotional raging and verbal outbursts and accusations are frequent occurrences, often motivated by psychological or physiological circumstances over which the individual has little control. Neurotransmitter changes, hormonal changes, or changes brought about by medication may be at the root of these events. The challenge for the counselor is to be able to distinguish the source of these outbursts, help the client work through them, and help the group in their understanding of the emotionality of recovery. The counselor must recognize when an outburst has gone beyond the cathartic to become a diatribe or a destructive force within the group. Outbursts involving physical danger to self or others cannot be tolerated under any circumstance in any group. The group leader must set clear guidelines forbidding physical violence of any sort and consequate any violations by removing the individual from the group. This dictum is especially crucial in today's drug culture with its frequently violence-laden episodes, and it presents a paradox. The task of counseling may be to change violent behaviors, but can those behaviors be changed if there is only a single response to violence—termination from treatment?

The group leader must be able to function from a nondefensive stance in the face of challenges and attacks from the group members, especially early in the life of the group. One of the common rejoinders to probing from group leaders is "You don't know how I feel. You've never been there." This difficult challenge is most often faced by nonrecovering counselors, but it also confronts counselors in recovery. Individuals addicted to drugs will challenge the experience and wisdom of group leaders in recovery whose dependency was alcoholism, for example. Usually these responses come forward as a way to divert attention away from painful and difficult issues needing resolution. Corey (1995) suggests challenges to the leader's authority and experience are often a significant part of the group member's movement toward autonomy. The precipitating factor for these challenges may be the transference phenomenon of projecting past events and past interactions onto current situations. Often counselors, especially beginning counselors, will retreat in the face of these challenges, with accompanying feelings of loss of personal and professional self-confidence. In reality, it is impossible for any counselor to know exactly what a group member is feeling. However, the leader has two allies in responding to this challenge: empathy and the power of the group members. Showing genuine concern and empathy is more helpful than a lot of talk when trying to convince the individual (and the group, for that matter) that the counselor really does understand. While the counselor may not share directly in the experience, he or she can relate to it and, more importantly, can guide individuals to solutions to the problems rather than simply reiterating the problems.

Although the counselor may not have had a similar experience, other group members might have. In that case, the leader should elicit sharing and support from the group members. Alex Levy directed Alpha House, founded in the early 1970s, as one of the first therapeutic communities serving individuals addicted to heroin. As a traditionally trained, nonrecovering counselor, he was the frequent target of attacks when he led groups. He would respond to the challenge "You don't know what I've been through; you don't know what I've suffered" with empathic agreement. Levy would continue with the gentle reminder that his job was not to go through the pain and suffering of addiction but to provide a support system that would allow clients to move beyond addiction into recovery. By dealing honestly and directly with challenges, as Corey suggests, Levy was able to maintain open lines of communication and affirm the importance and effectiveness of confronting sensitive issues in the group process. The support of the other therapeutic community residents was a powerful force vital in the mutual journey to recovery.

The Case of Heather

Heather was a 24-year-old rehabilitation counseling student on her internship. As part of her experience, she was sitting in on a counseling group, observing a skilled clinician conducting group therapy with individuals in treatment for dependence on crack cocaine. One afternoon the lead counselor was called away for a family emergency, and Heather volunteered to conduct the group. Twenty minutes into the session, one of the group members challenged her knowledge of crack dependency. Heather had been raised in an alcoholic home and was quick to assert that she knew the pain of dependancy firsthand. She was bewildered, hurt, and ultimately reduced to tears when her impassioned story of her own childhood problems was met with derision and anger.

Discussion   Questions: What did Heather do right? What did she do wrong? Is self-disclosure a good idea in the face of confrontation? Discuss some ways a group leader might respond to open challenges of the leader's authority and expertise.

It is important to understand the role of the power of the group leader and the power of the group. In all groups, both the members and the leader have considerable influence over the direction and activities of the group. In well-functioning, effective working groups that power is directed toward the completion of group objectives and goals. In other situations where conflict is present, group members (or even the leader!) may use their power for their own interests and concerns at the expense of the other group members (Zastrow, 1989). Power held by group members is both a function of the actual power held by the group member, based on the number of resources possessed by the member, and the perceptions of the other group members concerning the resources held by the member. A synergistic effect may eventuate. A group member with relatively few resources but with a strong standing in the group may be granted excess power by the group.

The classic paradigm for understanding the bases of power in groups was developed by French and Raven in 1968. Their model lists five bases of power in groups: reward, coercive, legitimate, referent, and expert power.

Individual group members who are perceived to possess *reward power* have the ability to dispense positive or negative consequence in response to a group member behavior. Group leaders have overt reward power, especially if their recommendation about an individual's behavior or progress in group will result in a positive change of status for the group member. In the outpatient dependency treatment, progress in group may lead to discharge. Reward power in correctional settings is especially tricky. Group members learn quickly that progress in group can lead to favorable outcomes in other parts of prison life, including changes in work or educational assignments, housing units, or institutional changes such as positive parole board recommendations. Consequently, counselors in correctional settings must continually evaluate group progress in tandem with other facets of the group member's overall performance. In all settings, reward power is held by group members as well, usually in the form of praise and support.

Discussion   Questions: Who has reward power in this classroom? How is that power utilized?

Coercive power is the perceived ability to dispense punishment or to remove positive consequences and, again, is held by the group leader and group members. The use of coercive power was a hallmark of many of the group activities in early therapeutic communities (TC) in a effort to expose TC residents to the consequences of their behavior, often for the first time. There is an important consideration, according to French and Raven, about the distinction between reward and coercive power. The positive nature of reward power will result in increased attraction between group members and the power holder. On the other hand, the negative consequences related to coercive power tend to reduce the attractiveness between group members and the holder of coercive power. Zastrow (1989) notes that coercive power tends to exacerbate rather than settle conflict, while reward power, used legitimately, will result in positive gains. However, if reward power is seen as being used in a manipulative fashion by the leader or one of the members, the group is apt to respond negatively.

Discussion Who has coercive power in this classroom? How is it utilized?
Questions: Has anyone been influenced by reward or coercive power? How did you feel about what happened?

Legitimate power is power conferred by virtue of assignment, electioxn, or appointment. Designated group leaders have a legitimate power base as a consequence of their job roles. Group members may have legitimate power as a result of decisions made by the group or as a result of appointment by the group leader. For example, a group member may be designated to perform special activities (i.e., leading a particular discussion section), thus according that member legitimate power with respect to the appointed task. Zastrow (1989) notes that legitimate power has limited scope, and efforts to exercise power beyond the designated range of power will be met by resistence from the group members.

Discussion Who in the classroom holds legitimate power in this setting?
Questions: In other settings? Does the legitimate power from one setting tend to transfer over to other settings? In what circumstances?

Referent power is power that is assigned to a group participant by other members, based on a display of attractive qualities and behaviors desired by the group members. Thus, referent power is akin to charisma. Referent power is the base of power for individuals who are highly regarded in peer self-help fellowship meetings, and displays of referent power are an explicit and forceful part of peer self-help. In AA meetings, individuals with lengthy histories of recovery are called upon to share their stories of success, and newer members are encouraged to emulate these respected elders. Much of the power of AA sponsorship is grounded in referent power, too. As Zastrow (1989) points out, in ambiguous situations, such as the to-drink-or-not-to-drink crisis faced by many individuals in recovery, the wisdom, beliefs, and values of the group and the sponsor can be a valuable sustaining force.

The perception that a group member has special knowledge or expertise confers *expert power* on that individual. This type of power is typically obtained through education and experience, and counselors serving as group leaders automatically have expert power. Group members may have expert power depending on the education and experience they bring to the group. For example, individuals dependent on certain drug types may be regarded as having expert power about the effects of that drug and related recovery issues. Individuals who have relapsed and who are participating in group treatment for the second or third time may have expert power conferred on them by the first-timers in the group. Unfortunately, these members who are repeating treatment may be perceived as expert, but they may not have the skills, values, and attitudes that will be helpful to the group. They may have as much to learn and gain from the group experience as the newer members. Expert power has a very constrained range of authority limited to the specific area of concern. Attempts to use expert power outside that range will reduce the impact of the power and the credibility of the expert.

Discussion   Who possesses expert power in this classroom? In what areas?
Questions: What happens when individuals with expert power try to exceed the bounds of their power?

CHARACTERISTICS IMPORTANT
FOR GROUP LEADERSHIP

The literature identifies a number of personal and professional characteristics pertinent to group leaders. Corey (1995) notes that counselors must be (1) emotionally present, (2) self-confident and possessed of personal power, (3) courageous and comfortable with risk taking, (4) self-confrontive, (5) sincere and authentic, (6) in touch with their own identity, (7) devoted to and enthusiastic about group process, and (8) creative and inventive. A number of these issues have special significance for doing group work in dependency treatment settings. Having a strong sense of personal identity implies personal understanding and insight about values, beliefs, goals, and attitudes. Group leaders, perhaps more so than individual counselors, must be aware of their feelings and attitudes about a variety of sensitive issues. For instance, group leaders must be clear on their personal beliefs about drug and alcohol use, incest, gender issues, racial issues, and sexual choice issues. The self-awareness that the leader brings to the group is indispensable. Fixed perceptions and opinions will be carefully scrutinized by group members. Closely linked is a sense of "personal honesty," as Yalom (1985) asserts. The leader has a clear model-setting role that requires honesty about strengths and weaknesses, risk taking, self-confrontation, and self-disclosure. In particular, honesty about personal drug and alcohol use is fundamental. Leaders need not be abstinent from legal drugs and alcohol if they do not have a history of dependency or abuse. However, they must have a rational, well-conceptualized, and insightful understanding of their own use patterns, for they will surely be questioned about their beliefs. Finally, group work requires a higher level of stamina and energy to attend to all of the members and their participation in group activities. Groups are highly complex, and creativity and attention are required to deal with all of the issues and problems.

SUMMARY

Group counseling is a primary treatment modality in substance abuse and dependence rehabilitation, largely attributable to the influence of the peer self-help movement. Additionally, group counseling is highly valued as a microcosm of society and as a cost-efficient and staff-efficient way to serve large groups of clients.

While many argue that group counseling is an effective treatment model, others have questioned its effectiveness and, in particular, the long-term effectiveness of groups employing verbal confrontation strategies. Criticisms have been leveled at the passive nature of didactic groups and the use of groups as standardized treatment, discounting the importance of individualized care. Counselors must acquire a basic understanding of group dynamics and leadership skills before attempting group counseling.

Four broad types of groups are seen in substance abuse counseling. Counseling groups focus on intrapsychic change and usually deal with recovery experiences and relationship issues. Didactic groups aim to impart information, often through the use of videotapes and other media. Peer self-help groups are voluntary groups serving individuals with common problems. Alcoholics Anonymous is the most ubiquitous. Many agencies host peer self-help groups. Self-improvement groups combine elements of counseling and didactic groups, seeking to bring about intrapsychic change by teaching new behaviors and skills.

Certain elements must be in place for group counseling to be effective. The group must be a safe and secure haven where new ideas can be explored and new risks taken. Instilling hope and a sense of optimism for the future is vitally important and is often accompanied by an altruistic spirit from the group members. All groups strive to develop a strong sense of cohesion as they deal with the universality of their problems. Both vicarious learning and interpersonal learning make significant contributions to the success of a group.

All groups go through similar stages of group development. In the definitive stage group members are looking for structure and information about the group, while in the transition stage they explore their position and power in the group. The action stage is characterized by the emergence of interdependence among group members, moving in contrast to the independent action formerly seen. This leads to the working stage, distinguished by a high level of group activity and productivity. The termination stage signifies an ending for group members and may be especially significant for individuals with drug and alcohol problems. Many agencies have developed formal termination rituals to assist clients in making the transition to a newfound recovery status.

Successful group leadership starts with defining the goals and objectives of the group and developing an awareness of the unique and specific characteristics of group members. The clinical goals of the group can be reached only if sufficient attention is directed toward the logistics of the group and the format of group activities. Groups that are centered on activities, a trait of self-improvement groups, begin with an introduction of the activity and the tasks of the group, followed by the conducting of the activity. After the activity is completed, group members should share their experiences and process their feelings about the activity. Both the leader and the group should explore ways that the activity will generalize and be applicable to the real world. Finally, the group leader should summarize the events of the group activity.

Both trait and position approaches have been used to examine leadership styles. Authoritarian leaders tend to dominate the group, compared to democratic leaders who rely heavily on member input and information. Laissez–faire leaders tend to offer minimal direction and guidance. Confrontational leaders rely on confrontation of negative behaviors and continuing defense mechanisms, a strategy often employed but with little empirical evidence of long-term success. Charismatic leaders rely on the strength of their personal characteristics to be successful in group leadership.

While most groups have designated leaders, any member of the group may perform group leadership duties depending on the situation. Group task activities promote the ongoing functioning of the group and include the day-to-day practical tasks that need to be accomplished. Maintenance activities focus on the interpersonal, cohesion, and morale-building needs of the group. Designated group leaders have the responsibility for providing direction to the group and keeping it on task. Other qualities important for group leadership in substance abuse settings include tolerance and nondefensiveness. The group leader possesses significant power in the group, but the group itself is powerful. Power bases include reward power, coercive power, legitimate power, referent power, and expert power.

The personal and professional characteristics important for group leadership include the ability to be emotionally present with the group, self-confident, and courageous. Group leaders must be willing to be self-confrontive of their own behaviors, attitudes, and beliefs and be sincere and authentic in their role, remaining in touch with self. Group leadership is demanding, therapeutic work, requiring a strong belief in the group process and creativeness and inventiveness for success.

7

Family Counseling

CHAPTER 7 OUTLINE

WHAT IS A FAMILY?

Family issues have been a concern in dependence treatment from the earliest days. The chapters in the *Big Book,* the formation of Al-Anon and Al-Ateen, and the early inclusions of family issues in the treatment process attest to the impact of dependence on the family. However, while family issues have always been paramount concerns, the definitions of family and the impacts of dependence have continually expanded.

Definitions of who and what constitutes a *family* have shifted dramatically during the past 50 years. During the earliest days of dependence treatment, family typically meant the family of origin or the birth family. This family was viewed in very traditional ways: The members were Mom and Dad and the naturally born children, and it included the transmission of both genetic and cultural/environmental information from parents to children. The nuclear family is viewed as mother, father, and children, too, but the children may have different origins. Some may be the offspring of both parents, and others may be adopted. In any case, this is the family in which individuals are raised—it is the nucleus of their belief system about and understanding of the family process. For many—indeed, most—individuals, family of origin and nuclear family are synonymous. However, the intergenerational transmission of genetic, biological family material and the intergenerational transmission of cultural, attitudinal, and behavioral material may have significant impact on the development of the dependence process.

For some ethnic groups, especially Native Americans, Asian Americans, and African Americans, the extended family plays an important role. The extended family is a large, complex family that includes the nuclear family and assorted other individuals or groups. Usually the extended family is consanguineous, having the same ancestor or ancestors and therefore directly identifiable ancestors, such as great-grandparents. For other extended families, the pattern of descent is more amorphous but still related to a common blood relative. This is commonly seen among Native American groups who may view their tribe or clan or a series of households in a geographic locale as the extended family. However, in other situations, nonblood relatives may be included in the extended family. In the African-American community, for example, the terms *aunt* or *auntie* are names of endearment reserved for a respected, revered older female acquaintance who may not be related to the family by blood but who has significant influence and respect within the family.

Most Euro-American families are oriented toward the nuclear family, although great pride may come from the ability to trace their ancestry through several generations. Many Italian-American extended families are quite closely knit, involving three or four generations, with great respect paid to the elder members. Similarly, Asian-American families are tightly bonded across generations. The "Chinatowns," "Japan Towns," and "Little Italys" in America's cities are testaments to the importance and power of group and family solidarity within these ethnic groups. The notion of extended family is important for many reasons. First, the extended family can play a significant role in the transmission of the dependence process, both through genetic and cultural/behavioral modes. Second, the extended family can serve as fertile ground for the progression of codependency. In large, complex extended families, finding a willing, although often unsuspecting, codependent may be relatively easy. Finally, the extended family can serve as a significant support system in the recovery process. Extended families frequently contain multiple resources of time, energy, and nurturing not available in smaller families.

Other definitions of family have developed as divorce rates in society have changed. Stepfamilies include children not born to one of the parents. Blended families are variants of stepfamilies in which both parents bring a set of children to the new family.

The multiple problems of single-parent families in which one parent is either temporarily or permanently absent have been extensively examined in the popular press. For the rehabilitation practitioner, issues about single-parent families go beyond the problem stage to include concerns about the recovery process. Recovery is a complex, often frustrating process, requiring the expenditure of significant amounts of time, energy, and support that may not be readily available. Moreover, both societal attitudes and family therapy models tend to presuppose the importance of a family in which both parents are present.

Surrogate families may replace or provide support besides that provided by traditional families. For many individuals who are separated or disenfranchised from their families of origin, surrogate families may be their *only* family. These families are often based in religion or recovery. Some may have strict rules about inclusion and participation, while others may be more free-flowing in form.

Alternative families is a term used to describe families whose membership does not fit within the generally accepted cultural bounds. They encompass families in which both parental figures are of the same gender; families in which the parents are not married to each other; families in which other relatives (i.e., grandparents, aunts, uncles) serve in parental roles; and families in which no parental figure is present. It has been suggested by one group of authors that alternative families headed by grandparents are increasing largely due to drug- and alcohol-related issues, including parental abuse and dependence, parental incarceration, child neglect and abuse, and parental death due to AIDS and violence (Pinson–Millburn et al., 1996). They noted that both the grandparents and the children in these alternative families are at increased risk for both physical and mental health problems. Thus, while grandparent-led families may present a short-term solution to keeping the family intact, long-term, multigenerational consequences may result.

Treatment concerns with alternative families involve the traditional focus of many family therapy models toward two-parent, mother-and-father-headed families besides more practical concerns about the availability of financial support for treatment services. Many public and private sources of medical coverage recognize only legally sanctioned marriages for purposes of determining who is an eligible beneficiary for support. Consequently, adolescents growing up in a gay alternative family or an unmarried alternative family may not have coverage for dependence treatment because of insurance regulations.

The essential question to be asked of all clients is "Who is your family?" The rehabilitation practitioner must guard against preconceived personal notions about family and its influence.

Discussion
Question: Who constitutes your family right now?

HOW DO FAMILIES FUNCTION?

Families are the foundational structures of society. Within the safety of family individuals learn basic and complex skills, test roles and responsibilities, and receive reactions about performance and possibilities. Consequently, a family is not just a collection of individuals housed under one roof, but it is a dynamic, evolving, synergistic system made up, according to Murray Bowen, of a series of interlocking relationships, well-developed rules and regulations, and self-correcting mechanisms (Goldenberg & Goldenberg, 1996).

The family system as a whole is constructed of a collection of subsystems of infinite variety and form. One, and only one, subsystem within families is autonomous and impenetrable: the parental subsystem. Other subsystems and their membership wax and wane according to the needs and development of the family and the individuals within the family. All of the children of a family may band together in sibling subsystems; all males (father and male children) may join a male subsystem; older family members may belong to a family subsystem separate from younger members. Within families where dependence is present, the nondependent family members may form a subsystem closed to the dependent family members. Any family member may belong to or drop out of a subsystem anytime.

Boundaries separate subsystems from the system and from each other. Also, they separate individuals from each other and from subsystems and serve as demarcation lines between the family and the outside world. Families that have boundaries that are easily crossed and permeable are said to operate using an open system. Open systems are characterized by a high degree of information flow within the family and between the family and the outside world, and they are adaptable to changes and stress. Conversely, closed system families usually have very rigid boundaries, little information flow, and a tendency to become disorganized and dysfunctional in the face of changes and stress, a characteristic known as entropy. It is readily apparent that families in which dependence is bound away as a shameful, secretive issue are headed for disorganization and dysfunction.

It is an axiom of systems theory that all systems, whether open or closed, continually and automatically seek homeostasis. This state of equilibrium and balance is vital to the continuation of the family system in the face of the multiple pressures, threats, and stresses experienced on a daily basis. Individuals tend to perceive life events in terms of linear causality: One event leads to another event, nonreciprocally. However, families experience circular causality, in which multiple positive and negative forces act on the system, subsystems, and individuals simultaneously. One way all families deal with the circular forces of life and the need to maintain homeostasis is to develop a complex set of rules and roles. Some family rules are overt, specific, and known to all members:

Bedtime is 10:00 P.M. for children under 12.

Teenage curfew is 11:00 P.M. on weekday nights.

No TV until homework is done.

Only Mom and Dad can withdraw money from the bank account.

Other family rules may be covert, but usually all family members have an awareness of them:

Don't bother Dad while he is watching the basketball game.

Older children are responsible for watching younger children.

The development of a series of covert rules is one of many usually futile strategies families may use to deal with dependence:

Don't talk about Dad's drinking with outsiders.

Mom is ill with one of her migraines, not hungover.

Hide the liquor so Dad can't get drunk.

Teenage drinking is okay; just be thankful it's not drugs.

Discussion Questions: What rules exist in your family? Are they overt or covert?

Family roles serve to define status and development in the family and to create an organized, hierarchical power structure within the family. As with rules, some roles may be explicit, and others may be more implicit. As society has changed, roles have transformed as well. In the past Mom may have been the stay-at-home nurturer, Dad the working disciplinarian ("Just wait till your father gets home!!!"), and children had extended periods of dependence. In today's double-income, latchkey environment, many family roles are being redefined. However, the precepts of history and tradition may impose structures, attitudes, and expectations that may no longer be either valid or sustainable.

Discussion Questions: What are the roles in your family? What changes have occurred in your family over the years?

For rules and roles to serve their purpose, intricate patterns of communication are developed. Methods of conducting day-to-day activities, problem solving, negotiation, and conciliation are continually evolving to permit families to perform the tasks of life. According to Hanna and Brown, all communication, whether verbal or nonverbal, has both content and process functions. The content part of the communication is the specific message being transmitted; the process part of the communication defines the relationship between the message sender and the recipient and conveys stated and unstated expectations of performance. In functional families with open patterns of communication, expecting a high degree of congruence between the content and process sections of communication is reasonable. However, in dysfunctional families where dependence is present, there may exist a significant dichotomy between content and process.

The communication patterns, family rules and roles, and the nature of the family system and subsystems combine to formulate the family paradigm, temperament, and identity. The family paradigm is the model of how the family views the world, including their shared, internalized perceptions about the external environment and their role and potential success in it (Goldenberg & Goldenberg, 1996). Some families operate from the premise that the world is a comfortable place with orderly, predictable, and trustworthy characteristics. These families value individual opinion, operate democratically, and enjoy (or at least cope well with) the challenges of daily living, displaying high levels of adaptability and cohesion (Fenell & Weinhold, 1989). Other families may view the world as threatening, hostile, and unpredictable. Their interactions are characterized by rigid boundaries, strict rules and roles, and banding together to deal with external dangers. In their research, Kantor and Lehr (1975) identified a third family paradigm type: the random family. These families are essentially unorganized; few rules and roles exist, boundaries are blurred and easily crossed (Goldenberg and Goldenberg, 1996), and the family operates more on an intuitive level. None of the family paradigm types ensures successful functioning in the world, nor does any type imply dysfunctionality. Constantine's research (1986) suggests that families with closed systems and randomly modeled families may be less successful in coping with high-stress events. Moreover, even families who see their environment as comfortable and trustworthy may be overwhelmed by the sudden stresses of a crack cocaine addiction in the family or a long-term alcoholism problem.

Just as different individuals have different energy levels and response styles, so do families. Family temperament refers to the manner in which the family responds to both internal and external demands, solves problems, and conducts normal, regular daily activities. Some families have high energy levels, close interactional levels, and a broad repertoire of behaviors. Other families may be more conservative in energy expenditure and the range of depth of interactional levels. "Family identity is the family's subjective sense of its own continuity over time, its present situation, and its character" (Steinglass, Bennett, Wolin, & Reiss, 1987, p. 58). While family temperament might be characterized as a family's psychological emotional sense of self, family identity is the family's cognitive perception of its existence and is closely analogous to concepts of individual ego identity. Consequently, it would be expected that families with a strong family identity would be more resilient in the face of threats imposed by drug or alcohol problems. However, just like individuals, these families are not immune to drug and alcohol problems and their challenges.

Just like individuals, also, families must accomplish a series of developmental tasks as part of the life of the family, and failure to accomplish those tasks will lead to family dysfunctions. The success of development and growth within the family is typified by the family's ability to cope with the continuous and discontinuous changes of the family's life cycle. Continuous changes are those changes that are normal and expected episodes in the life of the family. They include marriage, planned pregnancies, children's matriculation and graduation from school, and similar events. While all change brings disruption to the family, most families can cope with continuous changes easily because changes in the family system are necessary to its vitality. Discontinuous changes are unplanned, unexpected events that are both sudden and disruptive to the daily functioning of the family and include events such as sudden death, divorce, accidents, and the like. Some ordinarily continuous changes may become discontinuous in nature if sufficient planning or preparation has not occurred. Unplanned pregnancies, early graduation from high school, early retirement, and so forth are some examples. All families have difficulty coping with discontinuous changes, and some families may never again return to their level of pre-change functioning. The ability to cope with change positively is a good indicator of family health and stability.

The classic work in family development was first postulated by Evelyn Duvall in 1977 and later expanded in collaboration with Miller in 1985. This model suggested that the traditional, average American family went through eight developmental stages:

1. Married couples without children (about 2 years)
2. Childbearing families (2.5 years)
3. Families with preschool children (3.5 years)
4. Families with children (7 years)
5. Families with teenagers (7 years)
6. Families as launching centers (first to last child leaves home; 8 years)
7. Middle-aged parents (empty nest to retirement; 15 years)
8. Aging family (retirement to death of both spouses; 15+ years)

This model depicts the movement of the family through time and plots both the stages and chronology of family development. Descriptive rather than explanatory in nature, it suggests that both individuals and families must accomplish a series of development tasks and that there is a close interplay between individual development and family development. For example, in the married couple first stage, the individuals must make the transition from independence to interdependence and as a couple makes a commitment to shared life as a family. Similarly, in later stages family members must learn to cope with changes from both the individual and family perspective. Consequently, the failure of individuals to accomplish developmental tasks will influence the family, and the failure of the family to accomplish developmental tasks will influence the individual family members. Family dysfunction may indicate that either individuals and/or the family are at a developmental impasse. While this classic work offers a utilitarian analysis of family development, it has been criticized of late for failing to incorporate issues related to alternative families and families at lower socioeconomic levels. Feminists have criticized it for its assumptions of a two-parent, male-headed family structure and its orderly two-year transition from marriage to birth of the first child.

This model also fails to address the developmental changes and disruptions that happen in families where divorce and remarriage occur. At the time of Duvall's initial development of the model in the 1950s and 1960s, divorce was a relatively rare event. In the 1990s nearly one in four marriages ends in divorce, and the rate in families where dependence is present is thought to be significantly higher (Steinglass et al., 1987). The evidence is clear that divorce has powerful disruptive effects on both the family and individuals. The adult family members may have trouble reconciling their own feelings of failure, abandonment, despair and loss; children may be confused, angry, or guilty, depending on their level of psychological development. If a remarriage occurs, the new family must go through a period of resolution, stabilization, and resumption of family life. An entire new set of rules, roles, and communication patterns must be established, and a new family identity must develop. This can be a painful time of exploration, discovery, frustration, and challenge for everyone in the new family and for the members of the former families.

Duvall's model fails to address the developmental issues facing alternative families, notably families headed by a single, female parent. Nearly one in three single-female-headed families exists below the poverty line, and many female heads of household suffer from depression and stress and may be at higher risk of the development of drug or alcohol problems. While no causal evidence proves a connection between single parenthood and drug or alcohol problems, these women and their families clearly have fewer resources, fewer options, and greater life pressures. Members of these "unorganized families" have limited power and control over life circumstances, typically little or no health insurance, and are more dependent on social welfare systems. Additionally, the children lack important role models with the absence of a responsible male parental figure in the home. More teenage pregnancies occur in these families, further altering the already skewed family developmental process that may exist. Consequently, while these families may be most in need of dependence prevention and intervention services, they may be the least likely families to receive those services.

THE IDEAL ROLES OF THE FAMILY

It is not just rhetoric to suggest that the family represents the foundation of society. It is within the bounds of the family that individuals learn the rules, regulations, social structure, and mores and behaviors that will carry them through life. Brown (1988) has identified a series of ideal roles for the family to provide maximum benefit to children as they struggle to find their identity. The first and most basic role is the provision of safety and security. Families are bound by law—but, more important, by societal standards—to provide a safe, secure environment. Consider then, the trauma imposed upon the child who is abandoned at birth because Mother is addicted to crack cocaine or the daily violence thrust upon the child born in an environment where abuse and neglect go hand in hand with drug or alcohol dependence. Not every home must be surrounded by a white picket fence, but every home must provide a place where the growing child can feel safe and secure from the ravages of the world.

Nurturing is the next ideal role of the family and includes both physical and emotional components. Food, basic sustenance, meets the physical need of people, but emotional nurturing expressed through love and affection is equally vital. The family is responsible for providing a place of core focus, too. The family and home become an environment where identity develops, bonding happens, and initial social skills develop. The family environment is the setting where standards are taught and values are learned. However, if the child does not feel safe, secure, nurtured, and bonded to the family, is it reasonable to expect that a value system can develop? The prerequisite for valuing may be having a sense of one's own value.

As the foundation of society, the family is the first place where an individual learns a sense of organization, both about self and the world. Boundaries, hierarchies, and patterns of interaction are developed, tested, analyzed, and reviewed. However, the child growing up in a home where roles are confused, boundaries are either too rigid or nonexistent, and inappropriate behaviors are tolerated—in short, an alcoholic home—is unlikely to develop much of a sense of personal or world organization. Tied closely to this notion is the role of the family serving as a basic social system. Robert Fulgham (1990) wrote, "Everything I learned, I learned in kindergarten." Perhaps it would have been more accurate to suggest that everything important for learning occurs not in kindergarten but in the years before kindergarten. Learning how to share with, negotiate with, and occasionally conflict with others begins with sibling and parental interaction. It is during these early years that people learn a fundamental social system model, including relationship and communication skills. However, as Wegscheider-Cruse and Cruse (1990) point out so cogently, growing up in an alcoholic home may cause role development more attuned to survival in a chaotic environment than in developing a basic life model.

The family is the environment where indispensable elements of culture, language, and symbols are transmitted. Through learning the history and extended relationships of the family, the child develops a sense of place in society. Perhaps even more important for our concerns, the family is the environment where the child first learns about styles and types of drug- and alcohol-consuming behaviors. The evidence is clear that individuals who have early, positive experiences with alcohol, either through ritual or food-related events, are less likely to develop later alcohol abuse or dependence problems.

Finally, the family provides the environment where individuals develop a sense, both conscious and unconscious, of the vital role of homeostasis in family life. All families establish a point of balance, a norm for the operation of the family. Family members develop a sense of the importance of congruent role patterns and perceptions to allow the family to remain in equilibrium. Even in the face of threats imposed by drug or alcohol dependence within the family, all members will strive to overcome disequilibrium. It is because of this determination that families can cope with the tremendous pressures of drug addiction and alcoholism. Paradoxically, it is because of the tendency toward homeostasis that families may be unable to develop new strategies to deal with the addictive behaviors of its members.

What happens to the ideal roles of the family when dependence is introduced? This question has no easy answer, in large part because of the variability in dependence. Alcohol dependence in adults is often a long, slowly developing process around which most of the models of family problems are based. Alcohol dependence or alcohol abuse problems among adolescents can develop very quickly. Researchers are now investigating neural response to alcohol, and evidence suggests that the adolescent brain responds much more quickly and dramatically to alcohol than the adult brain. Crack cocaine dependence can develop quite suddenly among adults and adolescents, resulting in addiction developing in months or even weeks, unlike the long-term dependence process in alcoholism. Indeed, one of the common familial responses to crack cocaine addiction is bewilderment. Unlike long-term dependencies that often have an entire series of warning signs about the progression of the dependence, crack addiction can come about so suddenly that both the family and the dependent individual are unprepared for the devastating consequences. Heroin dependence can occur quite rapidly, too, and the warning signs may be different as well. Often individuals who become dependent on heroin are disengaged from their families because of the high levels of criminal activity and societal disapproval of heroin dependence. This disengagement may result from familial rejection of the dependent individual because of the consumption of an illegal, morally stigmatizing drug and the criminal behaviors necessary to support an expensive drug habit. The disengagement may be initiated by the dependent family member trying to conceal the addiction from other family members who may voice disapproval about the drug consumption or the lifestyle necessary to support the dependence.

Discussion Question: What are some dependence progressions seen by class members?

The myriad variables associated with the different types of dependence patterns make it difficult to postulate a single model that accounts for or describes the process of psychoactive substance dependence in families. Nonetheless, experience confirms that the dependence process comes to occupy a dominant focus of the family's life. Stephanie Brown (1985) argues this point eloquently in her discussion of alcoholism as the "central organizing principle" of family life. Brown asserts that alcohol and drinking behaviors become the central focus of family and individual life both for the alcoholic individual and other family members and that denial of the drinking behavior and alcoholism become the primary cognitive focus for the entire family. Finding opportunities to drink and worrying about the availability of alcohol dominate the alcoholic individual's life. Nondrinking social and recreational activities are abandoned, and nonalcohol-centered relationships are relinquished, according to Brown. The alcoholic, and later the family, relinquishes physical and emotional ties to the general community (Buelow, 1995).

Brown argues that the family becomes deeply enmeshed in the alcoholism process to the extent that family members develop the same behavioral and cognitive distortions as the alcoholic. All develop *alcoholic thinking*, a system of core beliefs and illusions of control maintained by defense mechanisms such as denial, rationalization, and minimization. The drive toward homeostasis requires that all family members shift their thinking and behavior to conform to the ability to deny the alcoholism while simultaneously permitting the alcoholic behavior to continue. At varying times different family members will try to assume personal control of the family; ultimately, everyone feels responsible for the continuation of the alcoholic behavior and guilty about not being able to control the problems.

Initially the family environment involves control. The alcoholic claims, "I can control my drinking." The family adopts a variety of strategies, beginning with personal denial ("There's no problem"). Next, family members may make minimal attempts to control alcoholic behavior by limiting the quantity or potency of alcohol in the house—for example, allowing only beer. Finally, they try overt control, such as pouring the alcohol down the drain. Incoming objective data and information that conflicts with the family's homeostatic control mechanisms and needs are rejected, ignored, denied, or altered to fit the family's developing alcoholism-based paradigms and identity. Much energy is expended in futile attempts to manage the ways in which others perceive and respond to the family, resulting in increased levels of anxiety, stress, and depression.

Discussion   Question: What control efforts have been seen by class members in alcoholic situations?

When control efforts deteriorate completely, the family may be left in a state of complete chaos. Schedules and routines become nonexistent; roles and rules become fragmented; and the family life is full of surprises. This inconsistency and unpredictability are very damaging to the development of the family and especially to the development of the children (Buelow, 1995). Children may find it impossible to succeed in normal developmental tasks when the rules and roles of the environment are in constant flux. Vacillating standards of authority and continuous redrawing of boundaries coupled with constantly changing truths and explanations for behavior create a milieu in which children cannot hope to predict and be responsible for the interpersonal consequences of behavior. As the chaos continues, the sober parent may attempt to assume both parental roles, or one of the children may take on a parental role. Unfortunately, neither of these strategies is an adequate replacement for the guidance, support, and nurturing found in two-parent homes. The family atmosphere is constantly in a state of tension, and the stress increases proportionately to the expanding dissonance between reality and denial. Outbursts of rage, violence, and anger are common; shame, emotional anguish, physical pain, public embarrassment, and withdrawal from the structures of society are just as common.

CODEPENDENCY:
A MATTER OF DEFINITION

Everyone who has ever worked in the dependence treatment field, or for that matter has picked up a self-help text at the local bookstore, has come across the construct of codependency. Originally conceptualized as coalcoholism (Whitfield, 1987) and later broadened and called *enabling,* codependency has become the broad term to describe the behaviors that occur when family members become so involved with the life of their dependent family member that negative consequences override the positive benefits of the relationship. However, the term has become so broad, encompassing so many behaviors and "addictions" that establishment of sound diagnostic criteria and treatment protocols has been extremely difficult. Indeed, some contend that codependency does not exist as a discrete clinical construct but describes a constellation of behaviors associated with the stress of trying to live in a family where dependence is present.

Therefore, before a discussion of codependency as a construct can be attempted, certain characteristics and elements of disorders in general must be considered. For most physical and psychiatric disorders, a taxonomy has been established through scientific investigation and analysis. A taxonomy allows researchers and treatment practitioners to agree on a classification system to describe the disorder and to develop universal criteria that distinguish the disorder from other similar disorders. In turn, a taxonomy allows the creation of disorder boundaries so that treatment practitioners can gauge the severity of cases and progress toward recovery.

The classification of clients is an important characteristic of a taxonomy, addressing the question of who is included in the population of individuals with the disorder and who is excluded. Stratification of cases is important, too. For example, are there acute cases of codependency, and are there chronic cases? How is a long-term case differentiated from a short-term case?

Another element of taxonomic classification is the establishment of diagnostic standards. Diagnostic standards allow practitioners to differentiate a disorder from other, similar disorders and to develop adequate treatment plans and outcome measures. In considering diagnostic criteria, it must be determined if a given disorder is conjunctive or disjunctive in nature. Conjunctive disorders must have all diagnostic elements if a diagnosis is to be rendered. For example, if a disorder has three diagnostic criteria, and the disorder is a conjunctive disorder, then all three criteria must be present for a diagnosis to be made. Many physical medicine diagnoses are conjunctive in nature, and in general people understand conjunctive classifications relatively easily because many activities of life are conjunctive in nature. Obtaining a driver's license is a conjunctive activity, for example. To get a driver's license a person must be a certain age, pass a written test, pass a vision test, and pass a driving test. Meeting only some of these criteria would prevent the possibility of obtaining a license.

Disjunctive disorders must present some, but not all, of the criteria for a diagnosis to be made. Many psychiatric disorders classified in the *Diagnostic and Statistical Manual, Revision 4* are disjunctive in nature. For example, psychoactive drug dependence is diagnosed if three or more indicators exist. Informal, man-on-the-street diagnoses are often disjunctive, particularly with respect to psychoactive chemicals. A person may be labeled an alcoholic because he or she drinks in the morning or becomes physically abusive after drinking. Similarly, disjunctive criteria can be used inappropriately to rule out a disorder. It is commonly believed that drinking only beer cannot lead to alcoholism.

Discussion Questions: What are some disjunctive criteria used appropriately or inappropriately to diagnose psychoactive substance abuse or dependence? What are some disjunctive criteria used to diagnose codependency?

Creation of diagnostic criteria allows treatment professionals to distinguish one disorder from another and to determine how the disorder is transmitted. Further, it can be determined if a disorder is related to other disorders. These are all-important characteristics of concern with codependency. Some families display significant codependency patterns with very negative outcomes; other families cope very differently with dependency problems. What is it about either of these families that causes them to act and react in the ways they do? Why do some seemingly high-risk families exhibit codependency patterns while others do not?

Finally, creation of diagnostic classification standards allows for the development of prevention strategies. If the parameters of a disorder can be identified, then determining the strategies important in preventing the disorder is theoretically possible.

Taxonomic classification permits a greater understanding of treatment possibilities, including the establishment of a theoretical foundation for treatment. Today, treatment strategies for codependence are seemingly as numerous as the many definitions of the disorder. Little attention has been given to whether the disorder is of psychological, behavioral, educational, developmental, or interpersonal origin. Similarly, scant attention has been given to the theoretical foundation of treatment strategies, largely because no foundation for the cause of the disorder exists. Often this has led to inappropriate or "one-size-fits-all" treatment with no consideration of the unique needs and problems of the family in designing the treatment plan. This is not to suggest that common themes do not exist between families where codependency exists. There are common themes, but without a theoretical foundation for codependency treatment, it has become too easy to rely on simple strategies for the common themes rather than addressing the much more complex issues presented by unique family needs.

Training of professionals is another area of concern. Because codependency is so vaguely defined, it is unclear which professionals should provide care, in what setting, and with what credentials. Should training be offered in graduate schools or in certification programs? Is there a prerequisite to training in codependency, such as a degree in social work, rehabilitation, psychology, or counseling? Finally, what is the role of recovering individuals in the treatment process? Questions arise about the quality of recovery, length of recovery, and the type of dependence experienced by the person or family in recovery. Families in treatment may voice concern about codependency groups led by individuals who are recovering from their own dependencies. Questions may arise about the quality of recovery. Traditionally chronological markers have been used to judge recovery; two years of recovery is considered the minimum, but empirical data does not support this. For some individuals or families, two years might be the right amount of time in recovery, whereas for others it may not be nearly enough. Still others may experience "quality recovery" in a far shorter time. Therefore, is chronology an adequate marker at all? Adoption of this standard makes the assumption that everyone *can* experience quality recovery, but logic dictates this is not the case. Some individuals and families may bring premorbid conditions to the recovery process that make quality recovery impossible. Individuals with severe preexisting personality disorders may not be good candidates to lead codependency recovery groups.

The purposes of research include proving that disorders exist, identifying differing treatment options, and showing that varying treatment options result in different responses and outcomes. To demonstrate valid differences between treatment approaches, research must be conducted empirically using random samples, blind selection, and controlled design, and the results should be disseminated in the professional literature. All these factors are important to permit replicability of the studies and methodologies and to allow other treatment professionals to adopt the treatment techniques. A substantial body of information about codependency exists, both in the popular literature and the media, and in the professional literature. However, virtually all of the studies in the literature are conceptual or anecdotal in nature, with few extant objective studies that address treatment outcomes or scientifically based theory development. While there is a need for conceptually based, qualitative descriptions of codependence and its treatment, the reality is that definitions, treatment strategies, and concepts are nearly as numerous as the authors writing about them. Until objective, replicable research is conducted and published, identifying reliable and valid prevention, diagnostic, and treatment strategies will be difficult if not impossible.

Finally, there is a growing, practical concern about developing a scientifically valid definition for codependency and its prevention, diagnosis, and treatment. Increasingly, both private and public funders of dependence treatment are demanding greater selectivity in treatment admission, diagnosis, and levels of care. Treatment must be based on an accurate diagnosis of client problems and planned in such a way to deliver an effective outcome in the most efficacious manner. Many insurers are limiting the number of available treatment days or episodes, and they are requiring that all treatment be based on diagnostic criteria from the *Diagnostic and Statistical Manual of Mental Disorders* (DSM-IV), the American Society of Addiction Medicine (ASAM) diagnostic and levels of care standards, or the guidelines of the *International Classification of Diseases* (ICD-10). However, codependency is not a recognized disorder under any of these classification systems. Some treatment centers have offered codependency treatment services to families by wrapping the cost of these services into the overall costs of individual care. Other centers have diagnosed family members, often inappropriately, with psychiatric diagnoses to bill for family codependency services. Adjustment disorders of adulthood or childhood and depressive disorder diagnoses have been used in this way. Unfortunately, neither one of these practices will hold up to either financial or clinical services audits, and both are ethically questionable. Still other facilities have opted to provide codependency family services without cost. While this is a laudable practice, it usually represents a significant financial and energy commitment by the facility, and it may not be affordable over the long term.

Current Definitions of Codependence

Disease Codependency is a disease in which the primary compulsion is to act in a way that satisfies the dependent. It is a primary progressive and chronic disease that stands between the afflicted person and his or her ability to act out of free choice rather than to just react, or behave in the way he or she learned in order to survive in a sick situation (Rogers Memorial Hospital, 1988).

Behavioral Codependency is a behavioral pattern with its own rules about not feeling, talking, or trusting, often learned when growing up in a family where a relative is chemically dependent (Kramer Communications, 1990).

Personality Codependency can be defined as a recognizable pattern of fixed personality traits rooted in the internalized shame resulting from the abandonment that naturally happens to everyone in a dysfunctional family system (Bradshaw, 1988).

Neuroses "The spouse of the alcoholic often behaves in a way that has been described as codependent. A *codependent* spouse is one who, out of the neurotic need to preserve the marriage, is unwilling to seriously challange [*sic*] the drug-dependent partner's dysfunctional behavior. Thus, the codependent partner helps to perpetuate the presenting problem of dependence or addiction" (Fenell & Weinhold, 1989, p. 14).

Addiction "Codependence is, indeed, a disease that has many forms and expressions and that grows out of a disease process that is inherent in the system in which we live. This is the addictive process. The addictive process is an unhealthy and abnormal disease process, whose assumptions, beliefs, behaviors, and lack of spirituality lead to a process of nonliving that is progressively death-oriented. This basic disease, from which spring the subdiseases of codependence and alcoholism, is tacitly and openly supported by the society in which we live.

I also believe that trying to generate definitions from a rational, logical premise is actually a manifestation of the disease process. I want to avoid that sort of analysis" (Schaef, 1986).

What can we glean about codependence from these definitions? First, codependence is a disorder based on relationships (usually family). A solitary individual cannot be codependent, but adoption of a solitary lifestyle may be a symptom of codependence as the codependent withdraws from participation in the hurtful relationship. Second, codependence is a constellation of events, a pattern of responses and an ongoing process. It is not a singular event or something that you "get" and then recover from. Third, codependence is a function of society or some similar larger sense of organization. While it is manifest in the family, it is a part of the larger social fabric. Beyond these three commonalities, little agreement is found. Some argue that codependence is based in a relationship in which drug or alcohol dependence is found. Others, notably Bradshaw (1988), suggest that codependence is usually found in dysfunctional families, and still others argue that codependence is an addiction itself or a component of the addictive process that is affecting the dependent family member.

In 1986 Timmon Cermak sought to reduce the ambiguity in definitions of codependence by proposing diagnostic criteria for codependency, emulating the *Diagnostic and Statistical Manual of Mental Disorders* model. The following are his criteria for codependent personality disorder:

1. The continual investment of self-esteem in the ability to influence and control others on the face of obvious adverse consequences.

2. The assumption of responsibility for meeting others' needs to the exclusion of one's own needs.

3. Anxiety and boundary distortions in situations of intimacy and separation.

4. Enmeshment in relationships with personality-disordered, drug-dependent, and impulse-disordered individuals.

5. Three or more of the following features:
   —Excessive reliance on denial
   —Constriction of emotions
   —Depression
   —Anxiety
   —Hypervigilence
   —Compulsions
   —Substance abuse

—Recurrent physical or sexual abuse

—Primary relationship with an active substance abuser for at least two years without seeking help (Cermak, 1986)

Cermak's criteria offer a comprehensive, more specific analysis of the co-dependency construct than earlier (or subsequent) definitions. They specify specific behaviors associated with codependency and offer more objective standards of measurement for those behaviors. As with many other definitions, they limit codependent behavior to relationships with individuals who have dependence disorders and acknowledge that one outcome associated with codependency may be the development of a dependence disorder by the codependent individual.

However, several questions remain unanswered by Cermak's criteria. It is unclear if a causal relationship exists between codependency and the related behaviors. Indeed, does the codependency occur first, or do individuals who become codependent have preexisting personality or psychological difficulties exacerbated by involvement in a dependent relationship? It is equally unclear from these criteria if codependency represents a specific psychological disorder or if it is simply a collection of disjunctive symptoms and behaviors that appear in varying fashion from individual to individual. In a review of the psychological, rehabilitation, and self-help literature, Miller (1992) concluded that Cermak's criteria reflected current conceptual thinking about the symptoms and behaviors related to codependency but found little empirical validation of the existence of a specific, consistent codependency disorder across individuals. Giermyski and Williams (1986) have suggested that codependency may be an analog of dependency, with less stringent, ambiguous specifications and more diffuse boundaries of inclusion and exclusion. The greatest support for codependency as a unique, specific disorder appears in the anecdotally and conceptually based self-help literature, with limited empirical examination of codependency in the professional psychology, social work, or rehabilitation press. This may in part reflect the ambiguity and uncertainty of construct definitions or the difficulties encountered by professionals in treating this population, difficulties enhanced by lack of a clear definition and base from which to build a treatment plan.

Discussion Question: Define *codependency*. (Students should form small groups and attempt to come up with a comprehensive definition of codependency that will survive scientific scrutiny.)

THE WEGSCHEIDER-CRUSE MODEL OF FAMILY DYSFUNCTION

Perhaps the most famous and utilized model of family dysfunction in families where alcoholism is present is the model first espoused by Sharon Wegscheider-Cruse in 1981 and later expanded in 1985. Drawing upon the earlier work of Virginia Satir's scheme of faulty communication styles (Bandler, Grinder, &

Satir, 1976) Wegscheider-Cruse proposed that alcoholic families respond to alcoholism in the family in similar ways and that ultimately the family assumes a group of roles in an attempt to restore homeostasis to the family. The families go through progressive stages of denial, bargaining, disorganization and chaos, and reorganization with the problem present. If these efforts fail, the family may resort to escape or total reorganization without the dependent family member. The denial stage is typified by (1) the dependent family member's denial of drinking behaviors and problems ("I don't have a drinking problem"; "I can control my drinking") and (2) family members' denials of alcohol-related problems ("He's really a good provider and father, but he's having a tough time with his job right now"; "She doesn't drink anything but white wine, so how could she have a drinking problem?"; "The family physician prescribed that medication, so it must be okay"). It is in this stage that family members begin to practice Claudia Black's (1982) three-pronged code of alcoholic families: *Don't feel. Don't think. Don't talk.* This code serves as the basis of family internal interactions and for their relations with the external world. As the alcoholism progresses and as the family's coping mechanisms grow less effective, the power of the code deepens. Also, it is in this denial stage that the alcoholic family member may begin to blame the other family members for causing family problems, resulting in significant feelings of guilt and shame for all.

As the drinking continues, and the denial begins to fail as a defense mechanism, families frequently turn to bargaining to control the drinking behavior and growing family problems. The children may agree to act good in return for greater parental control or concealment of alcohol problems. Family entrance into therapy is a frequent occurrence during this stage, often under the guise of marital problems or problems with a child. Part of the bargain may be an implicit agreement that the alcohol problems will not be discussed in therapy. Consequently, the therapist begins treatment with the family at a disadvantage and is forced to be clairvoyant about the presence of an alcohol problem. This is especially unfortunate, as the data suggest that individuals with mild to moderate, early-stage alcoholism problems may be more amenable to treatment and recovery (Zweben & Barrett, 1993). The alcoholic family member usually has fewer medical and psychological problems related to alcohol consumption, and the family has experienced less stress and discord. Occasionally, the family may enter therapy because of an identified drug or alcohol problem of one of the adolescent children. Often these families are reluctant to enter treatment and resistant to total family participation, believing that they are being forced into treatment by the courts, the school system, or a state family and children's services agency (Trepper et al., 1993). More cogently, their reluctance and resistance may be based on an unwillingness to expose longstanding parental drinking or drug-taking problems. In either situation, the therapist must take care to create an environment that will allow the discussion of an unacknowledged parental alcoholism problem. Many long-term, severe problems could have been averted if therapists had been savvy enough to investigate the presence of alcoholism problems where none were thought to exist.

Discussion   What are some clues that might suggest the presence of a
Question: parental alcoholism problem?

   Disorganization and chaos form the next stage in the progress of alcoholism within the family, characterized by the emergence of legitimate external threats to the safety and homeostasis of the family. Financial, legal, medical,
and employment problems begin to occur, and the family becomes more engaged in maintaining the secrecy of the alcohol problem, isolating itself from
the outside world and its sources of input and help (Brown, 1985). School
problems often begin for the children as they expend huge amounts of psy-
chic and physical energy trying to cope with the anxiety-provoking dissonance they experience at home. Conversely, some children may begin to excel
in school as a way to cope with the disorder and chaos in their home lives.
Crisis avoidance and crisis resolution become the driving forces in the family's
existence as they completely reorganize around the existence of alcoholism in
the family. When the maintenance of homeostasis fails, the family begins to
take on a series of new roles in a frantic effort to bring the family back into
balance. In many ways these roles become a way of surviving an otherwise totally chaotic and destructive environment. At this point they adopt the roles
of *chief enabler, hero, scapegoat, mascot* (or *clown*), and *lost child* (Wegscheider-
Cruse, 1981).
   The *chief enabler* role is usually assumed by the nondrinking spouse whose
overriding concern becomes the smooth functioning of the family. This individual tries to assume complete control of the family and its dynamic, and
planning and rescuing become paramount activities. In fact, so much effort
may be expended in these activities that little if any concern is felt or expressed
about personal physical and mental health or about the issues of family members other than the drinking spouse. Children may miss significant developmental milestones because the nondrinking parent's behavior is oriented solely
toward controlling the impact of alcoholism on the family environment.
Thwarted efforts to control the uncontrollable saddle the enabling spouse with
continuous worry and anxiety, guilt, control needs, fear of the worst, and low
self-esteem. It is common for these individuals to experience significant stress-
related physical and emotional problems, including depression, somatic complaints, hypertension, and anxiety-related disorders. The data suggest that chief
enablers may be at risk for developing dependencies of their own, often to
medications prescribed to control psychiatric symptoms or sleep disorders.
Nevertheless, the role of chief enabler is not without its secondary gain benefits. The spousal role of chief enabler carries an illusion of nearly total control
and power, especially if the children in the family are still young. Nothing is
delegated, and all responsibility is assumed for everything. Consequently children may be denied the opportunity to participate in normal autonomy- or
identity-seeking developmental activities for fear of upsetting the delicate family balance. Of course, this results in further complications later in the lives of
these children as they cope with their developmental deficiencies. The role of
chief enabler may result in considerable community and family admiration for

the enabler's hard work, perseverance, and self-sacrifice in the face of over-whelming odds.

The *hero* child is often the oldest child. This individual assumes the duty of looking good and doing good to promote the myth of family health and sta-bility. This individual will often be a superachiever in school and community life and may share many characteristics of the chief enabler with whom cross-generational alliances may be established. However, at times an adversarial re-lationship may follow with the chief enabler when disagreement occurs about how to restore and maintain family balance. As adults, because of their de-velopment losses, these individuals may continue their superachieving ways rigidly and mirthlessly, all the while mourning their lost childhood.

It is the *scapegoat's* responsibility to deflect attention away from the alco-holism of the parent through negative acting out behaviors. Thus, the focus of outside examination of family problems centers on this child's defiance and irresponsibility (Fisher and Harrison, 1997) and not on the alcoholic parent or the enabling parent. Usually this role is filled by a middle male child who becomes at high risk for both adolescent and adult chemical dependency problems because of his behaviors, relationships, and associations. Frequently the problems of the scapegoat will be the impetus for family participation in therapy, with the scapegoat child serving as the identified patient. This is one situation where therapist exploration of the total family drinking and drug-consuming behavior is vital.

The *mascot* has the task of diverting family and external attention and family tensions away from alcoholism. Often mischievous or clownlike in action, this child may be diagnosed as hyperactive or immature and is at significant risk for the development of adult chemical dependency problems because of poorly de-veloped self-control mechanisms and lack of mature means of getting attention.

The *lost child* is often seen as shy, withdrawn, isolated, and requiring or seek-ing limited family attention (Fisher & Harrison, 1997). Often a later birth order child born when the progression of the parental alcoholism was well established, this child may be excluded from any understanding of functional family dynam-ics. The withdrawal and avoidance may be survival skills needed for an individual trapped in a chaotic environment where disorganization is the norm. Moreover, the family may see this child's needs as inconsequential because of all of the fam-ily havoc. Unfortunately the reclusive personality development that happens with these children results in low feelings of self-worth, lovableness, and an in-ability to deal with normal social situations and interactions.

Family members may persist throughout the life of the family in these symbiotic roles in a vain effort to restore some form of normalcy and home-ostasis. Other family members may make an effort to escape bedlam and dys-function. Attempts to escape the alcoholism are common for the entire family, often by moving to a new locale. Known as the "geographic cure," the family may believe that moving to a new state where the economy or culture is dif-ferent or the liquor laws are more severe will fix the family problems. On an individual level, children may seek to escape by running away, and spouses may pursue relief through separation and divorce (Dittrich, 1993; Steinglass, 1987).

Long episodes of separation and reconciliation may result as both spouses and family members struggle with issues of blame, shame, and guilt. When divorce does occur, it too may be accompanied by significant guilt, shame, and a pervading sense of failure. Often the divorced codependent spouse will enter another relationship with another dependent person. This may be an attempt to "get it right" the second time, or it may be due to the codependency needs of the divorced spouse. These marriages usually fail as well.

WHY FAMILIES ENTER COUNSELING

The choice for families to enter counseling is more complex than the decision for an individual to enter counseling. As Prochaska, DiClemente, and Norcross (1992) have suggested, entrance into the therapeutic process is typically catalyzed by the individual's desire to take action about a problem after going through contemplation and precontemplation stages. A family's decision to enter and participate in therapy may not be so straightforward. Some family members may be aware of the need to take action to deal with family problems; others may still be contemplating choices; and others may be in a precontemplative stage. Within alcoholic families it is common to see the nondrinking spouse ready to take action while the drinking spouse remains in denial, with no interest in changing. The children in the family may either take one parent's side or may be totally confused by the strife they see around them.

For many families, a sense of loss may be the precipitating event for entrance to therapy. The loss may be a real, physical, often personal loss, such as the death of a child, or the loss of health and well-being because of an alcohol-related accident. Job loss, financial loss, or loss of freedom related to arrest may be important precipitating events, too. The loss may be current or anticipated, or it may be the anniversary of a loss that stimulates therapy entrance. For other families an impending sense of loss may be the precipitating event. These families may be experiencing developmental dysynchrony, a feeling that the family is out of step with the normal and expected family developmental stages. Intense interpersonal conflict in the household causes some families to enter treatment. These are often families for whom coping strategies of any kind have failed. Finally, court or family services mandates may force some families into therapy. Mandated therapy poses tricky problems for both the family and the therapist. Very early in the first session the counselor should resolve the issue of how the family feels about being forced to participate in therapy. Some members may be bitter and resentful, others may be anxious about potential revelations, and still others may be either secretly or openly relieved about the possibility of change. The entire therapeutic process and any potential family change may hinge upon resolution of conflicting feelings about mandated treatment.

Discussion What are some strategies a counselor might use to explore and
Question: resolve differing feelings about mandated therapy?

Frequently symptoms evidenced by children are the presenting problem that initiate therapy. School problems, abuse problems, truancy problems, or drug and alcohol problems may result in the child being the identified symptom bearer and, consequently, the identified patient. Problems central to the adults in the family may also hasten therapy entrance. These include money problems, sexual problems, marital relationship problems, and occasionally, though less often than would be expected, spouse abuse problems. Generally the possibility of a dependence problem is mentioned only rarely, and the therapist must divine the impact of drugs and alcohol on the functioning of the family. Regrettably, many counselors fail this test of clairvoyance (or avoid exploring the issue altogether), and everyone is confused and bewildered later when the family therapeutic process flounders.

Some families do enter treatment because of a family alcohol or drug-dependence process, often as part of aftercare or as part of the ongoing treatment process. As in other situations some may enter therapy voluntarily, while others are coerced or mandated into treatment. The same caveats and concerns about differing individual perceptions apply to these families. They may enter therapy admitting the presence of a drug and alcohol dependence, but they may not be happy about it or universally willing to work on the problem. Importantly, the perceptions of family members of entrance to therapy will have substantial impact on their progress. Some families will enter therapy believing nothing is wrong with any of them as individuals but that the family system has broken down. Another stance may be to target one family member as the person with the problem, but, because of the family's insistence on keeping secrets from outsiders (in this case the counselor), the problem person may not be the alcohol- or drug-dependent person. The importance of keeping family secrets sometimes leads families to blame everyone in the family for causing problems, thereby diverting attention away from the drinking behavior and forcing the counselor to sift through the myriad family problems to get at the core dependency problem. Coerced or mandated families will often assert that nothing is wrong with the family; they are simply victims of a bureaucratic system forcing them to participate in counseling neither wanted nor needed. Finally, some families are absolutely clueless about being referred to or mandated to participate in counseling. As opposed to openly resistant clients, this group will claim, "We don't know why we are here."

ASSESSING DEPENDENCE
PROBLEMS IN FAMILIES

No matter what the family perceptions, the counselor is confronted with a daunting assessment and diagnostic task. Families come to counseling very interested in content issues: explaining why they are in counseling and looking for the counselor to repair the family damage. Rather than focusing on this often obfuscating content, the counselor must attend to the process dynamics of the family interactions. Who talks to whom? Who sits together? Who sits apart? Who talks and who remains silent? What is the message of body language? This battle of content versus process is one that will be waged throughout the family counseling process. Dealing with concrete content issues is easier than the painful issues of rebuilding and reshaping family interactions.

Assessing the dynamics of family interactions goes beyond observations of behaviors. Several assessment scales have been developed to analyze family interactions, including the Family Drinking Survey (Whitfield, 1987), the Family Environment Scale (Moos & Moos, 1986), and the Circumplex Model (Olson, 1986).

Whitfield's Family Drinking Survey is a 31-item inventory that assesses two factors. First, the survey examines the respondent's perception of drinking behaviors and related problems within the family and the perceptions of the impact of the drinking behavior (Has a family member ever failed to remember what occurred during a drinking period? Is your family having financial difficulties because of drinking?). Second, it examines the emotional and behavioral impact of the drinking behavior on the respondent, asking questions such as these:

> 2. Do you feel sorry for yourself and frequently indulge in self-pity because of what you feel alcohol is doing to your family?

★ ★ ★

> 12. Have you ever tried to control the drinker's behavior by hiding the car keys, pouring liquor down the drain, etc.?

The Family Drinking Survey is completed in paper and pencil format by answering *yes* or *no* to 31 items written at a middle school reading comprehension level. Whitfield asserts that *yes* responses to two questions indicate the "good probability" that a drinking problem exists in the family. Affirmative answers to four or more questions signify a "definite indication" that someone in the family has a drinking problem. Users of the Family Drinking Survey will note its similarity in format and content to Selzer's (1971) Michigan Alcohol Screening Test (MAST). This survey is especially useful in unmasking differing family perceptions of the impact of alcohol on the family. However, because secrecy may be a well-ingrained rule, some families may not answer the questions candidly or truthfully.

The Family Environment Scale is a 90-item true-false scale that "attempts to assess the impact of the family environment on individual and family functioning" (Goldenberg & Goldenberg, 1996, p. 345). Each member completes the scale according to how the family functions in real life and according to an ideal perception of the family. The responses from family members are averaged, and the combined grouping provides a schema for understanding how the family interacts. The measure contains 10 subscales: Cohesion, Expressiveness, Conflict, Independence, Achievement Orientation, Intellectual-Cultural Orientation, Active Recreational Orientation, Moral-Religious Emphasis, Organization, and Control. Subscale scores are depicted in a bar graph. The subscales Cohesion, Expressiveness, and Conflict illustrate the family's interpersonal interaction style. The next five subscales (Independence, Achievement Orientation, Intellectual–Cultural Orientation, Active Recreational Orientation, Moral–Religious Emphasis) characterize the family's growth and development along social/cultural/morality lines. The Organization and Control subscales offer a glimpse of the family's structure and its roles and rules. The comprehensive nature of the Family Environment scale, its ease of use, and its graphic illustration of family dynamics make it usable with families where dependence may be present.

The Circumplex Model, developed by Olson and his associates, examines family interactions as measured by its adaptability and cohesion. This model asserts that balance on the two constructs is ideal and that extremes on either or both constructs exemplify family dysfunction. As with the Family Environment Scale, family members complete the 20-item Family Adaptability and Cohesion Evaluation Scale (FACES III), indicating their present view of the family and then offering their "ideal" view of family functioning. In families with excessive cohesion, as might be seen in families where alcoholism is present, the lives of the families are intricately intertwined, with diffuse boundaries and confused division between separation and togetherness. This cohesion promotes the destructive keeping of secrets, exclusion of outside input and interaction, and maintenance of the destructive status quo (Herbert, 1989). Often these are families with low levels of adaptability unable to respond to the need for change, growth, and development.

Families in which dependence has resulted in a significant degree of disorganization are characterized by low levels of cohesion. It is likely that families in which a sudden onset of dependence has occurred may fit into this family type. Alcoholism tends to be a long-term family problem resulting in enmeshment to protect the family from the outside. Crack cocaine dependence, conversely, can have a sudden, rapid onset with disastrous consequences for family cohesion. Families with a history of cohesive interactions may find themselves torn asunder by the conflicting and unfamiliar feelings associated with suddenly being plunged into the morass of crack dependence. In this situation it is important for family boundaries to remain diffuse and clear to allow for continued communication and interaction by family members while simultaneously remaining firm but flexible to permit support for each other and the dependent family member (Goldenberg & Goldenberg, 1996).

Adaptability is another key issue. Olson (1986) asserts that families with high scores on the adaptability construct are characterized by too much change, a lack of rules, and unpredictability, a type seen in families where economic, unemployment, and legal pressures may have destroyed the family sense of organization. Families with low levels of adaptability (typified by rigid rules and roles) may have great difficulty responding to the demands of sudden onset dependence. Interestingly, families with low scores on this construct may be challenged by the need to respond and to adapt to the sobriety of the dependent family member. Having developed rigid rules and roles designed to protect themselves from the consequences of the dependent (and codependent) behavior, the family may struggle to cope with the changes caused by the recovery process. Family members who interacted with each other in very stylized, self-protective ways may now be forced to talk, to share, and to trust. For some families, these changes may be too difficult, and the recovery process may be sabotaged trying to restore the dependency-based homeostasis.

Information generated from the FACES III questionnaires are depicted graphically on the Circumplex Model grid that illustrates the family identity and temperament for the family and the counselor. Families may be classified according to one of 16 family systems. This information is useful in depicting both current family functioning and the direction for needed change. The Circumplex Model has been the subject of ongoing refinement and validity studies and has been examined for reliability with many different types of families.

Other less formalized methods of data collection may offer valuable information about family interactions. Often the initial contact for family therapy will have been made by a distressed family member, and the intake data should give at least one perception of the family struggles. Personal data from other family members must be collected for comparison and contrast. Herbert (1989) notes that two views exist about the collection of family data. Some theorists have suggested that family members should be seen individually, allowing them to express their own unique views about personal problems and the depth and influence of family problems. Others suggest that families be seen as a group beginning with the initial interview. Starting with the innocuous task of collecting basic demographic information, the counselor can move to more sensitive areas of concern that impact the entire family. An advantage of this latter approach is the counselor's ability to observe nonverbal behavior and interaction when sensitive topics are broached. These observations may be vitally crucial with families who have developed a strict and well-controlled sense of secrecy and isolation.

Family photograph albums and videotape collections may provide a rich source of information about family dynamics. Who appears with whom in photographs and, perhaps more important, who does not appear in these photos may provide significant clues about family interaction. Young children may be reluctant to discuss family problems in a family group interview format, or they may find the group too boring or beyond their developmental scope. In these situations counselors may take young children aside and ask them to draw a picture of their family. This strategy removes potential distractions and disruptions, and the resultant drawing may reveal significant information about their families through their art. Color, placement, and inclusion and exclusion are important variables to examine collaboratively with a trained art therapist. Lawson, Peterson, and Lawson (1983) describe several art therapy assessment strategies for use with families where alcoholism is present. They note that both conjoint and individual drawings can reveal much information about family perceptions and dynamics.

Asking families to diagram their family structure can provide clues about family membership, alliances, and participation. While diagraming can be an informal process, two formal diagraming models have been developed and are in wide use. Minuchin's (Minuchin & Fishman, 1981) Mapping strategy was developed for use by structural therapists to depict family interactional patterns, boundaries, and alliances. A straightforward group of symbols illustrates such structural concepts as coalitions, detours, alliances, involvement, and so forth. This diagraming model is of greatest use in helping counselors understand family boundary concerns.

A more extensively developed and widely used diagraming model is the Genogram model first conceptualized by Murray Bowen (Bowen, 1978). Genograms provide a diagrammatic representation of the patterns and influences of the family through several generations of the nuclear family, including the families of origin of the parents and children and the extended family. A partial set of genogram symbols is seen in Figure 7.1.

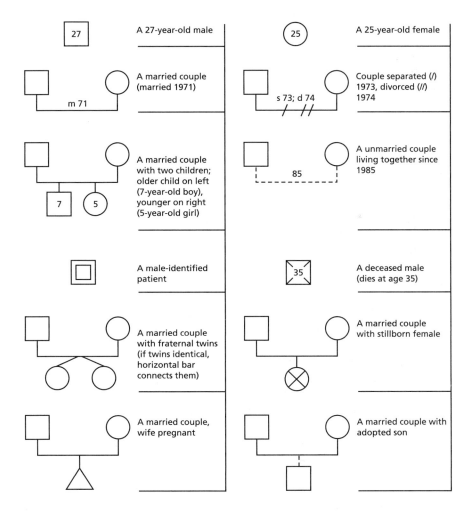

FIGURE 7.1 Commonly used genogram symbols.

SOURCE: Goldenberg & Goldenberg, 1996, p. 182

It is Bowen's contention that unresolved family emotional issues will be repeated from generation to generation and that distinct patterns of family interactions will continually recur. This feature of problem and pattern recurrence is especially critical for dependence-bearing families where multigenerational transmission of dependence is present but hidden. The genogram objectifies family information and makes it more accessible and available, consequently allowing both the counselor and the family to trace patterns and history and to examine multigenerational, genetic, and cultural influences on family development. Greater understandings of the cross-generational emotional underpinnings of the family become more apparent to all. As Goldenberg and Goldenberg (1996) point out, the genogram is not a static document, but it reflects ongoing family changes and development. As counseling progresses, it is common for family members to recall and/or be willing to reveal additional information, changing the structure and information of the genogram. The genogram can be a potent force in helping the counselor build rapport with the family. By working with family members in the construction of the genogram, the counselor can become actively involved in helping the family describe and understand its history. In doing so, the counselor moves from the role of outsider to a sharer of the family's background and development.

Discussion   Create a genogram for your family, including three generations.
Question: Be prepared to discuss your genogram in class.

Collection of assessment data from families incorporates both modernist and postmodernist trends. The objective information generated by instruments such as the Circumplex Model and the Family Environment Scale is in the best modernist tradition of the collection of data and reliance on objective, empirical information to make decisions. Families, however, are more than a linear series of data points. From a postmodern viewpoint, the information gleaned from interviews, recollections, family history and family perceptions, and even photographs provide fundamental knowledge not tapped by more objective, standardized measures. Essential family realities exist as family and social constructs based in history and set in social experiences. Indeed, counselor perceptions of the family may be more a reflection of the process of inquiry about the dynamics of the family rather than a reflection of extruded or deduced facts.

FAMILY COUNSELING PRACTICES

Entering a counseling relationship with a family is significantly more complex than entering an individual counseling relationship both for the counselor and the family members. In many ways initiating family counseling is similar to the beginning of group therapy, except that the group has been an intact group for a long time and has established a clear set of group norms, expectations, and behaviors. Just as in individual counseling, one of the first tasks a counselor faces is the establishment of a relationship and the building of rapport, a counseling strategy Minuchin (Minuchin & Fishman, 1981) calls "joining." Nevertheless, unlike individual counseling, the counselor must establish a relationship and build rapport with all of the family members, not just a single individual. Family counselors cannot be seen by the family as taking a side, and they must strive to identify and understand the unique roles, problems, and dilemmas encountered both by each family member individually and the family as a whole. Indeed, taking an individual family member's side is a two-edged sword. In some instances the nonfavored family members may display resistant behaviors, refusing to participate in the counseling process. It is equally plausible that the family might join with the counselor in the favoritism in an effort to scapegoat another family member or to divert attention away from secret problems. Third, the nonfavored participants may form a coalition to dissuade the counselor from the perceived inappropriate stance, again altering the focus of counseling toward process issues and away from the goals of counseling.

Connecting with the family is both an attitude and a skill. It implies that all family members and their points of view are equally accepted and respected for now they see life and perform the tasks of living, problem solving, and interacting. Haley (1976, cited in Lawson, Peterson, & Lawson, 1983) calls this the "social stage" of family counseling and a time for all to become comfortable with and sensitized to the new counseling environment. It is a time for validation of the importance of all family members and a time to acknowledge the experience and action of the family. Identification of family strengths and affirmation of the family can be a very consequential process. "Focusing on the family's strengths and resources contributes to the development of self-confidence, inspires hope, and enhances growth within the family" (Hanna & Brown, 1995).

The next phase of counseling deals with the identification of the problem that brought the family to counseling. At first glance the problem may seem obvious—alcohol or drug dependence—but it is important to remember that each family member will have a unique perception of the problem and its implications. The reality for many families embroiled in dependence problems is that they have expended all of their energy talking about and attacking what they perceive as "the problem" without truly addressing the issues that are destroying the family. One way the counselor can aid the family is through a period of education. Most families come to counseling with limited knowledge of dependence and its impacts. Often their knowledge has been gained through observations of those around them, from the popular media or from folktales and folklore. The dispelling of myth and presentations of facts and data about dependence can help clarify the family's perception of their issues. It may help them understand that they are not alone or unique in their problems and that there is hope for family recovery. The outcome of this problem and education phase of family counseling, suggests Steinglass and his colleagues (1987), is to relabel dependence as a family, not an individual, problem.

Discussion Question: What are some of the myths and folklore that families bring to the counseling relationship?

By the time they get to counseling, families have generally been through repeated barriers of frustration. Many families will be confused and demoralized because they have been trying so hard for so long without making any progress. All of their efforts lead not to change but to more frustration. They do not understand that undirected, nonfocused effort is a futile exercise; change requires more than effort and intention, and this is where the counselor comes in. The task of counseling at this point is to engage the family in the hope of change through goal-directed, action-oriented effort. It includes strengthening the family by helping them refocus on the existence of the family apart from the dependence. Families need to learn how their past behaviors and efforts supported the dependence/codependence process, but, more cogently, they must learn detachment from and avoidance of negative experiences. They must also learn effective self-protection and self-limiting strategies. What is and is not controlled and controllable by the family are important concerns. Frequently families in dependence relationships try to control factors, behaviors, and actions that are beyond their sphere of influence, and they neglect to control what *can* be controlled. Consequently, they begin to see themselves as buffeted by the fate, out of family internal control, and victimized by forces outside their control. Helping the family gain a sense of an internal locus of control is essential to the counseling process. Lazarus (1981) points out that counseling participants who have a sense of victimization and lack of control are much more difficult to treat and are less likely to be successful. Beck and his colleagues (1993) argue that individuals who are dependent must develop a set of control beliefs ("I can enjoy life without using drugs") to replace their addictive or dependence beliefs ("I can enjoy life *only* when I use drugs"). The same is true for families.

Discussion Question: What are some family dependence beliefs and control beliefs?

Part of the dilemma of providing counseling to families recovering from dependence/codependence is helping them avoid the pitfalls inherent in the recovery process. Helping family members let go of the trauma and pain of the past is central to change. When the dependent person enters and completes treatment successfully, the family dynamics will undergo significant change. A formerly nonparticipating, pain-causing family member returns to the family fold a new, in-recovery person. The entire family is thrust into a period of role readjustment, emotional uncertainty, and new, often unfamiliar communication and behavior patterns (O'Farrell, 1995). While family members may be pleased at the changes in the dependent person, they may need help in resolving and forgiving the pain of the past and in responding to the changes swirling about them. Failure to reach resolution may result in the recovery process being inadvertently sabotaged. Alternatively, family members may bury their feelings of resentment and pain, only to have those feelings resur-face later in life. Many problems encountered by Adult Children of Alcoholics stem from their inability to deal with and resolve the pain of growing up in a dependence-based relationship even after the dependent family member is in recovery.

Going too fast, too soon by setting recovery expectations too high is an-other common pitfall. Many families will equate abstinence with recovery. When relationship and behavior changes develop slowly and a return to fam-ily homeostasis is slow in coming, they may become frustrated or bewildered. As Steinglass (1987) notes, the transition from being what he calls a wet alco-holic family to a dry family results in a period of instability and uncertainty. Counselors must take into account the impact of recovery on the family sys-tem so that the newly sought homeostasis will be positive and beneficial (Fisher & Harrison, 1997).

Discussion   What are some signs that a family might be trying to proceed
Question: too fast?

UNIQUE ETHICAL AND PROFESSIONAL
CONCERNS ABOUT WORKING
WITH FAMILIES

Counseling families who are enmeshed in dependence/codependence rela-tionships requires a paradigmatic shift in thinking for the counselor. The con-cern shifts from what is best for the client to what is best for the client, the family, and the individual family members. Unfortunately the best individual solutions for the identified client, the family, and the individual family mem-bers are not always mutually compatible. The counselor faces difficult choices with a complex set of intricate decisions and no easy answers. Goldenberg and Goldenberg (1996) ask the question of to whom does the counselor owe loy-alty and responsibility, noting this is more than "academic hairsplitting" (p. 397). Grosser and Paul (1971) differentiate between situations in which family therapy is required to help an identified client in overcoming a specific problem versus a family or relationship problem without a clear distinction about who is the identified patient. In this latter situation, most akin to coun-seling dependent families, they note that the counselor must consider all fam-ily members equally in need of counseling as "each one has contributed to the creation and persistence of the family problem" (p. 125).

Apart from this basic question of loyalty and responsibility, family coun-selors are confronted with a series of other conflicts. Morrison, Layton, and Newman (1982; cited in Goldenberg and Goldenberg, 1996) identified three additional conflicts: (1) how to handle family secrets, (2) the use of di-agnostic labels, and (3) the ability of the counselor to increase or decrease family conflict.

Handling family secrets can be potentially explosive and destructive to the family. Infidelities, spouse abuse, sexual problems, financial difficulties, and illegal drug use or illegal activities may be divulged during counseling. The counselor must take care to ensure the safety and well-being of all family members, while respecting individual rights to confidentiality and privacy. Some secrets cannot be ignored or dismissed by the counselor. Most states require that any disclosure of child abuse be reported to the appropriate state authorities. Given the very high rate of incest in dependent families (Glover, Janikowski, & Benshoff, 1995) and the high rates of violence associated with dependence, the disclosure of child abuse is very common. As part of the intake/assessment process, counselors are duty bound to inform families of the legal responsibility to disclose information about child abuse.

In today's managed care, insurance-driven health care systems, diagnostic labels may be the key to the counseling room. Is it reasonable or ethical to assign a diagnostic label to family members so they that can be seen in counseling and so that the costs of counseling will be reimbursed to the agency? There is an argument that family members need counseling and that they may have certain pathological characteristics as a result of the family dysfunction. However, is that pathology a result of the family dysfunction, or is the pathology reflective of inherent psychological characteristics of the individuals? The practice of assigning a supposedly "benign" label such as *adjustment disorder* (American Psychiatric Association, 1994) is fraught with a variety of problems. Clearly, it is unethical to diagnose a disorder that does not exist or for which there is only minimal evidence, and it is likely to be considered fraudulent professional behavior by professional accreditation bodies and state regulatory agencies. Improper diagnostic labeling can have lifelong consequences for family members. Officially recorded diagnoses follow people through life and may affect future job seeking, school acceptance, or, in the case of continued family problems, lead to divorce, litigation, or child-custody battles. One solution to this dilemma has been to "blend in" the costs of family counseling with the cost of individual care for the identified dependent patient.

The counselor in a family counseling relationship has substantial power, advertently or inadvertently, to alter family stability. The here and now, active, solution-oriented focus of family counseling may bring explosive issues to the surface. Even information-gathering techniques such as mapping or genograms may uncover dangerous family secrets; other more active techniques such as family sculpting or paradoxical interventions can be especially threatening if ill-conceived or inappropriately timed.

At one time or another during the counseling process, nearly every family member will attempt to get the counselor to take sides. Haley (1963) and Zuk (1971) assert that neutrality and impartiality is impossible and unavoidable in the family therapy process. No matter how impartially the counselor attempts to act in the counseling relationship, some member or some coalition of the family may view the therapist as acting favorably or unfavorably. Even the most innocuous statement may be seized upon by a family member as validation or invalidation of that family member's position. Zuk points out that the issue is not that of impartiality. Rather, he notes, "By judicious siding, the therapist can tip the balance in favor of more productive relating, or at least disrupt a pattern of pathogenic relating" (p. 219). Counselors must avoid consistently aligning with one part of the family; the inevitable result will be to force the other individuals to band together to defend their position or to flee the counseling process, either literally or symbolically. Similarly, adopting a continually neutral stance may force the family into guessing what the counselor thinks "is right." Many counselors deal with issues of partiality by refusing to see individual members except during the family session, thus avoiding the impression of sharing secrets or otherwise aligning with select family members.

Special issues may arise with drug- and alcohol-dependent families in counseling concerning informed consent and confidentiality. Informed consent implies that all participants in the therapeutic process have been fully informed of the reasons for participating in counseling, the course of the counseling relationship, and the ultimate goals or objectives of counseling. However, many families enter counseling for dependency problems under some form of duress or coercion. Sometimes the dependent family member may be pressured to enter counseling by threats or intimidation from other family members or from some external force such as an employer, a family welfare agency, or the courts. Similarly, the entire family may be required to enter treatment by the edict of an agency or the criminal justice system. Some treatment agencies may require the families of individual counseling clients to participate in family counseling as a condition of admission of the dependent individuals. Can involuntary, coerced entrance into the counseling relationship truly be informed? Can family counseling be successful if any or all of the participants feel they were coerced into the counseling relationship?

Discussion   Discuss some strategies to deal with the issue of involuntary,
Question: coerced participation in family counseling.

Broadly speaking, privileged communication and rights to confidentiality protect a client from disclosure of confidences discussed in counseling in a court of law or with other outside agencies (Fenell & Weinhold, 1989). This raises several issues of concern. First it must be established who exactly is the client. Is the client the individual with the identified dependency problem or the individual who first sought counseling, perhaps the spouse of the dependent individual? Is the entire family the client? As noted above, rights to confidentiality and privileged communication may not apply in all situations. Counselors are required by every state to disclose instances of child abuse to the appropriate state agency. In many states they may be required to report threats of harm to self or others. Judicial mandates may force the counselor to report acts of criminal behavior, particularly if the family is required to enter family counseling by the courts. Holding the title of counselor may not protect the counselor or the family from unwanted disclosure, especially if the counselor does not possess either academic or professional credentials. Despite the continuing proliferation of national, state, and professional credentialing organizations, uncertainty remains about who is entitled to the privilege. Traditionally the courts have acknowledged the sanctity of the counselor-client relationship. However, counselors need to become aware of their own state laws concerning the disclosure of confidential information.

Finally, just as in any counseling situation, counselors engaged in family counseling must continually examine their own values, beliefs, and attitudes. However, family counseling presents several unique issues. Margolin (1982) suggests three specific values that may cause difficulties for family counselors: divorce, extramarital affairs, and family gender roles, especially as they apply to women. Other value-laden matters with families in which dependence is a problem may include the types of drugs abused within the family, child abuse, spouse abuse, AIDS, and illegal activities. The counselor must continuously be aware of the impact of values and attitudes on the counseling relationship. Being able to adopt a flexible, hope-instilling, and supportive stance with families is imperative for the counselor, despite the issues the family brings to counseling (Hanna & Brown, 1995). If the counselor cannot adopt this type of stance, the family should be referred to another counselor or facility.

Discussion Question: What are some values and attitudes possessed by students that might hinder or support the family counseling relationship?

SUMMARY

Family issues have been a concern in drug and alcohol dependency treatment since the earliest days. While most early models focused on treatment issues seen in traditional families (i.e., nuclear families or families of origin), the ever-growing array of new family types and models requires a careful examination of what *family* means to the client.

Most family treatment models rely on a systems approach, viewing the family as an interactive system with functioning subsystems. Boundaries are the invisible demarcations between family systems and the other system and the world. Open systems have easily crossed boundaries and high levels of information exchange; closed systems have rigid boundaries and little information exchange and often become dysfunctional through entropy. All families seek to maintain homeostasis when confronted by the multiple forces of the family, society, and the environment. Most systems in the physical world operate in a linear fashion; the impact of and response to multiple forces sets up complex circular causality forces for the family. Families operate according to a well-defined set of rules and roles with enduring patterns of communication and behavior. Each individual family establishes its unique family paradigm, family temperament, and family identity.

Family development is effected by continuous and discontinuous changes. The ideal family provides a well-defined series of roles in its functioning. Safety and security, nurturing, provision of a core focus, the elucidation and promotion of standards and values, a sense of organization, social system development, and cultural transmission are essential tasks of successful families. The introduction of alcohol or drugs into the family system disrupts the developmental processes of the family.

Many family problems are conceptualized in terms of the codependency that emerges in the family. Although codependency has developed a significant following, empirically based examinations of the phenomenon are inconsistent. Codependency is fraught with definitional problems, lacking a taxonomy of the disorder, a classification system for clients and diagnostic standards, formal professional training, and a clear, consistent body of research.

Numerous models of codependency appear in the literature. The Disease Model, arguably the most popular, suggests that families go through the same addictive disease process as the alcoholic or drug addict. Other models draw upon behavioral, personality, neurosis, or addiction constructs as their basis. Cermak's model of codependency sets forth a scheme based on DSM II-R codification. Wegscheider-Cruse postulates the existence of a family typology in codependence, including the chief enabler, the hero, the mascot, the scapegoat, and the lost child. Her model has enjoyed great popularity.

Families enter counseling for diverse reasons. Some experience a sense of loss, and others enter because they have a sense that something is not right in the family development, a condition referred to as developmental dysynchrony. Interpersonal conflict is a common precipitator for treatment entrance, and many families are mandated to enter treatment by the courts or child welfare agencies. No matter the catalyst for treatment participation, most families are initially loathe to discuss drug and alcohol dependence and may seek to conceal it from the counselor.

Assessing family issues requires attention to both the content and process of the family's participation in treatment. Rather than the usual intake and assessment processes, it is preferable to use a combination of standardized assessment devices, formal and informal data collection strategies, and tools and observational methods. Mapping and genograms are two family therapy strategies often used to assess the family.

Successful family counseling depends on the ability of the counselor to join the family. Problem identification is important because often the true problems confronting the family differ from the presenting problem. For families involved in dependence problems, education is often the first and most necessary step. After learning about and developing insight about their dependence problems, families need to learn empowerment skills to regain control of the family and their individual lives.

Family counselors face significant ethical and professional concerns, including dealing with issues of loyalty and responsibility and responding to family secrets. Diagnostic labeling of family members can also become an issue of concern. Working with families may impose different standards of confidentiality and informed consent, and family counselors must attend carefully to the impact of their own values, beliefs, and attitudes.

8

Treatment

CHAPTER 8 OUTLINE

A holistic model of rehabilitation and recovery begins with the premise that all life events are interconnected and interwoven and that prolonged imbalances in any single area of life will cause a total life imbalance. Psychoactive substance dependence and its countless influences on psychological, physiological, interpersonal, vocational, and social elements of life result in a dramatic life imbalance. Recovery, then, must focus on a recentering of the individual's life and lifestyle. It is neither a short nor easy process, and it rests on a continuum of care with multiple facets. Recovery resources, including treatment programs and peer self-help programs, are examined in this chapter.

TREATMENT PROGRAMS

Before the 1970s very few alcoholism treatment facilities and almost no treatment services for drug addiction existed in the United States. Most treatment programs for individuals with alcoholism problems were based in hospitals and offered detoxification services, followed by outpatient therapy and referral to Alcoholics Anonymous. Some specialized treatment services existed that utilized AA concepts for long-term treatment, typically offering services on a free or low-cost basis. Often residents of these programs were supported through family contributions, private charitable contributions, or through work performed at the facility. Public financing or insurance financing of treatment was virtually nonexistent. A nexus of events in the late sixties and early seventies resulted in the establishment of the dependency treatment model in use today. The crucial milestones included the following:

1. The rising social consciousness of the 1960s and increased public awareness and concern about drug and alcohol problems

2. The passage of the Hughes Act and the accompanying establishment of the National Institute of Alcoholism and Alcohol Abuse and the National Institute of Drug Abuse

3. The expansion of the National Council on Alcoholism, particularly in the industrial sector

4. Growing industrial and business concern about the impact of alcohol and drugs on the workforce

5. The development of private nonprofit and proprietary alcoholism treatment centers

6. Dole and Nyswander's 1965 discovery of the utility of methadone for treating heroin addiction

7. Passage by Congress of the Federal Narcotic Rehabilitation Act, designating opiate addiction as a disease rather than a crime (Dickman, 1985; Winger, Hofmann, & Woods, 1992)

From this convergence of laws, events, social movements, and public awareness blossomed the dependency treatment movement. States established agencies to fund and support drug and alcohol treatment services, although often with separate bureaucracies and mandates. Nonprofit agencies were created, often as part of the community mental health center system or as a department within a general care or psychiatric hospital, and toward the end of the 1970s private for-profit facilities began to grow as an important part of the treatment scene.

From the earliest days treatment centered around the "disease" concept of alcoholism that undergirded the Minnesota Model of Chemical Dependency Treatment, the dominant model of dependency treatment in the United States for the past 25 to 30 years (Doweiko, 1996; Fisher & Harrison, 1997; Jung, 1994; Miller & Hester, 1995). The disease concept asserts that alcoholism is a treatable disease with specific etiology, symptoms, progression, and outcome. Recovery from alcoholism is possible only through abstinence. Originally conceptualized as an innovative new strategy for treating alcoholism dependence in the 1950s (Doweiko, 1996), the Minnesota Model embraced and expanded upon the disease concept, and Minnesota Model programs have become the essence of treatment. The model is characterized by abstinence; a strong emphasis on AA programming; a combination of didactic, education, and psychotherapeutic approaches; and the widespread use of confrontation as a counseling strategy (Miller et al., 1995). It emphasized a continuum of care including detoxification, inpatient and outpatient services, and aftercare services, including AA participation. For the first time it brought together treatment professionals from a variety of disciplines including medicine, psychology, counseling, social work, and recreation, and it stressed the need for standardization of treatment (Doweiko, 1996). While the Minnesota Model was developed for alcoholism treatment, it became the paradigm for treating all forms of dependency, despite the reality that little research existed concerning its efficacy with dependencies other than alcohol. During the early treatment development years (1970s) the principal drugs of abuse and dependency were alcohol and heroin, both sedating chemicals. Marijuana and hallucinogenic drugs were the drugs of choice for adolescents. Inhalant use, mostly as glue sniffing, emerged as a problem in the 1970s, although treatment protocols were nonexistent (Goldberg, 1997). Cocaine was little known outside a limited circle of users and was not thought to be addicting. Of course, crack cocaine and many synthetic designer drugs of the 1980s and 1990s were completely unknown. Nevertheless, the Minnesota Model has maintained its preeminence in all forms of dependency treatment in the United States.

TREATMENT RESOURCES

Detoxification

The first contact with treatment for many individuals with dependency disorders is through detoxification. Detoxification is a brief period of palliative care designed to provide support for clients who have just discontinued the use of dependency-causing chemicals. It is available in three forms: medical detoxification, social model detoxification, and self-detoxification.

Medical detoxification is warranted when medical indicators suggest the client may be in potential life jeopardy and is usually mandatory for individuals with a long history of alcohol dependence. Indicators for medical detoxification include increased or unstable vital signs (blood pressure, pulse and respiratory rates, temperature), history of long-term drinking or drug ingestion involving large quantities of alcohol or drugs, the presence of severe physical or neurological discomfort including delirium tremens and hallucinations, and a history of prior medical problems. Individuals with chronic alcohol dependency history often have compromised cardiovascular, respiratory, and gastrointestinal systems related directly to their alcohol consumption and to its accompanying lifestyle. Always done in a hospital setting, medical detoxification includes 24-hour nursing care and physician supervision. Frequently minor tranquilizers from the benzodiazepine group (e.g., Xanax, Librium, Valium) are administered in decreasing dosages to reduce the danger of seizures and the discomfort of withdrawal (Fisher & Harrison, 1997), although some strict Minnesota Model facilities may eschew the use of psychotropic medications completely. Vitamin therapy is usually initiated to treat nutritional problems; vitamin B-1, thiamine, is recommended for treatment of cognitive and neurological disorders and to prevent long-term neurological sequellae (Rone et al., 1995).

Medical detoxification is absolutely indicated for individuals with a dependency on benzodiazepine medications (Ativan, Librium, Xanax, Valium, etc.). Although these drugs are often viewed benignly, unsupervised withdrawal from them can result in severe, acute neurological reactions, including fatal seizures (Fishbein & Pease, 1996; Goldberg, 1997).

Social detoxification is appropriate for individuals whose withdrawal problems are less severe and who can be managed in a nonmedical setting. Usually social detox is accomplished in a nonmedical setting residential facility, and it may be done on an outpatient basis. Despite the lurid depictions in the popular media, individuals who are addicted to heroin are good candidates for social detoxification. Psychotropic medications are rarely used in this model. Palliative care is provided through over-the-counter medications, vitamins, monitoring of progress, rest, and nutrition. In both social and medical detox, clients are introduced to treatment through participation in counseling and didactic groups, and individual counseling.

As the phrase implies, *self-detoxification* is unmanaged, unsupervised detoxification, often called "going cold turkey." Most individuals with dependency problems have tried one or more episodes of self-detoxification with generally negative results. The lack of supportive care, appropriate medication, and a structured regimen mitigate against successful self-detoxification in most cases.

Detoxification is just the first phase of comprehensive dependency treatment, and Doweiko (1996) questions if it should be considered treatment at all. As a stand-alone experience, detoxification is probably not treatment but simply a "drying out," rejuvenating experience or an opportunity to avoid consequences from spouses, employers, or the police for negative activities. Also, after detoxification, individuals with dependency problems may quickly revert to former destructive behaviors without follow-up treatment. To be effective, detoxification must be linked closely to a continuum of care, and its role as a gateway to treatment is its biggest advantage. Other important considerations in medical and social detoxification include prevention of an instantaneous relapse as seen in self-detoxification and the availability of resources to deal with medical and psychological emergencies. Social detoxification facilities are less costly to operate than medical detoxification facilities. Lengths of stay in both types of formal detoxification range from three to five days, although withdrawal from benzodiazepines and barbiturates may take considerably longer because of their neurotoxic effects.

Residential Treatment

Residential treatment for psychoactive dependency treatment takes a variety of forms: medical and social setting residential facilities, halfway houses, and therapeutic communities. The best-known inpatient settings are variously called Minnesota Model Facilities, 28-day programs, inpatient rehabilitation facilities, or inpatient programs. The term *inpatient program* will be used to distinguish these programs from other types of residential programs. The Betty Ford Center and Hazelden are two of the most visible inpatient programs, although hundreds of programs operate across the country. As the name implies, inpatient programs offer services on a residential basis. Services may be offered in a medical setting or in a social setting. Medical setting inpatient programs may be housed in a hospital or on the campus of a medical center and are characterized by round-the-clock nursing care and extensive physician supervision of treatment. Many hospitals converted empty medical-surgical beds to dependency treatment beds as a way to recoup lost revenues in the last decade, with varying results.

Discussion   What are the concerns in converting a medical-surgical bed to
Question: a dependency treatment bed in a community hospital?

Social setting inpatient programs, also referred to as freestanding programs, offer inpatient programming in a community-based setting with lower levels of direct medical care available to residents. Consequently these programs are much less expensive to operate than medical setting programs. Both social setting and medical setting facilities are operated by profit-making (called proprietary) companies and not-for-profit facilities. During the 1980s and continuing into the 1990s the trend has been toward corporate ownership of multiple facilities as a way to reduce costs and maximize services. Multifacility groups are usually owned and managed by health care, psychiatric care, or dependency treatment companies, although some chains have been the property of such diverse organizations as the Avon Corporation. Inpatient programs are funded by insurance coverage, state grants, medicaid, and private payment. Costs for a single inpatient stay can range up to $500 a day in medical setting facilities.

Historically inpatient programs have been known as 28-day programs for their customary length of stay, although many programs have decreased their treatment length in response to eternal economic pressures from funding organizations. Indeed, no research evidence suggests that 28 days was the appropriate or clinically needed length for the treatment of alcoholism. A perhaps apocryphal tale illustrates how inpatient programs came to be 28 days in length. According to this story, in the 1970s inpatient alcoholism program administrators and insurance company executives met to discuss insurance coverage for alcoholism care. Insurance carriers were willing to offer these benefits but wished to establish a standard length of stay for treatment, in conformity with other policies related to benefit coverage. The alcoholism program directors represented programs that ranged in duration from three to five weeks on average, and 28 days—four calendar weeks—was a satisfactory compromise for all. Unfortunately, no actuarial data was available from the insurance carriers, nor was outcome data available from the treatment providers showing that a 28-day length of stay was congruent with client needs.

Typically inpatient programs base their treatment on the disease concept, with abstinence from psychoactive chemicals as the explicit desired outcome for program graduates. Group therapy tends to be the emphasized treatment modality, although nearly all programs also provide individual counseling. Groups focus on psychological issues, and the strong educational component of many groups centers on teaching clients about the negative effects of drug- and alcohol-consuming behaviors. Inpatient programs view themselves as the starting point for the recovery process that is to be continued through aftercare counseling and continued participation in peer self-help fellowships. In fact, clients receive continued exposure to peer self-help ideas through group activities, bibliotherapy assignments, personal interaction, and participation in on-site and community-based fellowship meetings. In some areas of the country local AA councils designate AA treatment agency liaison volunteers whose task is to contact individuals in treatment and arrange a transition to participation in meetings in the client's home area after discharge. However, in its Sixth Tradition Alcoholics Anonymous forbids use of its name or logo by any outside organization:

> 6. An AA group ought never endorse, finance, or lend the AA name to any related facility or outside enterprise, lest problems of money, property, and prestige divert us from our primary purpose. (Alcoholics Anonymous World Services, Inc., 1976, p. 564)

While some inpatient programs may describe themselves as AA Model Programs, this is a self-claimed appellation and does not imply or reflect the endorsement of Alcoholics Anonymous.

Inpatient programs focus on the development and attainment of short-term goals while in treatment and the development of longer-term goals for completion after discharge. Since clients are in residence for an extended period, they are removed from the pressures and stresses of the drinking or drugging environment and have the opportunity to learn and experiment with new skills and behaviors in a safe, supportive milieu. Inpatient programs have multidisciplinary staffing patterns and bring multiple resources to bear on client problems. Additionally the intense staffing pattern means help and support are available on a 24-hour basis that may be especially important in the early days of sobriety, according to Doweiko (1996). Client anxieties, fears, and cravings may be at their worst in the very early hours of the morning, and the presence of staff support is instrumental in preventing drug and alcohol use. A strong sense of peer support and the peer teaching-learning emphasis of group counseling are hallmarks of inpatient programs.

Most inpatient programs operate a rigorous schedule of therapeutic activities, beginning in the early morning and ending late at night. Clients may start the day with a community group meeting to discuss the events of the day, followed by two or three counseling, didactic, or self-improvement groups in the morning. More groups and individual sessions are scheduled after lunch with structured recreation activities preceding dinner. Evenings are devoted to peer self-help group meetings. This intensive treatment regimen has been both praised and criticized. Inpatient programming is much more intensive and comprehensive than other forms of treatment. However, individualization of care may be sacrificed as clients are forced into a standardized, schedule-driven model. Moreover, the rigor of the schedule and the emphasis on didactic information may be overwhelming for some individuals whose impaired cognitive abilities have not fully recovered. Finally, the data suggest that inpatient programs are no more successful than outpatient programming or intensive outpatient programming (Fishbein & Pease, 1996). Despite this reality, a consensus in the literature asserts that inpatient programs are the treatment of choice for individuals who have failed multiple outpatient attempts at treatment, individuals with severe medical problems requiring medical management, and individuals with limited support systems and poor motivation toward recovery (Doweiko, 1996; Fisher & Harrison, 1997).

In 1972 Wolf Wolfensberger wrote the book *Normalization,* which asserted that individuals needing treatment services should receive those services in as close to a normal fashion as possible. From this work came the concept of the least restrictive environment, which suggests that clients should receive services in treatment environments that offer the least amount of restriction and the greatest possibility for success (Fisher & Harrison, 1997). Lamentably, inpatient programs are neither least restrictive nor do they offer the greatest possibility for success. They are more life intrusive and stigmatizing than other programs, and the artificiality of the environment may mean client learning and discovery may not transfer to the real world. Finally, great variety in the quality of care exists from program to program. Even the nature of the client population in a facility has an impact on the quality of care: Often there are few women, few older individuals, and few members of minority ethnic groups. The limitations may mean that some clients from minority groups may be isolated by not "fitting in" with the rest of the treatment population.

A *therapeutic community (TC)* is a long-term, residential, drug-free treatment program originally designed to treat drug addiction, which emphasizes peer self-help and confrontation of addiction and addictive behaviors

(Abadinsky, 1997). The therapeutic community movement began in the 1950s with the establishment of Synanon, a therapeutic community founded by Charles Dederich to treat individuals addicted to heroin (Bratter et al., 1985). The therapeutic community rubric encompasses a variety of program types, which have in common their long length of stay, high degree of program structure, focus on mutual self-help, employment of former addicts and program graduates as program staffers, and an emphasis on total behavioral change for clients (Fishbein & Pease, 1996, Goldberg, 1997). Typically prospective clients just do not walk in the front door and join a TC. Instead, they must go through a rigorous screening process conducted by individuals who were formerly addicted to drugs and staff members. By design, this screening process is aimed at separating individuals who truly want help and are willing to work diligently from those who are seeking a quick, easy, painless cure. Abadinsky describes the interview process as it was conducted during the formative years of Dayton Village, a prominent New York therapeutic community:

> The interview itself is demanding and traumatic: the prospect is ridiculed and required to accept his or her situation for what it is—'Don't try to con us, we're dope fiends, too'—and to admit that drug use is a symptom of being either stupid or a 'baby.' The prospect may be required to scream at the top of his or her lungs, 'Help me' or 'I need help.' (pp. 191–192).

He notes that intake admission procedures have become less confrontational and more professional in recent years, but the emphasis remains on selective admission of individuals committed to change.

Once enrolled in the program, clients find themselves in a highly structured, isolated environment with strict rules and regulations and equally strict consequences for deviations from accepted behaviors. Therapeutic communities are self-regulating, and senior residents are responsible for shaping and guiding the behavior of newer residents. Any resident can (and is expected to) correct the behavior of fellow residents (called "dropping a ticket") at any time. New residents are assigned to the most onerous, demeaning tasks (e.g., cleaning toilets), but they have the opportunity to perform more prestigious tasks as they display increased responsibility and progress (Abadinsky, 1997). Not surprisingly, a very high dropout rate occurs, especially during the early weeks and months of treatment (Doweiko, 1996; Goldberg, 1997) with as few as 25 percent of admitted residents completing treatment. Group participation is the fundamental treatment modality, using confrontational and encounter group strategies. As Lewis, Dana, and Blevins (1994) have noted, confrontation in group leads to compliance but not necessarily internalization of behavior change. The TC model seeks to first confront and then to force compliance through monitoring and regulation of behavior, in order to compel internalization of behavior change. One criticism of therapeutic communities has been that the behavior change that occurs within the TC does not transfer to the real world in part because TC residents have few opportunities to interact with the outside society. As long as the client is living in the confrontational, yet supportive, environment of the TC, the client can live and act in a productive drug-free manner. However, many TC residents relapse quickly when deprived of the TC's support. Synanon founder Dederich has asserted that therapeutic community membership is a lifelong obligation. It is ironic that the questionable confrontational and isolationist strategies used in long-term therapeutic communities undergird much of the philosophy driving the establishment of boot camps for youthful offenders.

Many early TCs were funded through federal or state grants or through fees for service. Today most TCs rely on the welfare-based income of their residents for economic survival, or they may operate small businesses staffed by program residents.

Empirical data about the success of therapeutic communities is equivocal and ambiguous at best. Dropout and relapse rates are high, and the isolation of TCs from both societal and professional structures has limited the measurement of client change. Many TCs have responded to criticisms and concerns about effectiveness by increasing educational and vocational programs for residents and increasing their involvement with the professional dependency treatment and mental health community. Individuals who are former addicts still occupy many treatment staff positions, but increasingly they hold counselor certification credentials earned through undergraduate and graduate training. Some TCs operate businesses that serve the joint functions of therapeutic milieu, vocational training site, community interface, and financial revenue generator. The client population for therapeutic communities has changed dramatically since the inception of the movement. Crack cocaine has replaced heroin as the addictive drug of choice, individuals are often abusing several drugs simultaneously, and addict behaviors have become increasingly violent and outside the structures of society. It is unclear how, or if, therapeutic communities will adapt to these new realities or if individuals with crack cocaine dependence problems can adapt to and succeed in the rigidly structured therapeutic community.

Residential rehabilitation programs are hybrids of inpatient programs and therapeutic communities. They range in length of stay from three to six months and emphasize confrontational and group-oriented strategies. Unlike TCs, however, they tend to have more of an orientation to participation of residents in society. Residents live in the program but work or go to school in the community. Thus, control is emphasized less and more emphasis is placed on decision making, judgment, and personal choice. Often residents of these programs are referred to them after release from incarceration or as part of the last phase of incarceration. Residents are expected to follow a strict set of guidelines, rules, and regulations and to participate in both treatment services and vocational and educational activities. Failure in the residential rehabilitation program, usually measured by a return to drug or alcohol use, may mean reincarceration to finish the remainder of the sentence. Urinalysis and Breathalyzer testing are key measures of resident performance. Residential rehabilitation programs employ professional staff and also recovering staff and are often part of a larger correctional, human service, or mental health service delivery system. They are funded by state or federal grants or fees for services and by resident fees deducted from paychecks or welfare checks.

Halfway houses are small residential programs designed to allow individuals with dependence problems to continue their preparedness for independent community living. Typically they are staffed by volunteers who are in recovery with a small paid staff and rely heavily on mutual peer support. Residents work in the community and pay rent for room and board. Evenings are spent in peer self-help meetings or other structured activities or attending individual and group counseling offered by community agencies. Halfway houses require residents to be clean and sober, and violations usually result in expulsion. They are not entry points to the treatment system but exit points for residents who often have been in one form of treatment or another for years. Unlike other residential programs, halfway houses have less stringent guidelines and are unlikely to be regulated by state or local licensing or credentialing bodies. Many are run by recovering individuals and funded through community and charitable support. The Oxford group is a loosely aligned group of halfway houses for individuals with alcoholism dependency that operates autonomous programs in cities across the country.

Aversion therapy programs are behaviorally based inpatient treatment programs for alcoholism. These programs were popular in the 1970s and 1980s, but they have declined in numbers in recent years despite impressive claims about success. Aversion programs pair alcohol consumption with nausea, electric shock, apnea, or imagery. Of these, nausea-alcohol pairing is the oldest and most frequently used (Rimmele, Howard, & Hilfrink, 1995). These programs utilize a basic behavioral strategy: The ingestion of alcohol is paired with the immediate and unavoidable consequence of nausea and emesis with the intended outcome focused on creating a complete psychological/physiological aversion to alcohol. Always conducted in an inpatient, medically managed environment, an initial course of aversion therapy requires a two-week length of stay. Following a lengthy and comprehensive medical history to rule out potential medical complications, patients (that is the correct appellation) participate in four to six treatment sessions. Preceding each session, a pharmaceutical is administered that causes general feelings of discomfort and immediate nausea and vomiting when alcohol is ingested. The patient is taken to the treatment room that is decorated to resemble a bar or tavern, and an array of the patient's favorite drinks are presented for mandatory consumption. The patient is directed by the attending nurse to begin and to continue to consume the drinks. Usually by the third or fourth drink the patient begins to regurgitate into a large bowl placed at the patient's side. Treatment continues until all of the drinks are consumed and expelled. Each of the succeeding sessions (scheduled every other day) is conducted in the same manner, but by the third or fourth session patients may begin to vomit at the mere sight of alcohol. After each session the patient returns to a private room with the now-filled emesis basin and rests in bed until he or she regains strength. Throughout the treatment session and the recovery period a nurse monitors the patient's vital signs to avoid an untoward medical crisis. On the alternate days when aversive conditioning treatments are not scheduled, patients participate in individual and group counseling sessions and bibliotherapy. AA modeled treatment strategies are less common in aversion therapy programs than in other types of dependency treatment. In part this stems from AA's insistence that individuals who are in any phase of recovery should not consume alcohol at all, even for therapeutic purposes. Instances have occurred in which individuals participating in aversion therapy programs were dissuaded from continuing their participation in aversion therapy by well-meaning AA members who saw aversion therapy as abstinence violation.

The inpatient phase of aversion therapy is followed by a series of booster sessions staggered over the year following treatment to reinforce the association between alcohol consumption and nausea. The patient returns to the hospital for a three-day stay during which an aversion session is conducted, and follow-up counseling and support are provided.

Because of the significant medical concerns associated with this form of therapy, it is never used in an outpatient or nonmedical setting. Some outpatient programs use Antabuse (Disulfiram) to control alcohol consumption and support a treatment goal of abstinence, incorrectly describing this process as aversion therapy. Antabuse is a pharmaceutical that causes nausea, vomiting, and a variety of other negative physiological changes shortly after alcohol is consumed. Some individuals are so sensitive to the effects of Antabuse that alcohol ingestion may be life threatening. Other individuals become so sensitized to the drug during a long-term course of maintenance therapy that even small amounts of alcohol or alcohol-like chemicals entering the body may cause a reaction. These individuals may find it necessary to stop using aftershave or abstain from eating products containing large amounts of vinegar (e.g., salad dressings) or other food products with a chemical similarity to alcohol. Fuller (1995) notes that Antabuse interacts with a variety of drugs, including many benzodiazepines, antidepression pharmaceuticals, and hypertension regulators, notably the alpha and beta blockers and vasodilators. Moreover, he cautions any potential alcohol-Antabuse reaction may exacerbate cardiovascular or cerebrovascular disease, pulmonary disease, diabetes, renal disease, and hepatic disease and notes that Antabuse therapy is contraindicated for individuals with these medical conditions.

Forrest (1985) describes a model for behavioral contracting with individuals with alcohol dependence in which the individual is prescribed a maintenance dose of daily Antabuse along with participation in outpatient counseling, peer self-help group involvement, and other support. In this context Antabuse becomes the agent through which abstinence is insured. Typically Antabuse-based therapy should be reserved for individuals who have failed repeatedly at other forms of therapy, and the initiation and continuation of Antabuse should be monitored carefully. At the beginning of therapy clients should report to the clinic for their daily Antabuse dosage and to take a Breathalyzer test. The unfortunate reality is that some individuals will not take their medication as scheduled without supervision and continue drinking. Because of the potential medical complications associated with Antabuse therapy, it should be initiated only in the most severe cases. Even then, the counselor should be aware that Antabuse is not a treatment in itself but a vehicle that will allow treatment to continue.

The Case of Isaac

Isaac was a middle-aged male with a long history of alcoholism. He was a graduate of several inpatient programs, but he always relapsed after several weeks or sometimes only several days. He was participating in an aftercare program involving outpatient counseling on a weekly basis and was hanging onto his recovery with his fingertips. He was working for the first time in years and attending AA. Nevertheless, both he and his counselor were fearful of the possibility of relapse. Consequently, Isaac and his counselor contracted for a daily regimen of Antabuse. Because the outpatient aftercare program was a social model program, it could neither store nor dispense the Antabuse, but Isaac and his counselor agreed that Isaac would stop at the program every morning to take his Antabuse in the presence of staff.

Several weeks into the Antabuse regimen the counselor went down the street to the local tavern to buy a pack of cigarettes. Unbeknownst to Isaac, the counselor spotted him at the far end of the bar downing a shot and a beer. The counselor returned to his office, confident that Isaac was about to become seriously ill and learn the error of his ways. The next morning Isaac appeared to take his Antabuse in an obviously chipper and upbeat mood. Upon questioning, he related that life was wonderful and that his day at work yesterday had been especially productive. As Isaac was about to pop into his mouth his two Antabuse tablets, reality dawned on the counselor, who asked, for the first time, to examine the white tablets. "Aspirin" was neatly embossed on each tablet.

Outpatient Treatment

Outpatient treatment for psychoactive substance dependence usually follows the traditional model of one hour of therapy one day a week for an extended period. In the past, outpatient treatment was unlimited or had very liberal limits imposed by funding groups. Now, however, insurance companies and state funding agencies increasingly impose upper limits on the number of outpatient visits per year or per policy. Historically, outpatient treatment served usually as either a precursor to inpatient treatment or aftercare to inpatient treatment, but outpatient treatment has become the most widely available and utilized, and often only, form of treatment modality for nearly all individuals. Unquestionably, outpatient treatment is less stigmatizing and less life intrusive than inpatient, and it is significantly less expensive. Family participation in counseling may be more likely if outpatient services are offered in the community during evening and weekend hours when all family members can participate and are not forced to lose job or classroom time. Moreover, outpatient treatment allows individuals to test out newly learned and acquired behaviors in the natural setting, resulting in immediate feedback about success or failure.

However, because individuals are not removed from the pressures of the drinking or drug-consuming environment, many feel that outpatient counseling is typified by a very high rate of missed appointments and a high rate of relapse. Since clients are seen only once a week for a brief period, rehabilitation professionals have a more limited view of clients and their behaviors and progress. Consequently, greater observational and analytical skills are required to track client improvement.

Discussion Question: What might be other advantages and disadvantages of outpatient treatment in the local area?

   Trying to reduce the disadvantages of outpatient treatment and maximize the advantages of inpatient programming, many agencies have implemented *intensive outpatient treatment programs*. Intensive outpatient programs (also called 4 × 4 × 4 programs) provide counseling services for 4 hours per day for 4 days per week for 4 weeks. So, they are cost-beneficial, less life intrusive, and less stigmatizing than inpatient treatment but more intensive and more effective at monitoring client behaviors than outpatient programs. Intensive programs rely on legal, vocational, or family mandates and sanctions for admission and participation, and many programs require daily urinalysis or Breathalyzer testing. A failed test means expulsion from the program and may result in job loss, family dissolution, or incarceration for the client. As clients participate in treatment for 4 hours at a time, counseling can be more intensive and multidimensional, and clients have expanded opportunities to explore new behaviors and risks within the safety of the program. Then they can try those behaviors in the natural environment and can report on their experiences at the next session. As with traditional outpatient counseling, clients can retain employment or remain in school as agencies operate day and evening programs to accommodate client work and school schedules. Intensive outpatient programs rely on the disease model and are group oriented in service delivery. Staffing usually consists of two primary counseling professionals per group, with ancillary support from other disciplines. Family therapy is an integral part of many intensive outpatient programs, and family members are encouraged to participate in family self-help programming while their family member is in treatment. Similarly, individuals in treatment are encouraged to attend AA or NA meetings during and after treatment. Intensive outpatient programs are popular with agencies, clients, and funding organizations and seem to hold great promise as a treatment modality. However, limited data exist to ascertain their effectiveness in comparison to inpatient or traditional outpatient counseling.

   The roots of *methadone maintenance* can be traced to 1965 when Dole and Nyswander published a classic paper in the *Journal of the American Medical Association,* describing the use of methadone to treat heroin addiction. Methadone is a synthetic narcotic that blocks the euphoria-producing action of heroin and blocks the addict's cravings for heroin. Dole and Nyswander's basic thesis was that individuals addicted to heroin suffer from a metabolic disorder or biochemical deficit that they self-medicate by heroin ingestion (Bratter, Pennacchia, & Gauya, 1985). Accordingly, they hypothesized that daily, closely monitored oral dosages of methadone accompanied by individual and group counseling would help addicts discontinue heroin use. From their earliest work, Dole and Nyswander viewed methadone as a corrective, not curative, treatment (Doweiko, 1996). Individuals on methadone maintenance programs must remain on those programs for life, and discontinuation of participation is thought to result in a return to heroin addiction. Estimates of the numbers of individuals participating in methadone maintenance approach 100,000 clients, with more than a third of methadone maintenance clients participating in New York City programs. Methadone distribution is regulated closely by the U.S. Food and Drug Administration and methadone can be dispensed by licensed clinics only. In theory, clinics are not just methadone distribution points; they should offer an array of counseling, vocational, and educational services, but many make little effort at providing comprehensive rehabilitation service.

Because methadone in administered orally (usually mixed with fruit juice), it eliminates the potential for contracting Acquired Immune Deficiency Syndrome (AIDS) through intravenous needle use. The narcotic blockade effect of each methadone dose lasts about 24 hours, much longer than the 2- to 4-hour effects of IV heroin ingestion. In the initial stages of treatment individuals participating in methadone programs must report to the clinic on a daily basis for their medication, and urinalysis is performed daily. Unlike Antabuse that as an alcohol antagonist causes physical discomfort if alcohol is ingested simultaneously, methadone is a narcotics agonist. Individuals on methadone can use heroin or other opiates without fear of becoming ill, but they will not experience any euphoric effects. Moreover, methadone is narcotic specific in its effect; users can consume barbiturates, alcohol, cocaine, and other drugs and obtain the intended effect while on methadone maintenance.

The use of methadone to treat heroin addiction is not without its critics. Some have questioned the morality of using one addictive substance to treat another addiction, especially when there may be no hope of ceasing treatment for the life of the client (Doweiko, 1996), and programs have been criticized for failing to provide needed support and rehabilitation services (Goldberg, 1997). Finally, some have noted that methadone programs may be captive victims of shifting political, health care, and financial vicissitudes, rising and falling in popularity capriciously, with limited concern for client benefits and outcomes.

PEER SELF-HELP GROUPS

If there is an ubiquitous element in dependence treatment, it is the prevalence of peer self-help group involvement. Probably every individual ever diagnosed with or considered dependent on psychoactive substances has been referred to Alcoholics Anonymous, Narcotics Anonymous, or one of the many other groups that have sprung up. Benshoff (1996) notes they provide guidance, support, sustenance, and solace to individuals seeking respite from a variety of dependence and abuse disorders. He goes on to assert that peer self-help groups are distinguished by their absence of formal professional leadership (in most cases) and acceptance of all who seek affiliation as long as the new member promises to change through participation in the structure and values of the group. While peer self-help groups have grown to become the most easily recognized and most widely acknowledged facet of the dependency movement, they are not and have never been treatment unto themselves. Rather, peer self-help groups serve as an adjunct to a comprehensive continuum of care available to individuals with dependency or abuse problems.

Alcoholics Anonymous

In 1935 a chance encounter brought together Dr. Bob Smith and Bill Wilson in the kitchen of the Smith home in Akron, Ohio. Both men were alcoholics who had tried a variety of unsuccessful approaches to sobriety and recovery. From that inauspicious beginning grew a fellowship numbering more than 1.7 million members in more than 89,000 groups in 150 countries worldwide (AA World Services, 1990; AA World Services, 1993). Indeed the date of the beginning of Alcoholics Anonymous—June 10, 1935—is the date of Dr. Bob's last drink and the beginning of his lasting sobriety.

AA's Third Tradition specifies the only criteria for AA membership: "a desire to quit drinking." No referral is necessary, no history is taken, no forms are completed, no dues are paid, and no treatment plans are developed. Participation is voluntary, not compulsory according to the tenets of AA, but the members are enjoined to live lives of rigorous honesty, especially concerning the unmanageability of alcoholism in their lives.

The 12 Steps are the foundation for individual participation in AA:

1. We admitted that we were powerless over alcohol—that our lives had become unmanageable.
2. Came to believe that a Power greater than ourselves could restore us to sanity.
3. Made a decision to turn our will and our lives over to God *as we understood him*.
4. Made a searching and fearless moral inventory of ourselves.
5. Admitted to God, to ourselves and to another human being the exact nature of our wrongs.
6. Were entirely ready to have God remove all these defects of character.
7. Humbly asked him to remove our shortcomings.
8. Made a list of all persons we had harmed and became willing to make amends to all of them.
9. Made direct amends to such people wherever possible, except when to do so would injure them or others.
10. Continued to take personal inventory and when we were wrong promptly admitted it.
11. Sought through prayer and meditation to improve our conscious contact with God *as we understood Him,* praying only for the knowledge of his will for us and the power to carry that out.
12. Having had a spiritual awakening as a result of these steps, we tried to carry this message to alcoholics and to practice these principles in all our affairs. (AA World Services, 1976. Reprinted with permission.)

From a counseling perspective, the 12 Steps incorporate important clinical issues, including problem recognition (Step 1), hope (Step 2), help seeking (Steps 3, 5, and 7), insight development (Steps 4, 6, and 10), restitution (Steps 8 and 9), stress reduction (Step 11), and adoption of a new consciousness and forms of behavior (Step 12) (McCrady & Delaney, 1995).

Discussion   What additional therapeutic elements are found in the 12
Question: Steps?

The 12 Steps are to be completed sequentially, starting with the first step regarded as the foundation. AA dogma holds that recovery cannot begin until the individual accepts the notion of powerlessness over alcohol, and the following steps reinforce the idea that alcohol consumption is an insane, egocentric behavior leading to self-harm and harm to others. There is no particular pattern of step completion, and many individuals continue to review and revisit the steps as a way of maintaining the recovery process (McCrady & Delaney, 1995). Central to the AA belief system is the concept that alcoholism is a lifelong process for which there is treatment leading to *remission* of the disease process through abstinence but not *cure*. "Consequently AA members refer to themselves as recover*ing* alcoholics, not recover*ed* alcoholics" (Benshoff, 1996, p. 59).

The local organization unit of Alcoholics Anonymous is the local group meeting. While most communities host several meetings a week, AA traditions assert that a group consists of two or three alcoholics gathered for sobriety. Thus spontaneous groups can and do occur—for example, at conferences and other gatherings. Groups take two forms: open and closed groups. Open groups are open to all comers, including longtime members and newcomers, alcoholic and nonalcoholic. Closed groups are individuals who self-identify as members of the fellowship of AA and serve as forums for the discussion of the unique and complex issues confronted in recovery. Often closed meetings focus on a deliberation of individual steps or AA traditions or beliefs. Groups are available to meet many needs: Newcomers groups are for AA beginners; Big Book Meetings center on the Bible of AA, *Alcoholics Anonymous;* Step and Tradition meetings feature the 12 Steps and 12 Traditions. In reaching beyond its traditional base of middle-aged, white, male membership, AA groups have been established to serve diverse segments of the population. There are women's groups, gay groups, business groups, Hispanic groups, physician groups, and so on. Meeting times and places are published in the newspaper, and often a local phone number will be included to provide information about meetings. Most AA meetings are held wherever free space can be obtained: Church basements, community centers, group halls, and public facilities are common sites for meetings. Chemical dependency treatment centers and detoxification centers will host meetings to expose individuals in treatment to the Fellowship of Alcoholics Anonymous. These meetings are conducted according to the tenets of AA and serve as a convenience to the host institution. Because AA tradition holds that any member can attend any meeting at any time, meetings in institutions are open to outsiders. This policy has been problematic at times for treatment centers that find they cannot control who participates and how they participate. Fortunately, most meetings held by treatment centers do not attract many outsiders.

Discussion Question: Identify local AA meetings. Select and attend an open meeting and write a one-page report about your experiences. Be prepared to discuss your experiences and feelings in class.

The work of local AA groups is guided by the 12 Traditions:

1. Our common welfare should come first; personal recovery depends upon AA unity.

2. From our group purpose there is but one ultimate authority—a loving God as He may express himself in our group conscience. Our leaders are but trusted servants; they do not govern.

3. The only requirement for AA membership is a desire to stop drinking.

4. Each group should be autonomous except in matters affecting other groups or AA as a whole.

5. Each group has but one primary purpose—to carry its message to the alcoholic who still suffers.

6. An AA group ought never endorse, finance, or lend the AA name to any related facility or outside enterprise, lest problems of money, property, and prestige divert us from our primary purpose.

7. Every AA group ought to be fully self-supporting, declining outside contributions.

8. Alcoholics Anonymous should remain forever nonprofessional, but our service centers may employ special workers.

9. AA, as such, ought never be organized; but we may create service boards or committees directly responsible to those they serve.

10. Alcoholics Anonymous has no opinion on outside issues; hence the AA name ought never be drawn into public controversy.

11. Our public relations policy is based on attraction rather than promotion; we need always maintain personal anonymity at the level of press, radio, and films.

12. Anonymity is the spiritual foundation of all our traditions, ever reminding us to place principles before personalities. (Alcoholics Anonymous World Services, 1976, p. 564. Reprinted by permission.)

Local groups elect officers on a rotating basis to administer the affairs of the local group. In larger metropolitan areas, groups may be affiliated with a regional service board. In turn, all groups look to the Alcoholics Anonymous General Service Board that is the "custodian of our AA Tradition and the receiver of voluntary AA contributions . . . (used to) . . . maintain our AA General Service Office at New York (Alcoholics Anonymous World Services, Inc., 1976, p. 567). The 21-member General Service Board includes both AA members (14) and nonalcoholic members (7) from the general population and functions not so much to lead the organization but to serve the fellowship. AA members of the General Service Board cannot hold positions of fiscal responsibility, such as the treasurer, a custom originating with Bill Wilson's early fears. Wilson believed that an individual who had relapsed could do great financial and moral damage to the fellowship. The primary tasks of the General Service Board include overall organizational oversight, publication and distribution of AA approved literature and paraphernalia, and acting as a clearinghouse for AA information. In addition, the General Service Board holds the biennial World Service Meeting to bring together AA members from throughout the world, "serving as a forum for the sharing of experience, strength, and hope" (Alcoholics Anonymous World Services, Inc., 1997 Winter/Spring, 1). The General Service Board is the only arm of AA that employs paid staff members. Rehabilitation professionals can obtain information from the General Service Board by subscribing to *About AA,* a twice-yearly, free publication aimed at providing information about AA to the professional treatment and rehabilitation community.

Every three years the General Service Board of AA conducts a survey of its members (Alcoholics Anonymous World Services, Inc., 1993). The 1992 random survey involved 6,500 participants, and the data reveal that the top reasons for coming to AA included contact with an AA member, self-motivation, treatment facility referral, and family motivation; members attend 2.5 meetings per week, and the majority of members were between the ages of 31 and 50, with the largest cohort in the 31 through 40 range (32 percent). The occupations of the members crossed the spectrum of job types, with the largest number of members (19 percent) employed in professional/technical areas. Slightly more than one-third of the respondents (35 percent) reported being sober for more than five years, and a similar number (34 percent) reported one to five years of sobriety, while just under one-third of the survey participants reported less than one year of sobriety (31 percent). A strong majority of respondents had a home group (83 percent), or a sponsor (78 percent), and they felt that counseling or treatment was instrumental in directing them toward AA (80 percent).

Discussion Question: Write to AA World Services, Inc., Box 459, Grand Central Station, New York, NY 10163 and request a subscription to *About AA.* Discuss the newsletter content in class. Was the information helpful and informative?

The principle of anonymity is the undergirding essence of AA. In 1957 Bill Wilson wrote, "Moved by the spirit of anonymity, we try to give up our natural desires for personal distinctions as AA members, both among our fellow alcoholics and before the general public. As we lay aside these very human aspirations . . . each of us takes part in the weaving of a protective mantle that covers our whole society and under which we may grow and work in unity" (Alcoholics Anonymous World Services, 1957).

The anonymity doctrine serves three basic purposes for the organization and the membership (Benshoff, 1996). First, it *focuses the attention of the newly recovering member on the process of recovery* and away from temptations of power, prestige, and grandiosity, seen by AA philosophy as contrary to successful abstinence. It is an axiom of AA that most, if not all, members have tried to control their drinking behavior through multiple strategies, failing to recognize that they were powerless over alcohol. Through anonymous participation in the fellowship, members can give up their ego-driven struggles. This is a stance that dates from the very founding of Alcoholics Anonymous. Both Bill Wilson and Bob Smith were successful in most aspects of their lives except their ability to control their drinking. Wilson was a stockbroker and businessman, and Smith was a physician. Both write eloquently about the destructive role alcohol played in their lifestyles, relationships, and vocational life, and both assert the importance of humility and surrender (Alcoholics Anonymous World Services, Inc., 1976).

Second, *anonymity provides a safe haven from the stigma attached to alcoholism.* While substantial progress has occurred in reducing that stigma in recent years, the negative social, vocational, familial, and personal consequences of alcoholism are difficult issues that confront many people. "Anonymity does not, however, provide an excuse or alibi for past irresponsible or harmful behaviors. Indeed, AA members are called throughout the 12 Steps to assume individual, personal responsibility for behavior, past and present" (Benshoff, 1996, p. 60).

Finally, *anonymity is the great equalizer in AA,* promoting participation from individuals from all walks of life. Members use their first names only in meetings, and AA Tradition 11 specifically cautions against personal identification even for benevolent purposes. AA is quick to separate itself from those who are seen as flaunting their recovery for personal gain or aggrandizement, stressing the importance of the development of a new, humble self-image free from the ego demands thought to lead to a return to drinking.

While anonymity simplifies participation, it is a significant negative factor affecting the development of an understanding of the efficacy of Alcoholics Anonymous and to evaluate successful outcomes. As Jung (1994) points out, because of the anonymity principle, it is impossible to conduct empirically rigorous investigations of the benefits of participation in AA. Researchers cannot determine who attends, for how long and how frequently, and to what end.

So scrupulous is AA about its name and image that it refuses to have its name associated with *any* organization, including alcoholism treatment centers, believing that doing so would separate the fellowship from its primary purpose. Contributions are not accepted from outside sources, and contributions from individual AA members are limited to $1,000 per year.

Discussion   What are the implications of accepting or refusing to accept
Question: outside contributions?

There is only one role in AA that separates one member from another—that of the sponsor. The sponsor is usually a longtime member of the fellowship with considerable recovery experience and a willingness and ability to share that experience in an ongoing manner (McCrady & Delaney, 1995). Sponsors provide information about a variety of issues including the workings of AA, how to avoid a relapse, the steps, meeting schedules. As part of their Twelfth Step work, sponsors are enjoined to be continuously available to their "pigeons" as sponsorees are called. McCrady and Delaney (1995) caution that sponsors should be of the same gender of the person being sponsored, but no formal guidelines exist for sponsorship. AA does not provide any training or guidance for sponsors except that which occurs vicariously through meeting participation, modeling others, and personal experiences from being sponsored.

Narcotics Anonymous

Narcotics Anonymous (NA) traces its history to the late 1940s and early 1950s when a group of individuals who were addicted to drugs and who were members of AA split from Alcoholics Anonymous and formed Addicts Anonymous. Recognizing the inherent problems and confusion in two similar organizations calling themselves AA, the group renamed itself Narcotics Anonymous. Today, there are nearly 20,000 NA groups meeting in 70 countries, including a membership that is predominately male and middle-aged. Unlike AA, Narcotics Anonymous does not complete comprehensive surveys of its membership, in part to protect the anonymity of NA members. While most AA members have a history of primary dependence on a legal drug, most NA members have been dependent on illegal drugs and thus would risk being identified or might be unwilling to honestly complete a survey.

The 12 Steps and 12 Traditions of Narcotics Anonymous are modeled closely on the 12 Steps and Traditions of Alcoholics Anonymous, a tribute to the roots of NA. However, Narcotics Anonymous departs from Alcoholics Anonymous in its emphasis on addiction to any chemical substance as the primary problem to be addressed as opposed to AA's focus on alcohol, although this distinction may be more semantic than real. From its earliest days, AA recognized the reality of cross-addiction to alcohol and other drugs, although there have been and still are local groups openly antagonistic to participation by individuals perceived as drug addicts. The very name Narcotics Anonymous may seem to exclude individuals whose drug addiction is to nonnarcotic drugs. The NA World Service Board of Trustees makes clear this is not the situation in Step One, which asserts that NA is concerned with powerlessness over addiction and not with specific drugs or drug types (Narcotics Anonymous World Services Board, 1997). Today many individuals participating in either AA or NA meetings have dual dependencies and are at home in either setting.

Cocaine Anonymous

Cocaine Anonymous (CA), founded in Los Angeles in 1982, has, like AA, a specific focus on a particular psychoactive drug. Even though the focus of CA is on cocaine addiction, the stated requirement for membership is a desire to stop using cocaine and *all other mind-altering chemicals*. CA claims about 50,000 members in 2000 groups in the United States, Canada, and Europe. The heritage of Cocaine Anonymous is explicit in the CA 12 Steps and 12 Traditions: They are exactly the same as the AA Steps and Traditions, except that CA is substituted for AA, and the phrase "cocaine and all other mind-altering substances" replaces "alcohol" in Step 1. In many ways the formation dates and the emphases of AA, NA, and CA reflect the history of psychoactive chemical dependence in this country and signal the emergence of treatment resources for particular substances. For example, from its inception, NA dealt primarily with addiction to opiate drugs, and its growth and development follows the growth and development of the therapeutic community model of heroin addiction treatment. If the development of Cocaine Anonymous is examined, an early emphasis on powder cocaine is revealed both in CA and in cocaine treatment (Washton, 1987). Later, as crack cocaine emerged on the abuse/dependence scene, there was a shift in treatment emphasis and an explicit statement by CA that the fellowship was open to individuals dependent on crack cocaine (Cocaine Anonymous World Services, Inc., 1997).

Other Peer Self-Help Groups

While groups that owe their heritage and structure to Alcoholics Anonymous dominate the peer self-help movement, other groups have emerged in recent years to offer an alternative format. *The Small Book: A Revolutionary Alternative for Overcoming Alcohol and Drug Dependence* (Trimpey, 1989) is the Bible of Rational Recovery (RR), a peer self-help model based on the principles of rational emotive therapy (RET) (Benshoff, 1996; McCrady & Delaney, 1995). Developed as an alternative to peer self-help programs based on the disease model, spirituality, and lifelong recovery, Rational Recovery emphasizes the use of rational cognitive processes and the rejection of self-defeating negative thought patterns to overcome dependence. RR postulates that self-esteem is central to abstinence from psychoactive chemicals and that, through the development and belief in self-esteem, empowers the individual to remain sober (McCrady and Delaney, 1995). Recently, Jack Trimpey, cofounder of Rational Recovery, has advanced the concept of the Addictive Voice Recognition Technique (AVRT) as a recovery strategy in the Structural Model of Addiction. (Rational Recovery Systems, 1997). The Structural Model of Addiction rejects the disease concept for unnecessarily complicating recovery and discouraging initiative. It suggests that the brain is divided into two structures. The *beast brain,* akin to Freud's id, is the center of physical pleasures and survival instincts and is the ruthless force driving the addictive state. Sitting atop the beast brain, according to RR is the cerebral cortex (also called the neocortex or *new brain*), the center of consciousness, language, thought, voluntary action, and problem solving. Through AVRT, Rational Recovery asserts that the cerebral cortex can prevail over the insatiable demands of the beast brain to continue the use of psychoactive, dependence-causing drugs.

Operated in a group format, Rational Recovery meetings are led by a coordinator who has experienced recovery through the AVRT method. Rational

Recovery Centers have been established in place of traditional treatment centers to teach the AVRT method of recovery. There are no dues or membership fees, but financial contributions are accepted at meetings. Rational Recovery sees itself as neither a support group nor counseling group but as an educational program where problems can be evaluated and a decision-making process can be learned.

The Secular Organizations for Sobriety (SOS) characterizes itself as "an alternative recovery program for those alcoholics or drug addicts who are uncomfortable with the spiritual content of widely available 12-Step programs" (Noelle, 1997, p. 1). As many as 1000 groups meet weekly in the United States, and the organization has been recognized as an alternative to AA or NA by at least two state correctional systems. Like Rational Recovery, SOS stresses rational, scientifically based decision making about dependence, but SOS also stresses the importance of peer support and the importance of lifelong total sobriety.

While AA and NA have been roundly criticized for being religious or quasireligious organizations, several peer self-help programs are unabashedly religious in their emphasis. Overcomers Outreach (OO) and Christians in Recovery are for individuals interested in a recovery program with a Christian context, while Jews in Recovery from Alcoholism and Drug Dependencies reaches out to Jews; the Substance Abuse Volunteer Effort (SAVE) targets members of the LDS (Mormon) church; and the Calix Society is a recovery organization for Roman Catholics (Homer & Dillon, 1997; McCrady & Delaney, 1995). Most of these organizations have developed step and tradition programs that are mirror images of the AA Steps.

Discussion   Discuss the advantages and disadvantages of peer self-help
Question: groups with a specific secular or religious emphasis.

Alcoholics Anonymous has been criticized for failing to be responsive to the needs of women. Often characterized as an organization founded by men, dominated in attendance by men, and focusing on male issues, traditional 12-Step programs have been perceived as insensitive to the needs of the growing numbers of women with dependency problems, estimated to be about a third of the total population at risk (Jung, 1994). In July 1976 Dr. Jean Kirkpatrick founded Women for Sobriety (WFS), a peer self-help program designed specifically to meet the needs of women with alcoholism problems. Kirkpatrick was a recovering alcoholic whose recovery was based in AA, but who felt that the special needs of women with dependency problems transcended the help offered by AA and other "traditional" self-help programs (Pabis-Mock, 1997). At the core of WFS is the "New Life Program," which promotes behavioral change through positive reinforcement, cognitive strategies centering on positive thinking, and wellness-promotion activities including meditation, nutrition, diet, exercise, and relaxation techniques. This philosophy is espoused in the Thirteen Statements:

"NEW LIFE" ACCEPTANCE PROGRAM

1. I have a life-threatening problem that once had me.
   I now take charge of my life. I accept the responsibility.

2. Negative thoughts destroy only myself.
   My first conscious sober act must be to remove negativity from my life.

3. Happiness is a habit I will develop.
   Happiness is created, not waited for.

4. Problems bother me only to the degree I permit them to.
   I now better understand my problems and do not permit problems to overwhelm me.

5. I am what I think.
   I am a capable, competent, caring, compassionate woman.

6. Life can be ordinary or it can be great.
   Greatness is mine by a conscious effort.

7. Love can change the course of my world.
   Caring becomes all-important.

8. The fundamental object of life is emotional and spiritual growth.
   Daily I put my life into a proper order, knowing which are the priorities.

9. The past is gone forever.
   No longer will I be victimized by the past. I am a new person.

10. All love given returns.
    I will learn to know that others love me.

11. Enthusiasm is my daily exercise.
    I treasure all moments of my new life.

12. I am a competent woman and have much to give life.
    This is what I am and I shall know it always.

13. I am responsible for myself and for my actions.
    I am in charge of my mind, my thoughts, and my life.
    (Women for Sobriety, Inc., 1997c. Reprinted by permission.)

Participants in the program are given the following directive: "To make the Program effective for you, arise each morning 15 minutes earlier than usual and go over the 13 Affirmations. Then begin to think about each one by itself. Take one Statement and use it consciously all day. At the end of the day review the use of it and what effects it had that day for you and your actions" (Women for Sobriety, Inc., 1997d).

In dramatic contrast to 12-Step programs, Women for Sobriety seeks to empower its members to develop new, richer, fuller lives. The program claims more than 300 groups, mostly in more populated urban areas. Each group is led by a certified moderator who is a recovering woman with well-established sobriety. Although founded to reach out to women with alcohol dependencies, women with other drug dependencies are found in the WFS membership. WFS is funded through proceeds from its literature sales, donations, and speaking fees paid to Kirkpatrick and other WFS leaders.

Discussion   Discuss and compare the 13 Statements of WFS with the 12
Question: Steps of AA.

THE EFFECTIVENESS OF TREATMENT
AND PEER SELF-HELP GROUPS

Organized treatment resources for individuals with dependency problems have
been widely available for just about a quarter-century; the oldest peer self-help
group, AA, has been in operation about 60 years, with the majority of other peer
self-help groups serving individuals for a far shorter time. What has been learned
about treatment or peer self-help group effectiveness during that time? Unfortunately, very little. Despite widespread popular support for and belief in peer self-
help programs, there is little evidence to support their effectiveness. In part this
is due to the unstructured nature of these programs and their emphasis on
anonymity. From a research perspective, the very nature of peer self-help programs makes it nearly impossible to track study participants over an extended period, to control treatment availability, and to control for extraneous variables that
may influence treatment. Because of the voluntary nature of peer self-help group
participation, it is impossible to randomly assign individuals to treatment and control groups. Thus, while it is known that some individuals benefit from participation in peer self-help groups, it cannot be said for certain that the benefit was an
effect of group participation or an interaction between participant characteristics
and the group process. Moreover, while little is known about the success of peer
self-help group members, even less is known about the recovery success of individuals who attend a few meetings and drop out or who attend meetings sporad-
ically (Benshoff, 1996). Logic suggests that some of these individuals will continue
in their dependencies, but some may enter a successful recovery period. Studies
examining AA participation have suggested that "successful" fellowship members
have a record of active participation and involvement in meetings (Emrick, 1987),
frequent participation (Hoffman, Harrison, & Bellille, 1983), and an external locus of control and strong affiliation needs (Ogborne and Glaser, 1981). McCrady
and Delaney (1995) report that no controlled studies have been conducted on
groups other than AA, and that the few controlled studies conducted using AA
members as participants have generally yielded mixed to negative results.

Analyses of standard treatment programs for dependencies have provided
scanty data at best. In a methodological study of 219 articles that examined a
variety of alcohol dependency treatment strategies and outcomes, Miller and a
team of researchers (Miller et al., 1995) uncovered few strategies that had positive outcomes. Indeed, some of the most cherished elements of traditional dependency treatment fared especially badly, including educational lectures and
films, confrontational counseling, psychotherapy, and general alcoholism counseling. Strategies with some positive support incorporated client-centered
counseling, cognitive behavioral strategies (especially behavior contracting and
behavioral self-control training), social skills training, and brief interventions.

The emphasis on inpatient treatment that has evolved in this country enjoys little empirical support but continues to have professional support and approval. Doweiko (1996) cites several studies that suggest that inpatient programs are no more likely to generate positive outcomes than outpatient programs and are uniformly less cost-effective. However, Doweiko asserts that "outpatient treatment programs are still viewed by many as inferior to treatment carried out in an inpatient setting" (p. 353). The literature contains a variety of clinical arguments, usually based on speculation or experience, that certain subgroups require inpatient treatment, including long-term addicts (Miller & Hester, 1986), individuals who are severely addicted and socially unstable (Miller & Hester, 1989), individuals dependent on cocaine, especially freebase or IV users (Washton, 1987), clients with poor levels of motivation or a history of frequent relapses (Fisher & Harrison, 1997), and individuals with limited social support and no stability in life functioning (Godley, Cronk, & Landrum, 1996). The efficacy of intensive outpatient programs was examined in a special issue of the *Journal of Addictive Diseases* in 1997. Campbell et al. (1997) found that participants in intensive outpatient treatment for crack cocaine showed improvement as measured by scores on the Addiction Severity Index, and they called for comparisons with standard outpatient and inpatient treatment groups. In another study Weinstein, Gottheil, and Sterling (1997) discovered that completion of a 12-week course of treatment resulted in lowered drug use and improved psychological functioning across intensive programming, individual outpatient treatment, or individual outpatient treatment augmented with group counseling. They suggested retention in treatment was an important variable for treatment success. Outcome differences between intensive outpatient samples and traditional outpatient samples at follow-up were not seen in a study conducted by McLellan and his colleagues (1997). However it was conceded that intensive outpatient participants presented for treatment with more severe medical, legal, employment, and psychiatric problems.

What is the counselor to do? With little to no empirical support for expensive, supposedly state-of-the-art inpatient programming; conflicting, often ambiguous and methodologically unsound support for peer self-help programs; and virtually no investigation of outpatient programs available, determining the appropriate treatment modality for individuals with dependence problems may seem difficult. However, perhaps the wrong question is being asked. Instead of attempting to determine the most effective treatment strategy, counselors should more closely examine the multiple treatment needs of clients and determine a course of treatment based on a continuum of care. As Miller and colleagues have suggested, there might not be a single treatment strategy that is adequate to the task of treating all individuals with dependency problems. Rather "the best hope lies in assembling a menu of effective alternatives, and then seeking a system for finding the right combination of elements for each individual" (Miller et al., 1995, p. 33).

SUMMARY

Few treatment programs existed prior to the 1960s when a series of events—federal legislation, increased societal and industrial awareness of alcohol problems, growing popularity of Alcoholics Anonymous, and professional organization development—served as the catalyst for the development of treatment services. The disease concept of alcoholism and the Minnesota Model of Chemical Dependency Treatment, characterized by abstinence, became and remain the dominant force for treatment of all forms of substance abuse and dependence.

The range of treatment resources begins with detoxification services, offered in either medical, social model, or self-detoxification settings. Residential treatment encompasses inpatient programs, therapeutic communities, residential rehabilitation programs, halfway houses, and aversion therapy programs. Inpatient programs evolved with strong ties to the disease concept and a significant reliance on AA and AA concepts. Programs are offered in both medical and social model setting and typically focus on short-term goal achievement along with establishing longer-term goals for recovery. Therapeutic communities were originally designed to treat heroin addiction. Using highly confrontational, group-based methods, TCs are largely self-regulating. Residential rehabilitation programs are a hybrid between inpatient programs and therapeutic communities, emphasizing community participation and integration. Usually staffed by professionals, they differ from halfway houses, which also stress community integration but are more likely to be staffed by individuals in recovery, often volunteers. Aversion therapy programs occupy a unique and rather small niche in the treatment world, offering behaviorally based, aversive conditioning approaches to alcoholism treatment.

The spectrum of outpatient models includes traditional outpatient counseling, intensive outpatient counseling, and methadone maintenance. Traditional outpatient counseling services often serve as a gateway for other services for many individuals seeking treatment, but these may be the only services available for many people. In an attempt to combine the advantages of outpatient counseling and inpatient services, intensive outpatient programs were conceptualized. More intensive services can be offered using this model, but it remains largely unproven in terms of success rates. Methadone maintenance programs exist solely for the provision of services to individuals who are addicted to heroin or other opiates.

Peer self-help groups are the ubiquitous element in dependence treatment. Alcoholics Anonymous is the prototypic peer self-help group. Founded in 1935, it is a voluntary organization whose criteria for membership is a desire to quit drinking. Based on principles contained in the 12 Steps and 12 Traditions, AA was modeled by Narcotics Anonymous and Cocaine Anonymous, as well as many other peer self-help groups. The steps and tradition embody many clinical concepts. Other peer self-help groups include Rational Recovery (RR), grounded in the theory of Rational Emotive Therapy, Secular Organizations for

Sobriety (SOS), and a number of others. One of the most interesting emergent groups is Women for Sobriety (WFS), founded in 1976 to meet the recovery needs of women. WFS stresses the importance of behavioral change, especially through becoming empowered and taking charge of life.

Although widely available and extremely popular, very little is known about the effectiveness of peer self-help groups. Research has been hampered by the unstructured nature of programs, anonymity principles, and the inability to control extraneous variables. Unfortunately, data are limited concerning the effectiveness of formal treatment programs as well. Inpatient programs enjoy popular and clinical anecdotal support but have little empirical support. Outpatient models are rarely examined in the literature. Perhaps the best treatment approach is an individualized approach combining the best available alternatives for each individual.

9

Assessment

ASSESSMENT CONCEPTS
AND TERMINOLOGY

Assessment may be defined as the process of identifying strengths and limitations of an individual in the context of optimal outcomes or client functioning. The potential outcomes for clients will vary markedly, depending on the
client, the nature of his or her disability, and the goals and resources of the
treatment agency. The assessment process should lead logically and directly into
the development of alternative service plans. These service plans ought to be
clear, behaviorally based plans of action founded on the information developed
through assessment.

Assessment entails gathering information from a variety of sources to help
make predictions about client outcomes and to assist clients with making decisions about their rehabilitation programs. Although prediction is a future-
oriented endeavor, assessment is also concerned with making a diagnosis of
current behavior or performance. The distinction is minor, however, because
the diagnosis of a present condition (e.g., alcoholism) implies a prediction of
what the individual will do in situations other than the assessment situation. At
its most basic level, assessment involves gathering information to answer three
basic questions:

1. What is the client's current level of functioning? Generally information is
   gathered about the client's major characteristics and abilities and organizing
   this information into categories of strengths, limitations, and preferences.

2. What goal or goals seem to be most appropriate for the client? Based on
   the client's current level of functioning, services of the agency, and community resources, alternative goals are tentatively identified and ultimately
   refined. The rehabilitation goal or goals result from a collaboration between the counselor and client and ought to result in optimal outcomes,
   capitalizing on client strengths, and minimizing or compensating for areas
   of deficit. They should also be consistent with client preferences.

3. What services and client activities are required to attain the goal or goals?
   Assessment should form the basis of a plan that integrates client data and
   environmental information with the goal or goals. Plans ought to be
   action-oriented, requiring clear behaviors on the part of the client and
   counselor and consist of successive, achievable subgoals that logically lead
   to the ultimate goal for the client.

Using this definition, it is clear that assessment is a comprehensive, ongoing
process that is intimately linked to substance abuse treatment and the client's
overall rehabilitation. The terms *evaluation, measurement,* and *tests* are closely related to assessment, and they have often been used interchangeably in the literature and by professionals in the field. These terms, however, have some
important distinctions: A client assessment may include an evaluation, which
in turn incorporates measurements produced by tests. Hence the terms move
from the very broad (assessment) to the very specific (test). Assessment, having

already been defined, may be considered a comprehensive component that underlies the entire rehabilitation process.

Evaluation is more specific, and it is understood to be a specialized component of the assessment process that entails the collection of information that describes and projects an individual's functioning level and behavior in a particular situation or situations of interest. Typical situations of interest in rehabilitation evaluations focus on such areas as medical/physical, psychological, social, educational, or vocational functioning. For example, a vocational evaluation would include an examination of the client's work and educational histories, using record reviews and interviews, the administration of vocational aptitude and interest tests, completion of work sample devices, and a determination of the client's job readiness. A psychological evaluation, on the other hand, would include a clinical interview to determine the client's current mental state, administration of intelligence and personality tests, and Diagnostic and Statistical Manual-IV diagnoses following the categories specified by Axes I, II, III, IV, and V. The type and extent of an evaluation will depend on the needs of the client and counselor, along with the resources of the party performing the evaluation.

Typically, evaluations incorporate both qualitative and quantitative information. Qualitative information consists of descriptions of client behaviors based on observations, interviews, and other sources of information such as letters, reports, and interactions with family members. Quantitative information describes client behaviors in terms of measurements, using numbers that have some reference for interpretation; common types of quantitative information include grade point averages from school transcripts, scores from tests of aptitude or achievement, and information from financial statements or earnings records.

The term *measurement* refers to the process of assigning a number to indicate the presence or amount of some attribute or trait possessed by the person. The most common tools for arriving at measurements are tests, observation instruments, rating scales, inventories, or other devices that facilitate quantification of attributes or traits. An example of obtaining a measurement is estimating a person's intelligence by using a test that produces an IQ score. Another example is using an inventory or rating scale to determine the level of a client's interest in a number of different occupations. The data produced by measurements may be at one of four levels: nominal, ordinal, interval, or ratio. Because of the widespread use of tests for quantification of human behavior (including substance abuse and addiction), it is important to understand what each level entails.

Nominal level measurements use numbers to classify or name elements based on their distinguishing characteristics—for example, assigning a number to a person based on gender (e.g., 1 = Male, 2 = Female) or categorizing clients seeking services based on the type of mental illness (e.g., the DSM-IV category for alcohol dependence is 303.90). Given its relatively low level of measurement, it isn't possible to perform mathematical operations such as addition or subtraction on nominal level data; however, it is permissible to use the data to arrive at frequencies.

Ordinal level measurements consist of ranking or ordering data within some class; scores can be scaled from highest to lowest or from most to least. Ordinal level measurements are more sophisticated than nominal level measurements in that they allow categorical data to be ranked on some dimension. For example, interest inventories may place interests into categories such as artistic, social, or business (i.e., nominal level) and then go beyond categorizing and order the level of interest from very high to very low. Generally, with ordinal level measures, negative numbers are never used, and the distances between ranks can vary, so the distance between 1 and 2 on the scale may not be the same as the distance between 3 and 4. Like nominal level measurements, you cannot perform any arithmetic operations on the data, other than counting.

Interval level measurements scale data as the same as ordinal data, but the intervals throughout the scale are equal. Hence, it is possible to add and subtract the data because the distances between any two numbers are of a set size. Examples of interval level data include temperature, calendar dates, or IQ scores. It is not possible, however, to multiply or divide interval level data because the scale has no absolute zero (0) point. If a zero point is used on an interval scale, it is determined arbitrarily or based on the size of the mean and standard deviation of a norm group. For example, a temperature reading of zero doesn't mean that there is an absence of temperature, nor would an IQ score of zero (if one could get a zero) mean an absence of intelligence.

Ratio level measurements are the most sophisticated. The difference between the ratio and interval level data is the presence of an absolute zero or true zero point. Examples of ratio level measurements include measuring height in inches or weight in pounds, or using a functional capacity evaluation to measure range of motion in degrees of movement. All mathematical functions may be applied to ratio level data. Unfortunately, very few psychological tests report scores at the ratio level; most will produce measures at nominal or ordinal levels.

The last, and most narrow, term to be defined is test. A *test* is an objective, standardized measure of a sample of behavior used to make predictions about behavior in other situations of interest (Anastasi, 1988). This behavior is thought to reflect traits that are predictive (e.g., intelligence, interests, personality). These are *hypothetical* "traits" that people are presumed to possess in differing degrees, such as levels of intelligence, aptitude, or even addiction. Tests are objective in that they should be free of any biases of the test administrator. In other words, the person administering and scoring the test should in no way influence its results. Tests are standardized in that they are administered, scored, and interpreted in a consistent manner, making meaningful interpretation possible. Typically, there are very prescribed steps in the way a test is given and interpreted. This allows for the comparison of test results to norm groups, which aids in the test's interpretation. For example, giving a test of math ability and allowing the client unlimited time and the use of paper and pencil would invalidate the test if it was normed on a group that had to complete the test in 15 minutes and do all the work in their heads.

INTAKE AND INITIAL INTERVIEWS

The initial stage of client assessment generally takes one of two forms: intake interviews and standardized tests, both of which are frequently used in combination. Intake procedures may be "home-made" (developed by the agency) or standardized, published interview protocols that guide the counselor in asking clients questions about their alcohol and drug use, family life, financial status, legal involvement, general health, and so on. Standardized tests may also be used to screen for substance abuse problems. Although there are biomedical-based tests such as mean corpuscular volume (MCV), most treatment facilities rely on one or more published self-report measures or tests for substance abuse.

The intake interview is typically one of the first activities in the rehabilitation process. Intake is a semistructured interview where the client and counselor construct the client's relevant history. Intake procedures will vary from program to program and incorporate the facility's needs for required documentation for meeting the requirements of funding sources, maintain accreditation, and track clients. Intake procedures focusing exclusively on substance abuse history tend to be overly narrow. It is important to recognize that substance abuse is a multi-determined, complex problem requiring a holistic assessment. When the complexity of the problem is ignored by assessing only the drug use, the treatment following assessment will be overly narrow and simplistic, with abstinence being viewed as health and nonabstinence as illness (Lewis, Dana, & Blevins, 1994). Comprehensive, multimodal treatment strategies are founded on comprehensive, multidimensional assessments. Therefore, substance abuse intake should follow a similar line of questioning as with any comprehensive rehabilitation intake procedure, with some additional information being gathered about substance use.

Because the intake interview occurs very early in the rehabilitation process, it often provides the first real opportunity for the counselor to build rapport with the client. The counselor should avoid a formal "grilling" of the client; rather, questions should be asked in a manner consistent with the counselor's listening skills, including good eye contact, attentive body language, and continuing paralinguistics (eg., huh huh). Further, the client should be informed of his or her rights as a recipient of services, especially the rights to privacy and confidentiality. In this way the counselor and client can begin building a relationship characterized by trust and support.

Rubin & Roessler (1995) recommended that the information processing questions used in interviews be separated into the categories of (1) physical, (2) educational-vocational, (3) psychosocial, (4) economic, and (5) personal vocational choice considerations. Obviously, there are many variations on this theme; the approach recommended by this text categorizes client information into (1) medical, (2) psychological, (3) personal-social, (4) educational, and (5) vocational realms.

I. MEDICAL

Determine Diagnoses. Ask questions to:

1. identify the client's primary medically diagnosed disability.
2. identify the client's secondary medically diagnosed disability (if any).
3. appraise the client's current general health status.

Determine Prognoses. Ask questions to:

1. identify current functional capacities, especially the functional limitations resulting from disability.
2. provide a realistic basis for tentative selection of rehabilitation objectives (related to functional capacities).
3. briefly describe any medical interventions that have been performed (e.g., surgery, physical therapy, drug treatments, etc.).
4. determine to what extent and by what means the disabling condition may be removed, corrected, or minimized by restoration services.

II. PSYCHOLOGICAL

Formal psychological evaluation and testing may not be needed in all cases, but informal psychological questioning is certainly involved in the planning of every rehabilitation program. This includes the study of the client's past behavior as well as conclusions drawn from observations of the client's current behavior during interviews and outside contacts. Types of information that may be included in this area are the following:

1. Information or confirmation of the client's abilities, aptitudes, achievements, and interests
2. Personality patterns that the client often demonstrates, such as locus of control, self-esteem, adjustment to disability, dependency
3. Evidence related to the client's capacities and abilities that are conspicuously absent, ambiguous, or contradictory

III. PERSONAL-SOCIAL

Social history is necessary for a holistic client picture. Social and family information are the background against which planning and treatment are predicted. There is no set form or procedure for taking social histories; however, the following information is generally included:

1. Early life and cultural climate of the home
2. Current family relationships (e.g., marital status, children, parents, siblings, other significant others)
3. Identification of the presence or lack of a support network
4. Economic information, such as sources of income, standard of living, major bills (depending on the client's situation, economic information could be a separate category)

5. Other questions that may be addressed are What individuals make up the immediate household? How does the disability affect family relationships? What is the family climate (discord or harmony)?

IV. EDUCATIONAL HISTORY

Include a brief description of the client's educational history in order to evaluate his or her current academic functioning and potential to engage in training that could range from remedial to advanced:

1. Final grade completed and when
2. Expressed (what the client says) and manifest (what the client does) attitudes toward education and possible future training
3. Favorite subjects (and why)
4. Extracurricular activities
5. Potential for future education and/or training

Standardized achievement tests of math, reading, and general learning ability are often used to augment interview questions. The client's educational history may also be used to indicate vocationally related interests and values.

V. VOCATIONAL HISTORY

Include a brief description of the client's work history in order to estimate current and potential vocational functioning. Minimally, ask questions addressing these areas:

1. Types of occupations in which the client has worked
2. Chronology of jobs within the past 15 years, include the job title, name of employer, length of employment at each job, and primary job duties
3. Reasons for leaving each job
4. Client's estimated relationships with supervisors and coworkers
5. Favorite and least favorite jobs and why
6. Work-related ambitions and goals

The work history may be used to examine any client skills that can be used in other occupations that are consistent with the limitations imposed by disability. As with the educational category, vocational questioning may be augmented by standardized aptitude and interest tests, and work samples and situational assessments designed to evaluate work aptitudes and tolerances. A complete understanding of a client's educational and work histories, aptitudes, skills, work habits, attitudes, interests, goals, and motivations is necessary for the rehabilitation counselor to solve the following problems: insufficient understanding of capacities and interests, lack of occupational information, selection of job objectives in line with abilities and transferable work skills, choice of and arrangement for an appropriate course of training, and locating and adjusting to a specific job.

The Case of Joe

At the time of his accident Joe was working as a traffic light installer. He suffered multiple electrical burns to his legs, right arm, and both hands from a 13,000-volt electrical burn while installing traffic lights. The pole he was placing for a stoplight touched a high-tension wire. His employer reports that Joe has been an average employee who has had some attendance problems and periods of poor performance. Joe has gone through a number of surgeries and physical therapy and at this time he is making excellent progress in his physical condition, with increasing stamina. Joe wears a prosthesis for his right leg and wears a special shoe on the left foot. He ambulates well with crutches and feels he will be able to walk unaided after he adjusts to the artificial limb. He continues with physical therapy and takes pain medication. The physical therapist has reported that he has missed a couple of morning appointments, but he works hard at his physical therapy.

School records show that Joe graduated from high school. He has two semesters' credits obtained as an electronics major in Technical College. Joe held a 2.8 GPA until he quit school in the middle of his third semester. Since he didn't attempt to do anything about his incomplete grades, his overall GPA was lowered to 1.6. Joe has indicated that he dropped out of school because his family was living on a minimal income for too long, so he returned to working full-time. Joe does not have a current driver's license.

You interviewed Joe at his home and noted that he drank a beer and smoked cigarettes during your scheduled interview. Joe seems to have come to grips with his physical disability and is determined to regain as much usefulness of his right hand as possible. He does resent his restricted ambulation at this time and vows to improve. He has set physical-performance goals that are clear and largely consistent with his disability. He wants very much to return to his former outdoor activities, such as camping and fishing. Joe currently is vague about his vocational goals, stating only that he knows he must return to work to support his family (he has a wife and two young children).

The preceding outline provides a basis for a comprehensive, generic intake assessment. When substance abuse is the primary or secondary diagnosis, or even suspected, it will be helpful to have additional questions that more fully explore the nature of the drug use. A typical intake form used in substance abuse treatment is shown in Figure 9.1. As indicated earlier, these questions are meant to augment, not replace, the more holistic intake questions outlined before.

The organization and content of intake interviews will certainly vary depending on the needs of the agency and the population that it serves. The interview is structured, generally following the content of the intake form, but the interview should not be so rigid as to ignore areas of concern as they arise. The interview should also be a collaborative effort, with both the counselor and client participating in the initial phases of both problem and goal identification. It is important that the intake interview be thorough and accurate because it will often provide the basis of developing a long-term rehabilitation plan. At the same time, counselors should avoid preconceptions and stereotypical

INTERVIEW DATE AND PLACE _____

INTERVIEW CONDUCTED BY _____

SIGNATURE OF INTERVIEWER _____

REFERRAL SOURCE _____

I. DEMOGRAPHIC INFORMATION

CLIENT NAME _____

FACILITY IDENTIFICATION NUMBER _____

DATE OF BIRTH AND AGE _____

GENDER _____

ETHNICITY _____

MARITAL STATUS _____

II. PRESENTING PROBLEM

PRIMARY PRESENTING PROBLEM _____

SERVICES BEING SOUGHT _____

SUBSTANCE USE HISTORY

PRIMARY DRUG OF USE _____

   AGE OF FIRST USE _____

   AGE REGULAR USE BEGAN _____

   DATE OF LAST USE _____

   MOST RECENT PATTERN OF USE (when, where, amount, associated
   events/triggers) _____

   MOST SEVERE PATTERN OF USE (when, where, amount, associated
   events/triggers) _____

   RELAPSE TRIGGERS (stress, free time, visual cues, associates)

   SIGNS/SYMPTOMS OF ABUSE/DEPENDENCE (tremors, craving, use
   to alleviate symptoms of withdrawal) _____

   WITHDRAWAL RISK (rate very low to very high) _____

SECONDARY DRUG OF USE _____

   AGE OF FIRST USE _____

   AGE REGULAR USE BEGAN _____

   DATE OF LAST USE _____

   MOST RECENT PATTERN OF USE (when, where, amount, associated
   events/triggers) _____

   MOST SEVERE PATTERN OF USE (when, where, amount, associated
   events/triggers) _____

continued

FIGURE 9.1 Substance Abuse/Dependence Intake Summary

RELAPSE TRIGGERS (stress, free time, visual cues, associates): _____

SIGNS/SYMPTOMS OF ABUSE/DEPENDENCE (tremors, craving, use to alleviate symptoms of withdrawal) _____

WITHDRAWAL RISK (rate very low to very high) _____
DRUG OF CHOICE _____
OTHER SUBSTANCES TAKEN WITHOUT HABITUAL USE _____

HISTORY OF SUBSTANCE ABUSE TREATMENT (where, when, and outcome) _____

III. PHYSICAL STATUS

NAME OF PRIMARY PHYSICIAN _____
DATE OF LAST EXAMINATION _____
MEDICAL HISTORY (major illnesses, hospitalizations, surgeries, major injuries/fractures) _____

CURRENT MEDICAL CONDITION (allergies, prescription medications taken, medical treatments) _____

TESTED FOR HIV, TUBERCULOSIS, OTHER COMMUNICABLE DISEASES? _____

IV. BEHAVIORAL/PSYCHOLOGICAL/SOCIAL ASSESSMENT

MENTAL STATUS

APPEARANCE _____
ORIENTED (TIME, PLACE) _____
MOOD/AFFECT _____
MEMORY (RECENT/REMOTE) _____
THOUGHT PROCESS/DELUSIONAL THINKING _____
CURRENT RISK TO SELF OR OTHERS? _____
HISTORY OF MENTAL HEALTH PROBLEMS (treatment, hospitalizations, medication) _____

FAMILY OF ORIGIN

FAMILY COMPOSITION (parents, sibilings, others) _____
PRIMARY LOCATION OF RESIDENCE DURING CHILDHOOD OR ADOLESCENCE _____
DESCRIPTION OF CHILDHOOD (abuse or neglect, substance abuse in the family) _____
RELIGIOUS/ETHNIC/CULTURAL BACKGROUND _____

continued

CURRENT FAMILY

NAME AND AGE OF SPOUSE/SIGNIFICANT OTHER _____

NAMES AND AGES OF DEPENDENT CHILDREN _____

DESCRIBE CURRENT LIVING ARRANGEMENTS _____

DESCRIBE CURRENT FAMILY RELATIONSHIPS/FUNCTIONING _____

ABUSE OR NEGLECT ISSUES? _____

DESCRIBE FINANCIAL STATUS _____

SOURCES OF SUPPORT (identify nature and extent of coping skills)

PEER/SUPPORT GROUP _____

RELIGIOUS INVOLVEMENT _____

SELF-HELP GROUP (AA, NA, other) _____

RECREATIONAL ACTIVITIES _____

OTHER SOURCES OF SUPPORT _____

LEGAL INVOLVEMENT

DUI CHARGES _____

OTHER ALCOHOL/DRUG-RELATED CHARGES AND DISPOSITIONS

_____

NON-ALCOHOL-DRUG CRIMINAL OR CIVIL CHARGES _____

PENDING LEGAL INVOLVEMENT OR COURT DATES _____

IS SUBSTANCE ABUSE TREATMENT MANDATED? _____

DESCRIBE CONDITIONS OF PAROLE, PROBATION, SUPERVISION

_____

_____

IV. TREATMENT RELATED CONSIDERATIONS

LEVEL AND NATURE OF MOTIVATION FOR TREATMENT _____

ISSUES OF INSIGHT OR DENIAL OF SUBSTANCE ABUSE/DEPENDENCE

ASSESSMENT OF SUPPORT SYSTEM _____

OTHER FACTORS AFFECTING TREATMENT _____

SUMMARY AND RECOMMENDATIONS FOR TREATMENT _____

_____

notions about their clients based only on information gleaned from the initial interview. Consequently, clients being interviewed at agencies specializing in substance abuse should not automatically be diagnosed as chemically dependent or alcoholic just because they were referred to the agency.

Discussion Question: What do you think are the strengths and limitations of qualitative information gained from interviews?

Role-Play: Pair up with another student; one person plays the part of Joe the disabled traffic light installer, the other plays the role of intake interviewer following the outlines provided for the intake and substance abuse interviews.

STANDARDIZED TESTS

Frequently, intake and interview procedures are augmented by the use of standardized psychological tests. In fact, there are a number of published interview instruments available that are designed especially for clients with substance abuse disabilities. These include the Comprehensive Drinker Profile (CDP; Miller & Marlatt, 1984), the Opiate Treatment Index (OTI; Darke, Hall, Wodak, Heather, & Ward, 1992), and the Addiction Severity Index (ASI; Fureman, Parikh, Bragg, & McLellan, 1990). Some of these protocols will contain scoreable items that are meant to aid in making a diagnosis of substance abuse or dependence.

True psychological tests are divided into a number of areas such as personality, intelligence, aptitude, achievement, and interests. Tests that address substance abuse or addiction fall within the personality realm and typically consist of self-report items that are answered true-false, agree-disagree, or some other format that describes information about the test taker's behaviors or feelings about himself or herself. There are a large number of substance abuse tests on the market, some focusing on alcohol, others that screen for substance abuse or dependence in general. The results of these and similar tests are interpreted in the light of data supporting their reliability and validity—concepts related to the test's objectivity and standardization.

Reliability Test reliability refers to the test's consistency in producing scores for a particular person. If test scores for one individual varied markedly with multiple administrations of the same test, the results would be useless since there would be no way to determine which score was accurate. Hence, reliability or consistency is a minimum requirement for a test to be useful. There are a number of different ways to examine a test's reliability; the most straightforward is the test-retest method. This approach simply gives the same test to the same group of people on two separate occasions. The scores of each administration are then correlated, and the correlation coefficient is an estimate of the test's consistency or reliability; in this case the reliability is an estimate of the amount of error that occurs in test scores over a particular time period. Other methods of examining reliability include alternate form, split-half, internal consistency (Kuder-Richardson formula), and inter-scorer. Each of these methods examines different aspects of the test's consistency and sources of error. With the exception of internal consistency, which produces coefficient alpha (α) , these methods produce the correlation coefficient r as an estimate of reliability. Both α and r may vary from 0 to + 1.0, with 0 indicating no consistency and + 1.0 indicating perfect (error-free) consistency. The closer the correlation coefficient is to + 1.0, the more consistent or reliable the test. Power (1991) characterized the level of reliability correlations as follows:

.80 to 1.0 = Very high correlation

.60 to .79 = Substantial correlation

.40 to .59 = Moderate correlation

.20 to .39 = Little correlation

.01 to .19 = Practically no correlation

Information on a test's reliability should always be presented in the test's manual. Generally, tests with reliability coefficients below .60 or .70 (depending on what trait is being measured) are not consistent enough to have practical value to the counselor.

Validity Validity refers to what a test purports to measure and how well it measures it. It is best to think of validity in terms of the test's intended use rather than the test itself. Tests vary in terms of the validity of their use—a test may be very valid for a particular purpose, moderately valid for related uses, and not valid at all for others. For example, a test of reading comprehension might be very valid for determining the grade level at which a client reads, moderately valid at predicting how well the client would do on job tasks that require extensive reading, and minimally valid in estimating a client's intelligence. To examine the validity of a test, we usually compare test performance (scores) with other independently observable facts about the behavior that we are interested in measuring. For example, a test used to diagnose substance abuse ought to be able to correctly classify people who have been diagnosed as having or not having a substance abuse disorder, using some external criteria, such as a psychologist's evaluation based on DSM-IV standards. This type of validity would be referred to as concurrent validity because it relates to classifying people in a group to which they currently belong. Other types of validity include predictive validity, which estimates a test's ability to make predictions about future performance or behavior; construct validity, which estimates the test's relationship to the construct or constructs it claims to measure; and content validity, or the test items' relationship to the content domain of interest. All of these types of validity involve examining the test's items or scores with external evidence tied to what the test purportedly measures.

Validity, because it is a more complex construct than reliability, is not generally estimated with a single statistic. Rather, validity should be examined in a number of ways, some of which may involve statistics such as a correlation coefficient. The ultimate level of a test's validity depends on how the counselor uses the test and the nature and extent of the evidence that supports that use. Although test manuals present information examining the test's reliability and validity, the test user is encouraged to use other sources of information to examine these properties. Professional journals on substance abuse will occasionally publish articles on tests; additionally, there are journals that are devoted to examining testing and evaluation in a wide spectrum of areas including substance abuse. Perhaps one of the better sources to consult is the *Buros Mental Measurement Yearbook,* a continuously updated source of independent reviews of many published tests. When examining these and other sources that describe test validity, the counselor should always keep in mind how he or she plans on using a particular test and look for evidence that supports or contradicts that use.

With the information on test reliability and validity in mind, the following is an overview of some of the most commonly used tests of substance abuse or dependence. The tests to be reviewed are the CAGE, Michigan Alcoholism Screening Test, the Substance Abuse Problem Checklist, the MacAndrew Alcoholism Scale, and the Substance Abuse Subtle Screening Inventory.

CAGE

The CAGE is probably the shortest self-report screening test for alcoholism in use today. It consists of only four items that ask the following questions about alcohol use: "Have you ever felt the need to **C**ut down?"; "Do you feel **A**nnoyed by people complaining about your drinking?"; "Do you ever feel **G**uilty about your drinking?"; and "Do you ever drink an **E**ye-opener in the morning to relieve the shakes?" (the acronym CAGE is taken from the first letters of the words cut, annoyed, guilty, and eye-opener). Two or more affirmative responses to the four items places the person in the potential problem drinker group. Using cut scores of two or more, the CAGE was able to correctly identify 75 percent of a group of people with a diagnosis of alcoholism, demonstrating that the CAGE has adequate sensitivity. Further, the CAGE showed excellent specificity by correctly classifying 96 percent of a nonalcoholic group (National Institute on Alcohol Abuse and Alcoholism, 1987).

Because of its straightforward, undisguised item content, the validity of the CAGE depends on the test-takers' honest responses to items. Essentially, the CAGE is a very quick, rough screening device that has found its best application in very busy settings such as emergency rooms or urgent care centers, where there is little time to interview people in depth (Allen, Eckardt, & Wallen, 1988). Positive results from the CAGE should be used to identify people who may be at risk for a drinking problem and could therefore benefit from a more thorough substance abuse evaluation.

Michigan Alcoholism Screening Test

The Michigan Alcoholism Screening Test (MAST) is one of the popular tests for alcoholism having been in use since 1971 (Selzer, 1971). It is a self-report inventory consisting of 24 scoreable items (one item is not scored) that are responded to by indicating either "Yes" or "No." All items deal with either drinking patterns; social, occupational, or medical aspects of drinking; or previous attempts at substance abuse treatment. Scoring items involves assigning weights from 0 to 5 to each item response, depending on the response's relationship to alcoholism. The majority of items have a weight of 2 if answered in the alcohol problem direction. Scores on the MAST may range from 0 to 53 with higher scores indicating alcohol problems. These are some examples of MAST items:

Does your wife, husband, a parent, or other near relative ever worry or complain about your drinking? (Item weight = 1)

Can you stop drinking without a struggle after one or two drinks? (Item weight = 2)

Have you ever attended a meeting of Alcoholics Anonymous? (Item weight = 5)

The MAST's results are evaluated in two ways: (1) sensitivity, or the percentage of positive item responses, which result in a diagnosis of alcoholism, and (2) specificity, or the percentage of negative item responses, which result in a nondiagnosis of alcoholism. A score of 20 on the MAST is considered to be indicative of severe alcoholism, but scores as low as 5 have been used to indicate alcoholic drinking. Four points is suggestive of alcoholic drinking, and 3 points or less is indicative of nonalcoholic drinking. Seltzer indicates that the MAST is very sensitive at the 5-point level and tends to find more people alcoholic than anticipated; however, he argues that the MAST is a screening device and should be sensitive at the lower levels.

The internal consistency of the MAST has been reported to be very high (alpha = .95). Miller (1976) has argued that its use has been consistently supported by empirical evaluations. Allen et al. (1988) indicated that studies on the MAST's validity found that it correctly classifying alcoholics and nonalcoholics with accuracy rates in the .80s and .90s.

An abbreviated version of the MAST has also been developed (Pokorny, Miller, & Kaplan, 1972). The Short Michigan Alcoholism Screening Test (SMAST) consists of 17 of the most discriminating items in the MAST. Scores on the SMAST have a high correlation with the MAST (r = .83), and it is considered to be very easy to use (Selzer, Vinokur, & Van Rooijen, 1974). Because it relies on fewer items but continues to use 20 points or more to indicate severe alcoholism, the SMAST is less likely to produce false positive results, or classifying nonalcoholics as alcoholics.

One of the major criticisms of both the MAST and SMAST is their susceptibility to a response bias or the ease in which results can be faked by participants who want to appear alcoholic or nonalcoholic. The scoring direction of each item is readily apparent, with even unsophisticated test takers being able to discern item direction (the alcoholic or nonalcoholic responses to items). Alcoholics who are in denial or problem drinkers who are defensive about their alcohol usage could easily choose their responses to make themselves appear nonalcoholic, just as nonabusers could manipulate responses to make themselves appear to be alcoholics if they so wished. Hence, like the CAGE, the validity of MAST and SMAST rests largely upon the honesty of the test-taker. Research on the honesty and accuracy of alcohol abusers' self-reports of their drinking and related behaviors indicates that there are certain conditions that increase the reliability and validity of responses. Generally, test results are more likely to be valid when the test is given in a clinical or research setting, when the client is not under the influence of alcohol, and when the client has been given assurances of confidentiality (Sobell & Sobell, 1990).

Substance Abuse Problem Checklist

The Substance Abuse Problem Checklist (SAPC), unlike the CAGE, MAST, or SMAST, focuses on more than just alcoholic drinking and includes items related to other drug use. It is a comprehensive self-report checklist consisting of 377 items addressing a variety of problematic behaviors. Items are grouped into eight categories:

1. Problems related to motivation for drug treatment
2. Health problems
3. Personality problems
4. Problems with social relationships
5. Job-related problems
6. Problems related to misuse of leisure time
7. Religious or spiritual problems
8. Legal problems

One of the advantages of the SAPC is its problem identification emphasis, which is beneficial to the development of treatment plans. According to Lewis, Dana, & Blevins (1994), the SAPC benefits clients by including them as an active collaborator in the treatment process, in addition to its use as a diagnostic and research tool. People taking the SAPC must be able to read and understand English; further, problem behaviors may be easily concealed by those wishing to do so, again calling into question the validity of test results of people who may consciously or unconsciously manipulate responses to obvious items.

MacAndrew Alcoholism Scale

The MacAndrew Alcoholism Scale was developed as a diagnostic device used for determining the presence and severity of alcoholism (MacAndrew, 1965). The 49 items that comprise the scale were taken directly from the Minnesota Multiphasic Personality Inventory (MMPI). The MMPI (currently revised as the MMPI-2) is the most widely used personality inventory in use to diagnose a variety of personality disorders or social and personal maladjustment (Power, 1991). All MacAndrew Scale items are answered either true or false and address a wide range of behaviors, most of which are not obviously linked to alcoholism. The test was developed, similar to the MMPI, using an empirical-criterion keying approach. MacAndrew examined the responses of 300 male alcoholic outpatients and 300 nonalcoholic male psychiatric outpatients to identify which MMPI items were able to distinguish between the two groups. Essentially, MacAndrew found that of the 567 MMPI items, 51 items were able to discriminate between the alcoholic and nonalcoholic groups; in other words, these items were consistently answered by the alcoholic group in one direction (either true or false) and consistently answered in the opposite direction by the nonalcoholic group. Two items were dropped from the scale because each had an obvious relationship with alcohol use, reducing the test to 49 items.

Each item is scored either 0 (indicating a nonalcoholic response) or 1 (indicating an alcoholic response), so scores may vary from 0 to 49. Total scores of

24 or more are generally considered to be at the threshold level, indicating the presence of an alcohol problem. Threshold or cut-score levels, however, may vary between 24 and 28 points, depending on such factors as treatment setting (Uecker, 1970), age (Friedrich & Loftsgard, 1978), and gender (Clopton & Klein, 1978). Since the MMPI was designed to screen for a wide variety of mental health–related problems, none of the items asks questions directly related to alcohol use. These are some examples of MacAndrew Alcoholism Scale items:

> My parents have often objected to the kind of people I went around with.
>
> I am certainly lacking in self-confidence.
>
> I readily become one hundred percent sold on a good idea.

In terms of the Scale's psychometric properties, its reliability has been shown to be good (MacAndrew, 1965), and numerous studies have demonstrated its ability to correctly classify alcoholic and nonalcoholic groups and even predict the development of alcoholism. Hoffman, Loper, & Kammeier (1974) examined the MacAndrew Scale scores of alcoholic men who had completed the MMPI an average of 13 years earlier, as part of their freshman entrance process into college. The scale was able to distinguish between those people who later sought alcoholism treatment and their non-alcoholic peers; the scale had a 72% accuracy rate using a cut score of 26 to classify participants. In general, the MacAndrew Scale doesn't measure the results of misusing alcohol; rather it seems to measure personality traits associated with, although not exclusive to, alcoholism. High scorers on the scale may be described as bold, self-confident, sociable, and somewhat rebellious. They may also be characterized as hedonistic, extroverted, and nonconforming. Further, these people are drawn to religion and use repression and faith to curb their defiant impulses (Finney, Smith, Skeeters, & Auvenshine, 1971), a trait that Alcoholics Anonymous support groups seem to capitalize on. MacAndrew (1981) argued that the high scores on the scale indicate a reward-seeking orientation, whereas low scores on the scale have an orientation to avoid punishment. Very low scores on the scale have in fact been found to be related to severe psychiatric diagnoses. People without alcoholic or psychiatric diagnoses tend to produce scores in the midrange level (Apfeldorf & Hunley, 1981).

Because of its focus on personality factors related to alcoholism, rather than directly addressing the consequences of alcoholic drinking, the MacAndrew Scale has been considered to be somewhat less valid than other paper-and-pencil devices. Nonetheless, its resistance to faking makes it an excellent tool when dealing with clients who are in denial or are defensive about their drinking behavior (Allen et al., 1988).

Substance Abuse Subtle Screening Instrument

The Substance Abuse Subtle Screening Instrument (SASSI), like the MacAndrew Scale, is designed to guard against response bias or faking (Miller, 1985). Unlike the MacAndrew Scale, the SASSI is meant to identify substance abuse in general, in addition to alcoholism. The SASSI is a self-report inventory with a purported fifth-grade reading difficulty. It consists of two divisions, the SASSI subtle items and the Risk Prediction Scales (RPS) for Alcohol and Other Drugs (also referred to as the Face Valid Alcohol and Face Valid Other Drug scales). The subtle items of the SASSI are 52 true-false questions that appear to be unrelated to substance use or abuse. The RPS contains 12 alcohol-related and 14 other drug-related items that directly address chemical use, so the items are referred to as "face valid" and depend on honest responses for valid results.

SASSI items were developed from a number of other tests, including the MMPI, the Psychological Screening Inventory, and the MAST, as well as other sources that were thought to produce items that differentiated between abusers and nonabusers. The 52 subtle items are related to a variety of behaviors pertaining to health, social interaction, emotional states, preferences, needs, interests, and values—all of which are answered with true or false. Here are some examples of SASSI's subtle items:

I have avoided people I did not wish to speak to.

I am a worrier.

I have had days, weeks, or months when I couldn't get much done because I just wasn't up to it.

The face valid items directly address alcohol and other drug-related behaviors and are responded to with Never, Once or Twice, Several Times, and Repeatedly. Here are some examples of face valid alcohol items:

Had drinks for lunch?

Argued with your family or friends because of drinking?

Become nervous or had the shakes after sobered up?

These are examples of face valid other drug items:

Taken drugs to improve your thinking and feeling?

Gotten really stoned or wiped out on drugs (more than just high)?

Spent your spare time in drug-related activities (e.g., talking about drugs, buying, selling, taking, etc.)?

Six subscales are produced by the SASSI items:

1. The Obvious Attributes Scale (OAT) measures openness and willingness to admit symptoms or problems or substance abuse.

2. The Subtle Attributes Scale (SAT) uses fake-resistant items to measure the predisposition to develop dependency on drugs and alcohol.

3. The Denial (DEN) identifies defensiveness to taking the SASSI—high scores indicate denial, while low scores are associated with feelings of worthlessness.

4. The Defensive Abuser versus Defensive Non–Abuser Scale (DEF) is used in conjunction with the Denial scale to determine if the person is a substance abuser, whether or not responses are those of a defensive nonabuser.

5. The Alcohol versus Drug Scale (ALD) indicates a preference for either alcohol or drugs.

6. The Family versus Controls Scale (FAM) is a preliminary measure of codependency, indicating how similar the test taker is to family members of alcohol and drug abusers.

Research has consistently supported the reliability and validity of the SASSI, especially when the six scales are used in conjunction with the two RPS or face valid scales. The test-retest reliability of the SASSI was reported to range from .76 (FAM) to .91 (SAT). Validity data on the SASSI indicated that of 459 substance dependent subjects, 88 percent were correctly classified, while 12 percent were incorrectly classified (Miller, 1985). Very similar results were reported for nonabusers: Of 249 subjects, 88 percent were correctly classified, and 12 percent were incorrectly classified. The SASSI is most valid when used with late-stage abusers who are already involved in treatment and therefore considered nondefensive; it was able to correctly identify 90 percent of this group. When used with early-stage abusers who are more defensive, the SASSI was able to correctly classify 80 percent of the group (Miller, 1985). In an independent study, DiNitto and Swabb (1991) were able to use the SASSI to correctly classify 87 percent of rehabilitation clientele who had primary or secondary substance abuse diagnoses. In a study of construct validity, the SASSI produced a correlation with the MacAndrew Alcoholism Scale of .87 (Cooper & Robinson, 1987); it should be noted that this result is expected because some of the SASSI items were borrowed from the MacAndrew Alcoholism Scale. Kerr (1994) in her review of the SASSI concluded, "The SASSI fits its population well; it does seem to accurately identify those who are denying or obscuring their substance abuse. . . ." (p. 251).

Discussion Questions: Which do you think is more helpful in understanding clients: qualitative information gained from interviews or quantitative information gained from standardized tests? Why?

DIAGNOSING SUBSTANCE ABUSE
AND DEPENDENCE

The ultimate diagnosis of substance abuse or dependence relies on the criteria set out in the *Diagnostic and Statistical Manual-IV* (DSM-IV), published by the American Psychiatric Association in 1994. The aim of the DSM-IV is to provide a useful and credible tool, supported by an extensive empirical foundation, to be used for clinical, research, and educational purposes. According to the American Psychiatric Association:

It (the DSM-IV) is used by psychiatrists, other physicians, psychologists, social workers, nurses, occupational and rehabilitation therapists, counselors, and other health and mental health professionals. DSM-IV must be useable across settings—inpatient, outpatient, partial hospital, consultation-liaison, clinic, private practice, and primary care, and with community populations. (p. xv)

The DSM-IV uses a multiaxial classification system to diagnosis any mental disorder. Each axis refers to a different domain of information that should be helpful in treatment planning and the prediction of outcomes. There are five axes used to make a comprehensive and systematic evaluation of the client.

Axis I—Clinical Disorders, Other Conditions That May Be a Focus of Clinical Attention

This axis includes the entire classification of mental disorders not attributable to personality disorders or mental retardation, plus other conditions that may be a focus of clinical attention. If a client has more than one condition, all disorders are listed under Axis I, with the principal disorder being listed first. The severity of the condition may be characterized as *mild* (few if any symptoms), *moderate* (symptoms or impairment greater than mild but less than severe), *severe* (excessive symptoms or symptoms resulting in marked social or occupational impairment), in *partial remission* (full criteria had been previously met but currently only some symptoms persist), in *full remission* (no longer any signs or symptoms of the disorder remain), or *prior history* (having a history of the criteria for a diagnosis, even when the person is considered to have recovered). If no Axis I condition exists, the diagnosis should be listed as No Diagnosis (V71.09) or deferred (799.9). Adult-onset substance use or abuse will be listed under Axis I, such as Alcohol Dependence (303.90), Alcohol Abuse (305.00), Amphetamine Dependence (304.40), or Cannabis Abuse (305.20).

Axis II—Personality Disorders and Mental Retardation

Axis II is used for the diagnosis of disorders with an onset in childhood or adolescence that persists in a stable form into adult life. It is very common for clients with substance abuse or dependence disorders to have such Axis II diagnoses as Dependent Personality (301.6) or Antisocial Personality (301.7). Axis II serves to ensure that the clinicians do not overlook the possible presence of a personality disorder or mental retardation that might be ignored because of the more pronounced symptoms or florid Axis I disorder.

Axis III—General Medical Conditions

Axis III is used to report any physical disorder relevant to understanding or managing the individual's mental disorder. It should be noted here that the separate axis for physical or general medical conditions doesn't imply that they are unrelated mental conditions; rather the purpose of the separate axis is to encourage thoroughness and facilitate communication between health care providers. For people with substance dependence disorders, it is common to find Axis III conditions such as Organic Brain Syndrome, Cirrhosis of the Liver, or Pancreatitus.

Axis IV—Psychosocial and Environmental Problems

Any psychosocial or environmental problems that affect the diagnosis or treatment of the client is listed on Axis IV. The problem should have occurred within one year of the evaluation and could include a variety of problems existing in such areas as work, school, support group, social environment, housing, finances, access to health care, and interactions with the legal system/crime. It is common to find Axis IV problems of DUI conviction, unemployment, or divorce when evaluating people with substance abuse or dependence disorders.

Axis V—Global Assessment of Functioning (GAF)

The GAF is the clinician's judgment of the overall functioning of the client. It is common for ratings to be made of both current functioning (at the time of the evaluation) and the highest functioning in the last year. A scale from 0 to 100, in increments of 10, is used to characterize the GAF:

   1 to 10 = Persistent danger to severely hurting self or others

   11 to 20 = Some danger to hurting self or others

   21 to 30 = Behavior influenced by delusions, hallucinations, or serious impairment in communication or judgment

   31 to 40 = Some impairment in reality testing or communication or major impairment in work, school, family relations, judgment, thinking, or mood

   41 to 50 = Serious symptoms

   51 to 60 = Moderate symptoms

   61 to 70 = Mild symptoms

   71 to 80 = Transient symptoms or expected reactions to stressors

   81 to 90 = Absent or minimal symptoms, good functioning in all areas

   91 to 100 = Superior functioning

   0 = Inadequate information

The DSM-IV recognizes an important issue in the conceptualization of mental disorders. The term "mental" disorder implies an unfortunate distinction or separation from "physical" disorders that is reductionist and overly simplistic. In reality, "there is much 'physical' in 'mental' disorders and much 'mental' in 'physical' disorders" (American Psychiatric Association, 1994, p. xxi). This is especially true for substance abuse and dependence, where the distinction between the disease/physical process and conscious/willful behavior is very blurred.

The DSM-IV sets out diagnostic criteria for every known mental disorder, including substance-related disorders. Substance disorders are grouped into 11 classes: alcohol; amphetamines or similarly acting sympathominetics; caffeine; cannabis; cocaine; hallucinogens; inhalants; nicotine; opioids; phencyclidine

(PCP) or similarly acting arylcyclohexylamines; and sedatives, hypnotics, or anxiolytics. Also included are sections on polysubstance dependence and other or unknown substance-related disorders. These disorders entail taking drugs of abuse, the side effects of prescribed drugs or medications, and exposure to toxins. The substance-related disorders are further subdivided into substance-use disorders (substance abuse and substance dependence) and substance-induced disorders (substance intoxication, withdrawal, delirium, persisting dementia, persisting amnestic, psychotic disorder, mood disorder, anxiety disorder, sexual dysfunction, and sleep disorder).

The types of information listed under each diagnosis are intended to systematically describe the disorder using nine categories: diagnostic features; subtypes and/or specifiers; recording procedures; associated features and disorders; specific culture, age, and gender features; prevalence; course; familial pattern; and differential diagnosis. For example, the following information is listed under 304.30 Cannabis Dependence (DSM-IV, 1994, pp. 215-221):

1. Diagnostic features include compulsive use that generally occurs without the development of physiological dependence, although tolerance to the effects of cannabis has been reported in many individuals who use chronically. Withdrawal from cannabis has never been shown to be clinically significant.

2. Subtypes and specifiers indicate that cannabis dependence may be specified with or without physiological dependence, early full or partial remission, sustained full or partial remission, and in a controlled environment.

3. No recording procedures are identified under cannabis dependence.

4. Associated features and disorders indicates that cannabis is often used with other drugs, especially nicotine, alcohol, and cocaine. Regular use is associated with mental lethargy and anhedonia (a loss of interest in or pleasure from activities). Laboratory tests usually are able to find cannabinoid metabolites, and cannabis smoke is highly irritating to the nasopharynx and bronchial lining, increasing the occurrence of chronic cough.

5. Specific culture, age, and gender features report that cannabis is probably the most widely used illicit drug and is among the first drugs of experimentation (often in teenagers). Cannabis disorders occur more often in males, and the prevalence is most common in the age group of 18 to 30 years.

6. Prevalence rates are based on a 1991 community survey in the United States and indicated that about ⅓ of the population have used marijuana one or more times during their lifetime; 10 percent used in the last year, and 5 percent used within the last month.

7. The course of cannabis dependence or abuse typically develops over an extended time period; however, few data are available on the long-term course of abuse or dependence.

8. The familial pattern of cannabis dependence or abuse is not presented.

9. Differential diagnosis notes that cannabis-induced disorders may be characterized by symptoms similar to a primary mental disorder (e.g., reported symptoms of anxiety are similar to a generalized anxiety disorder). Chronic cannabis use can produce symptoms mimicking dysthymia (mild, long-standing depression), and acute adverse reactions produce symptoms similar to panic disorder, major depressive disorder, delusional disorder, bipolar disorder, or schizophrenia-paranoid type.

In order to make a diagnosis under substance-related disorders, the clinician must use one of two classifications: Psychoactive Substance Dependence or Psychoactive Substance Abuse. The diagnostic criteria of dependence may be applied to all 11 classifications of substances. For a diagnosis of psychoactive substance dependence to be made, the client must demonstrate, within the past 12 months, a maladaptive pattern of substance use that leads to a significant impairment or distress, meeting three or more of the following seven criteria:

DSM-IV—The Seven Criteria for Psychoactive Substance Dependence

1. Tolerance, as defined by either of the following:
   a. A need for markedly increased amounts of the substance to achieve intoxication or desired effect
   b. Markedly diminished effect with continued use of the same amount of the substance

2. Withdrawal, as manifested by either of the following:
   a. The characteristic withdrawal syndrome for the substance . . .
   b. The same (or a closely related) substance is taken to relieve or avoid withdrawal symptoms

3. The substance is often taken in larger amounts or over a longer period than was intended.

4. There is a persistent desire or unsuccessful efforts to cut down or control substance use.

5. A great deal of time is spent in activities necessary to obtain the substance (e.g., visiting multiple doctors or driving long distances), use the substance (e.g., chain-smoking), or recover from its effects.

6. Important social, occupational, or recreational activities are given up or reduced because of substance use.

7. The substance use is continued despite knowledge of having a persistent or recurrent physical or psychological problem that is likely to have been caused or exacerbated by the use of the substance (e.g., current cocaine use despite recognition of cocaine-induced depression, or continued drinking despite recognition that an ulcer was made worse by alcohol consumption) (DSM-IV, 1994, p. 181).

The Case of Sandy

Sandy is a single female who lives alone. She injured her lower back at her job as a nurse's aide. She was transferring a 110-pound resident from a bed to a chair when she heard a popping sound and felt a sharp pain in her lower back. Sandy's treating physician, Dr. Loeback, diagnosed Sandy as having a herniated disc at the L4-5 level. After conservative treatment (rest, medication, and physical therapy) with no improvement, Dr. Loeback performed back surgery (a laminectomy). Sandy tolerated the procedure well but continues to report persistent lower back pain and occasional pain radiating into her right leg. Sandy is now receiving worker's compensation benefits, is not currently working, and spends all day at home watching TV and resting. She has refused to take prescription pain medication because she is afraid of becoming addicted; rather, when her back is "acting up," she prefers to drink a glass of wine, which she uses to wash down over-the-counter aspirin. Sandy says that this combination not only makes her back less painful, but it's good for her heart, too. Sandy soon discontinued taking aspirin because it upset her stomach, but she increased her wine consumption to two glasses a day. Her back pain persisted, and she is now "forced" to drink a bottle of wine over the course of a day. Sandy is now wondering if she should try taking prescription pain medication.

The DSM-IV sets out similar criteria for substance abuse, but it does not include criteria for tolerance, withdrawal, or a pattern of compulsive use. Rather, the client has demonstrated only harmful consequences of repeated use within the past 12 months. Harmful consequences include meeting at least one of the following criteria: (1) repeated failure to meet major role obligations at school, work, or at home (e.g., repeatedly missing work); (2) recurrent use in physically hazardous situations (e.g., drinking and driving); (3) multiple legal problems (e.g., arrests for substance-related disorderly conduct); and (4) continued use despite persistent or recurrent social and interpersonal problems that are caused or exacerbated by the effects of the drug. Further, to make a diagnosis of substance abuse, the client must never have met the criteria for substance dependence in the particular class of drug being evaluated.

Discussion Question: The DSM-IV diagnostic criteria assesses alcohol/drug dependence from a mental health perspective. Is this consistent or inconsistent with the disease model of alcoholism and addiction?

ASSESSMENT ISSUES FOR PEOPLE
WITH OTHER DISABILITIES

There are a number of factors that must be recognized when conducting substance abuse assessments with people with disabilities. When conducting a rehabilitation intake or interview, it is important to keep in mind that certain disability groups have higher than average rates of substance abuse. People with diagnoses of head or spinal cord injuries are typically young males, a group with higher rates of substance abuse; further, the onset of their disability may have resulted from behaviors while under the influence of alcohol or drugs. People with mental illness also have higher than expected rates of substance abuse. Because of the interrelationship between mental illness and substance abuse, this disability group is referred to as dually diagnosed. A common practice of people with dual diagnoses is to use street drugs to "self-treat" symptoms related to such problems as depression, schizophrenia, or bipolar disorders. Clients with learning disabilities also have higher rates of substance abuse due to stress caused by failure in school, lack of appropriate coping skills, and dysfunctional peer groups. People with mental retardation, however, have been found to have lower than average rates of substance abuse (Moore & Li, 1994).

The amount of drug use, in terms of what is considered to be acceptable use or abusive use, may vary, depending on the type of disability present. For example, certain coronary, kidney, respiratory or liver conditions will make the use of any psychoactive substance dangerous, and even minimal amounts of use is unacceptable unless it's under the direction of a physician.

Despite the complications that certain disabilities add to alcohol and drug use, many rehabilitation counselors are reluctant to examine the substance use of their clients. This may be due to enabling attitudes that cause the rehabilitation counselor to believe that drug use, if present, may be a minor problem in the face of a major physical disability. Another difficulty is caused by the necessity of prescription drugs use for treating certain kinds of disabilities. When disabilities cause chronic pain, the symptoms are commonly treated with the use of prescription narcotics. The rehabilitation of these clients is complicated when appropriate drug use becomes abusive or dependent in nature. Traditionally rehabilitation counselors do not receive training in substance abuse or dependence; hence, they may miss the signs and symptoms of a drug problem in their clients. Further, drug use may be masked by functional limitations associated with certain disabilities. For instance, slurred speech, imbalance, incoordination, and weight loss caused by drinking may be erroneously attributed to a client's disability. A study by DiNitto and Schwab (1993) of Texas rehabilitation clients found that undetected substance abuse is a substantial problem in rehabilitation clients. Using the Addictions Severity Index (ASI) to evaluate 86 rehabilitation clients with no substance abuse diagnosis, the authors found that 33 (38 percent) met the ASI criteria for alcohol or drug problems. Similar results were found with the SASSI, where 35 (25 percent) of 138 clients with no substance abuse diagnoses where classified as chemically dependent or chemical abusers.

Fortunately, rehabilitation counseling has begun to recognize substance abuse as an important rehabilitation issue. In 1990 over 23,000 (11 percent) of clients who were successfully closed from vocational rehabilitation services in the United States had primary diagnoses of substance abuse or dependence, with an additional 8000 (4 percent) having had secondary substance abuse disabilities (DiNitto & Schwab, 1993). In 1994 the Commission on Rehabilitation Counselor Certification (CRCC) formally recognized the significance of substance abuse to rehabilitation when it created a subcertification in substance abuse to the Certified Rehabilitation Counselor (CRC) credential.

Testing Issues

The use of standardized tests on people with disabilities is an issue that has received attention in the professional literature, as well as being singled out in the Rehabilitation Counselor Code of Ethics (Commission on Rehabilitation Counselor Certification, 1987). The code of ethics states, "Rehabilitation counselors shall promote the welfare of clients in the selection, utilization, and interpretation of assessment measures" (Commission on Rehabilitation Counselor Certification, 1987, p. 4). The specific rules under the assessment canon go on to indicate that caution must be used when evaluating and interpreting the performance of people with disabilities because they are not typically represented in the standardized norm groups of tests.

Regarding the use of standardized tests of substance abuse and dependence, test norms typically do not include disability populations for purposes of comparison or interpretation. This means that clients with disabilities are being compared to nondisabled norm groups, which may affect the meaning of test results. Further, the administration procedures for most tests require the client to read and respond to "paper-and-pencil-type" items. When administering tests that require reading, it is necessary to establish the reading difficulty of the test as well as the reading comprehension level of the client to ensure that the client is capable of understanding test items and completing the test correctly. People with mental retardation, learning disabilities, or attention deficit disorders are likely to have difficulty reading, understanding, or attending to written items, hence reducing their ability to correctly respond to test questions. These problems may be remedied by having someone read the test and record the client's oral responses, but this procedure would violate the test's standardization and the presence of the other person may alter the client responses, making the interpretation of results difficult. The rehabilitation counselor code of ethics cautions when it is necessary to make modifications for clients with disabilities, or when unusual behavior or irregularities occur during testing, the counselor must note these conditions and take them into account when interpreting test results (Commission on Rehabilitation Counselor Certification, 1987). In addition, it is important to note that many people with disabilities (including those with substance abuse or dependence) often have a past record of frustration and failure in academic or educational situations that may lead to "test anxiety" and the anticipation of failure when completing tests. High levels of test anxiety and a negative mind-set will make it difficult for clients to attend to test items and can adversely affect test performance.

Another limitation to the use of standardized tests on people with disabilities is the inferences drawn from certain types of test items. Tests such as the MacAndrew Alcoholism Scale and the SASSI rely on items derived, in part, from the MMPI. Like the MMPI, these items ask questions about behaviors such as loss of consciousness, shaking hands, feelings of fatigue that are indicative of a problems with substance abuse. The responses of clients with such disabilities as epilepsy, Parkinsonism, or chronic fatigue syndrome may be more accurately attributed to the presence of their disabilities rather than their personality or substance use.

In conclusion, the use of tests with people with disabilities is an important component of a comprehensive component. The interpretation of test results, however, must be done with caution. When the test user is required to violate the test's standardized procedure because of a client's disability, the use of published norm groups for the test's intrepretation is called into question. Further, the presence of a disability can alter the meaning of test scores, especially for those tests that attribute client responses to substance use or abuse, rather than the functional limitations of a disability. All of these factors must be considered and controlled for using standardized tests on clients with disabilities.

Discussion Questions: How do you feel about confronting someone with a physical disability about a suspected drinking or drug problem? Do you have any feelings of hesitancy? If so, where do those feelings come from?

SUMMARY

This chapter reviewed concepts basic to understanding assessment. Assessment was defined as a broad process of collecting client information throughout the rehabilitation process in an effort to identify functional limitations, goals, and services needed to achieve goals. Evaluation was a more focused component of assessment designed to address questions related to specific areas of client functioning; vocational, educational, psychological, and substance abuse are typical types of evaluations. Testing was the most specific term defined as an objective, standardized measure of a sample of behavior.

Intake interviews are usually the first type of assessment done, and the approach recommended by this text categorized client information into medical, psychological, personal-social, educational, and vocational realms. A typical initial interview outline was presented as a way to standardize the interview and gather information about client functioning in major life areas. A more focused substance abuse interview form was also presented to be used with clients with suspected substance abuse problems.

A review of the psychometric properties (reliability and validity) of tests was presented along with a review of the most popular paper-and-pencil tests of substance abuse. The CAGE is a very short initial screening measure designed to identify clients who may need a more thorough assessment. The Michigan Alcohol Screening Test (MAST) is probably one of the most widely used tests of alcoholism, but it is limited by its obvious items. The Substance Abuse Problem Checklist focuses on more than just alcoholic drinking and includes items related to other drug use. It is a comprehensive self-report checklist consisting of a large number of items addressing a variety of problematic behaviors. The MacAndrew Alcoholism Scale is an instrument based on the

Minnesota Multiphasic Personality Inventory (MMPI) and uses personality to assess the presence or severity of alcohol problems. The Substance Abuse Subtle Screening Instrument (SASSI), like the MacAndrew Scale, is designed to guard against response bias or faking. Unlike the MacAndrew Scale, the SASSI is meant to identify substance abuse in general in addition to alcoholism.

The ultimate diagnosis of substance abuse or dependence relies on the criteria set out in the *Diagnostic and Statistical Manual-IV* (DSM-IV); its purpose is to provide a useful and credible tool, supported by empirical foundation, to be used for clinical, research, and educational purposes. It uses a multiaxial classification system to diagnosis any mental disorder, including psychoactive substance abuse or dependence. Substance disorders are grouped into 11 classes: alcohol; amphetamine; caffeine; cannabis; cocaine; hallucinogens; inhalants; nicotine; opioids; phencyclidine (PCP); and sedatives, hypnotics, or anxiolytics. The diagnostic criteria for both dependence and abuse were presented.

The many assessment-related issues to consider when conducting substance abuse assessments with people with disabilities were examined. These factors included certain disability groups having higher than average rates of substance abuse; the amount of drug use in terms of what is considered to be acceptable use or abusive use, which vary depending on the type of disability present; and the difficulty encountered in diagnosing substance abuse in people with disabilities due to the masking effects of disability symptoms, enabling attitudes of health care professionals, and the inappropriateness of standardized testing procedures with people with disabilities.

10

Treatment Planning, Case Management, and Managed Care

CHAPTER 10 OUTLINE

TREATMENT PLANNING

Traditional substance abuse treatment planning typically involved the tasks of confronting the client's denial of substance abuse or dependence, educating him or her about the disease concept of addiction, inpatient counseling based on the 12-Step model (AA) of substance abuse, and referral to a 12-Step program, such as AA or Narcotics Anonymous (NA), for follow-up or aftercare. The treatment goal for all clients was always the same: lifetime abstinence from alcohol or psychoactive drugs (Morgan, 1996). According to Miller (1992), the substance abuse treatment field is in a state of transition. The old, uniform approach to treating all substance abuse clients that once dominated the field is on its way out, and treatment designed to meet the unique needs of the individual is gaining popularity.

Plan development in the field of rehabilitation has differed from traditional substance abuse treatment planning in that, in rehabilitation, goal selection and plan development are individualized and result in a written, signed document that incorporates both client and environmental information. The practice of putting the plan in writing has a long history in rehabilitation counseling; the Rehabilitation Act mandated the use of individualized written rehabilitation programs (IWRPs) in 1973. Each IWRP must be signed by both the counselor and the client and, at a minimum, contain the following:

1. The financial responsibilities for the services to be provided

2. Counselor and client responsibilities in the rehabilitation process

3. The long-term goal and intermediate objectives toward the goal

4. Services to be provided

5. Criteria and procedures for evaluating progress

6. An annual review for as long as the case is open

7. Closure information such as the reason for case closure and the client's status

These components are the essence of an organized, purposeful rehabilitation plan. Because of its detail and the active involvement of the client in its development, the rehabilitation plan requires considerable time and effort on the part of both the counselor and client and results in a unique document for each client (Wright, 1980).

Treatment plans are central to the rehabilitation process; the plan crystallizes the rehabilitation program, making clear the roles and responsibilities of the people involved, as well as the ultimate goal(s) and the steps to be taken to achieve them. In substance abuse treatment, an effective treatment plan should have, at a minimum, certain essential characteristics or elements that facilitate client success. These characteristics make the treatment plan, in both content and style, comprehensive, positive, realistic, sequential and specific, and measurable.

A *comprehensive* treatment plan should address all of the major needs of the client related to his or her rehabilitation. Although substance abuse rehabilitation in not meant to be a panacea or universal answer to all of the client's problems, neither should it be narrowly focused on just "resolving" the client's drinking or drug use problem. Comprehensive substance abuse treatment plans should be holistic; in addition to dealing with drug use, plans must address interrelated life areas such as physical health, emotional well-being, vocational functioning, family relationships, financial status, and leisure activities. For many clients, these areas are significantly and adversely affected by the client's substance abuse. Experience has shown that even after the reduction or cessation of substance abuse, clients can still benefit from help in these other areas. It is apparent that comprehensive treatment planning must integrate resources across disciplines and utilize multiple-service agencies. Therefore, treatment plans must not only articulate needed change but the agents of that change as well. A well-constructed, comprehensive treatment plan will serve as the central guide to all parties who are participating in the client's rehabilitation.

Treatment plans should be framed in *positive* terms, focusing on both client strengths and the solutions to their problems, rather than on client limitations and barriers to success. Plans that focus only on the limitations of clients and the barriers to goals are more likely to be discouraging, rather than encouraging, and result in failure. Treatment plans ought to respect client worth and dignity and avoid elements that may be stigmatizing or demeaning to clients. It is also important to remember that most substance abuse treatment involves the client giving up something—for example, the cessation of drug use, loss of lifestyle and coping mechanism, and loss of an excuse for being a victim or having a failure identity. Behavioral psychology has long held that when behaviors are extinguished, new ones rise to fill the void. It is important that when drinking or drug use behaviors are removed, new, positive, and functional behaviors should be identified and created. Treatment planning, therefore, should always emphasize the new behaviors, lifestyle, family functioning, and other gains that will be made with successful treatment.

Treatment plans must identify goals or objectives that are attainable or realistic in nature. *Realistic* goals are those that have a high probability of success, given adequate client motivation and professional participation. According to Egan (1990), a goal is realistic if (1) the resources necessary for its accomplishment are available to the client; (2) external circumstances do not prevent its accomplishments; (3) the goal is under the client's control—meaning that, although the client may use services or other sources of support, ultimately it is the client who has the power to change behavior and achieve the goal; and (4) the cost of accomplishing the goal isn't too high—meaning that the benefits of achieving the goal outweigh the costs to the client in changing.

Locke and Latham (1984) argued that the use of realistic goals helps clients in at least four ways: (1) they focus client attention and result on action, giving clients a vision toward which they can direct their energies and reduce aimless behavior; (2) they mobilize client energy and effort, beginning client movement; (3) they increase client persistence, prompting the client to do something and to work harder and longer because behavior is goal directed; and (4) goals motivate the client's search for strategies or a means to accomplish them.

The fourth component in treatment planning is the use of steps that are both *specific and sequential*. Treatment plans ought to clearly state the sequence of events that must logically occur in order to reach the desired behavior or goal. Plans that are too global or nonspecific (e.g., the client will use drugs less often or will achieve sobriety) result in unorganized and ineffective client behavior and in progress that is difficult to evaluate. Sequential steps leading toward a clearly defined goal ensure that client activities are purposeful and reinforcing. Creating success is an important first step for many clients who may have experienced multiple failures in their lives. Working toward a difficult, major life goal can be intimidating, especially for those people who have experienced past failures in trying to control their drug use behavior. When goals are broken down into sequential substeps, the client is allowed to develop a sense of mastery and encouragement as each subgoal is reached (Jarvis, Tebbutt, & Mattick, 1995). Typically, treatment plans should have timelines that provide checkpoints to evaluate client progress. There is, however, no such thing as a standard timeframe for every client; some things must be done immediately, others are midrange, and still others are long-term.

The progress and outcomes of treatment plans should be *measurable;* each goal, and its subgoals or objectives, should clearly identify the behavior that shall occur and how the desired change will be evaluated. Measuring progress is an important incentive to clients and ensures that the counselor is being accountable for the work done with clients. If possible, the plan should use quantifiable measures. If it isn't possible to use numbers to quantify progress, then establish some other clear and objective criteria for measuring progress. For instance, the goal of "drinking in moderation" could be operationalized by identifying the maximum number of drinks to be allowed in one sitting and

---

The Case of Ernest

Ernest was referred to intensive outpatient substance abuse treatment in part because of his third DUI conviction. He admits having problems recently both at home and on the job and feels that these stresses over the past four years contributed to his drinking. He admits that he has a problem with alcohol and that he's been using it as a way to cope with (or more precisely escape from) his problems. He has been open and honest with his counselor and with other people who attend his treatment groups about the nature and extent of his drinking problems and the other problems in his life. He is willing to work on both his drinking and personal problems and accept the help offered to him in treatment. He does not, however, want to commit to abstinence as a treatment goal. He states that he is 49 years old and feels that he was drinking responsibly from age 21 until he turned 45, when his drinking patterns changed. He wants a treatment plan that specifies controlled drinking at a level consistent with his preabuse habit (usually 1 or 2 drinks per day, never drinking more than 14 drinks in a week and never drinking more than 3 or 4 drinks in a sitting). He wants to try this plan for one month. If he can't follow it, Ernest states that he will have proved that he can no longer drink socially and will commit to abstinence as a goal.

the maximum total number of drinks per week. The goal of "getting a steady job in the food service field" could be measured by the number of job applications to be completed each week and the number of job interviews completed each month. The goal of reducing family discord could be measured by independent evaluations by each family member before (baseline) and after (follow-up) treatment or counseling.

Discussion Question: Traditional substance treatment planning had abstinence from alcohol or drug use for *every* client. What are the advantages and disadvantages, in terms of treatment planning, of this uniform treatment goal?

CASE MANAGEMENT

Definitions and Background

The implementation of a comprehensive treatment plan requires that it is monitored, evaluated for progress, and modified if needed; this process is commonly referred to as case management. Case management, in the broadest sense of the term, is the process of facilitating and coordinating the movement of each client through his or her rehabilitation program. Although related, case management should be distinguished from the term *caseload management,* which is the responsibility of the counselor for efficient management of the entire group of clients constituting the counselor's caseload. In other words, caseload management entails observation, tracking, and documentation relevant to all the clients carried by a particular counselor, whereas case management concerns the counselor's referral-coordination and monitoring efforts done to help each client move toward the rehabilitation goal (Wright, 1980).

There is a lack of consensus regarding the definition of case management because its practices have been applied in a number of social service fields and settings. Here are some examples of various case management definitions found in the literature:

"The counselor's capability to guide the client through the rehabilitation process from intake to case closure" (Roessler & Rubin, 1992, p. ix)

"A set of logical steps and a process of interaction within a service network which assures that a client receives services in a supportive, effective, efficient, and cost effective manner (Weil & Carls, 1985, p. 2)

"Reintegrating the mentally ill with the community" (Bagarozzi & Kurtz, 1983, p. 13)

"Helping people whose lives are unsatisfying or unproductive due to the presence of many problems which require assistance from several helpers at once" (Ballew & Mink, 1986, p. 3)

"Monitoring, tracking and providing support to a client, throughout the course of his/her treatment and after" (Ontario Ministry of Health, 1985)

"The counselor's managerial activities that facilitate the movement of each rehabilitant through the service process" (Wright, 1980)

"An approach to caring for the multiple needs of persons with chronic disabling conditions" (Johnson & Rubin, 1983)

"A creative and collaborative process involving skills in assessment, counseling, teaching, modeling, and advocacy that aims to enhance the optimum social functioning of clients" (Sullivan, Wolk, & Hartmann, 1992, p. 198)

Further complicating the issue is disagreement on who should perform case manager duties and how they should be trained (Austin, 1983; Bagarozzi & Kurtz, 1983; Patterson, 1957). Because it has been applied to differing client populations, with disparate problems and varying goals, there will likely be continued variance in defining the exact nature of case management. Despite these variations, case management is viewed as a flexible approach to dealing with many different client populations, problems, and settings and is particularly useful in addressing problems that are complex, intransigent, or persisting over long periods of time (Willenbring, Ridgely, Stinchfield, & Rose, 1991), all of which are characteristic of substance abuse disabilities. Willenbring et al., however, cautions:

> Vaguely conceptualized, case management can seem like a panacea, a solution for all complicated and protracted problems. Even worse, implementing case management may be used as a substitute for providing more definitive, but essential, services, such as housing, medical care, and alcohol and drug treatment. . . . Poorly conceptualized application of case management is also difficult to evaluate. . . . (p. 1)

Case management arose out of social work and the mental health fields as an attempt to deliver social services in an integrated and comprehensive way to clients with multiple, complex problems (Mejta et al., 1994). The deinstitutionalization movement that swept through mental institutions in the United States during the 1970s was meant to help people with disabilities by emphasizing freedom, independence, individuality, mobility, and a high degree of interaction with the general community (Shoenfeld, 1975). However, removal from the institution resulted in the need for close coordination, consisting of the identification of programs that could provide needed services, timely referral to those programs, and follow-up of service provision (Wright, 1980). Hence, by the late 1970s, case management became a formally recognized service for people with severe and persistent mental illness, and specific models of case management were being developed and evaluated beginning in the early 1980s (Rapp, 1996).

Case managementlike tasks for people with alcohol- or drug-related problems were historically carried out by a number of social service providers. Skid row mission workers, priests, church workers, court service workers, probation officers, and nurses would often provide outreach, assessment, referral/linkage, and follow-up to their clients or charges (Willenbring et al., 1991). Recently, there has been much interest in applying case management concepts, in a systematic way, to the field of alcohol and drug treatment.

Discussion Questions: What is more important to you as a student or human service professional: providing the treatment that will help your client cope with his/her drinking/drug problem or helping your client with coping with other problems that he/she faces at work, in the home, or in school? Is it possible to treat these two realms as mutually exclusive or independent from one another?

Case Management and Substance Abuse Treatment

Until the mid-1970s and early 1980s all substance abuse treatment was conducted based on one of three models: 12-Step Alcoholics Anonymous (AA), therapeutic community, or methadone maintenance for opiate addictions (Rotgers, Keller, & Morgenstern, 1996). People who were referred to substance abuse treatment were typically sent to 28-day, inpatient (residential) programs that would consist of detoxification, the provision of psychoeducational information about substance abuse, and "treatment" based on the 12-Step model of AA. Case management under this system was uniform and straightforward, requiring little of the treatment staff in the way of time, energy, or skill. Under this model, case management involved managing the client's inpatient stay so that individual, group, and family counseling could be provided in an orderly fashion, and, external to the treatment facility, the client would be linked up with a local AA or NA (Narcotics Anonymous) group.

The disease model has dominated substance abuse treatment, sanctioned by such eminent and powerful bodies as the American Medical Association, the American Psychiatric Association, and the World Health Organization. The model's limitations, however, have been identified—primarily its failure to attend to improving social functioning, life satisfaction, and enhanced employability. The classic disease model held that substance abuse and addiction was a primary condition that led to progressive secondary deterioration in important life domains such as employment, family relationships, mental health, and even spirituality (Jellinek, 1960). Since the disease was considered to be the cause of all of the client's problems, disease treatment and subsequent abstinence of use should logically and automatically lead to improvement in these other life areas. Many concerns, however, have been raised about the societal, organizational, and management implications of treatment based on a strict disease concept paradigm (Fingarette, 1988; Heather & Robertson, 1981, Peele, 1990). In practice many clients did not experience improvement in these life areas, even after treatment and abstinence. Siegal et al. (1995) noted that the clinical management or disease model approach to treatment has been criticized because it may not meaningfully address the myriad of problems that substance abuse clients often have and may even intensify many of the problems that it was meant to address. Sullivan, Wolk, and Hartmann (1992), however, argued that case management is an appropriate complement to traditional alcohol and drug treatment that can help address client outcomes in multiple life areas, in addition to helping maintain alcohol or drug abstinence.

Today, substance abuse treatment has become more varied and complex in nature. It has been characterized as a field in transition; transition resulting from the paradox of treatment being successful for many clients yet having little, if any, long-term benefit for other clients (Rotgers et al., 1996). Research has demonstrated that "traditional" substance abuse treatment focusing solely on achieving alcohol or drug abstinence has been ineffective with certain types of clients. Willenbring et al. (1991) identified the following groups as being less responsive to traditional alcohol and drug treatment:

> More severe forms of alcohol or drug dependence
>
> Coexisting medical or psychiatric conditions
>
> Severe disability in multiple areas of life
>
> Socioeconomic disadvantage
>
> Lack of formal educational accomplishment
>
> Unemployment and poverty
>
> Alienation from the larger society
>
> More extensive public service utilization
>
> Problems present for long periods (chronicity)
>
> Age, gender, and/or cultural differences (p. 5)

Siegal et al. (1995) argued that a case management approach can offer a clinical and/or programmatic enhancement to traditional substance abuse treatment. Siegal et al. believed that the addition of case management addresses at least three areas of concern for traditional substance abuse treatment. First, the role of the counselor in the disease model has been very directive. Because the counselor or treatment professional has assumed the responsibility for prescribing and implementing all therapeutic activities, the client has had a very restricted role in goal setting or planning his or her rehabilitation. This often resulted in the client having little ownership and investment in his or her rehabilitation or recovery program. Treatment was something done "to" clients rather than "with" clients. Second, treatment based on the disease model also focused on pathology and illness. This emphasis results in detailing the client's past failings and mistakes, so client limitations are well defined, but assets or strengths are all but ignored. Such an approach may alienate clients and cause them to drop out of treatment before they have had a chance to experience success. Third, substance abuse treatment has traditionally been delivered in hospitals or professional offices, making it more difficult for clients to access treatment and restricting the generalizability of treatment interventions; in other words, treatment has been separated from the normal course of clients' lives. These limitations are each countered by a case management approach because it emphasizes client involvement in treatment planning, focuses on client assets or strengths in planning, and often takes place in vivo with the counselor seeing clients in their homes or wherever services are being delivered.

Major Models of Case Management

There have been a large number of case management models developed, most of which evolved out of mental health treatment. Weil and Karls (1985) described four popular case management models: the generalist service broker, primary therapist, interdisciplinary team, and comprehensive service center models. The generalist service broker model involves a case manager controlling the entire case management process, assessing the need for particular services, and identifying the potential sources of those services. The client and/or family member is then given responsibility for obtaining the services. The primary therapist model relies on the client's therapist or counselor to provide case management services, along with therapy or counseling. The interdisciplinary team model uses several case managers as a team in which each specializes in a particular case management function. The comprehensive services center model uses centers to provide a wide variety of services to clients, and all services are orchestrated by the centers' staffs. Weil and Karls (1985) noted that the case management model selected by or for a client would depend on the client population's needs and the organization's and service network's resources.

Robinson and Bergman (1989) reviewed four case management models that have come to dominate the mental health field: the broker model, rehabilitation model, the Assertive Community Treatment (ACT) model, and the Strengths model. To investigate the effectiveness of these four models, and Rapp (1996) reviewed the research documenting client outcomes under each model.

The broker model conceptualizes the case manager as a "broker" of services, assessing client needs and identifying needed services and the sources of those services—and placing most of the responsibility on the client or a family member for actually obtaining them. According to Rapp (1996), there have been six studies evaluating programs based on the broker model; the results indicated that clients tend to do no better or worse on 12 of 20 indicators of client functioning. Rapp concluded that the broker model does not produce benefits for clients or reduce hospitalization rates.

The rehabilitation model emphasizes client goals and needs, rather than preestablished system goals. Case management under this model evaluates client skill deficits that act as barriers to achieve personal goals, then teaches the requisite skills for achieving goals. Only one study of the rehabilitation model was identified; it found increases in vocational functioning, leisure time activities, and independent living. However, no differences were found in the rate of hospitalization. Rapp (1996) concluded that there was insufficient data to form a conclusion on the effectiveness of the rehabilitation model.

The Assertive Community Treatment (ACT) model of case management stresses active involvement with clients to improve their level of functioning in the community. One of its hallmarks is the provision of case management services "in vivo" where the client lives or receives services instead of in the case manager's office. The model is meant to be proactive (anticipating needs and services rather than waiting for problems to arise), using individualized treatment and interventions provided directly by the case manager, who teaches clients about identifying and managing their symptoms and maintains small client-to-staff ratios. Rapp (1996) found 17 studies investigating the ACT model and concluded that it reduced client hospitalizations, and in no study did ACT clients fare worse than control groups. Uneven but promising results were also found on such variables as vocational functioning, independent living, and quality of life.

Finally, the Strengths model of case management is designed to capitalize on client strengths, rather than focusing on limitations or deficits. The case manager helps identify client strengths and actively creates personal and environmental situations where success can be reached and personal strength enhanced. This model holds that human behavior is significantly affected by the resources available to individuals, and that a pluralistic society values equal access to resources. The Strengths model stands on five principles: (1) facilitating the use of clients' strengths, abilities, and assets; (2) encouraging client control over the search for needed resources; (3) promoting the client and case manager/advocate relationship as primary; (4) viewing the community as a resource and not a barrier; and (5) advancing case management/advocacy as an active, assertive endeavor. Rapp (1996) identified six studies on the Strengths model of case management, all of which had consistently positive results. Although the research lacked experimental replication, Rapp argued that the promising results were resilient across studies and that the Strengths model produced positive outcomes in areas where the ACT model results were mixed (e.g., improved social functioning, leisure time, vocational functioning).

Components of Effective Case Management

Recently, case management approaches have been used in pilot programs with clients of substance abuse treatment programs, including veterans (Rapp & Chamberlain, 1985), intravenous drug users (Mejta & Bokos, 1992), opiate abusers at high risk for HIV (discussed in Mejta et al., 1994), and prison parolees (Inciardi, Isenberg, Lockwood, Martin, & Scarpitti, 1992). Overall, the results of these studies are encouraging, demonstrating that case management, when integrated with traditional substance abuse treatment, can improve client outcomes. Several authors (Agranoff, 1977; Austin, 1983; Levine & Fleming, 1985; Phillips, Kemper, & Applebaum, 1988; Willenbring et al., 1991) have concluded that case management approaches resulting in successful outcomes have a number of components in common, including assessment, planning, linkage, monitoring and evaluation, and client advocacy.

Assessment is understood to be the process of identifying client strengths and limitations in the context of optimal outcomes or client functioning. One of the dangers of assessment in the substance abuse field is the salience of client problems and the obstacles confronting them; this often results in an assessment that focuses solely on the substance abuse and its concomitant problems. Because client limitations are often very pronounced (e.g., poor or no vocational history, financial burdens, health problems, current uncontrolled substance use, unpredictable or unreliable behavior), client strengths are all but ignored. Regardless of the problems confronted by clients, it is important to also identify and even focus on client assets and resources that will encourage and help them during the course of their rehabilitation. Further, because of their similar problems, assessments of substance abuse clients may become uniform (in both style and content) and result in reports and recommendations that are highly similar from one client to the next. Good assessment procedures should result in a characterization of the client that is unique, using both quantitative (e.g., tests) and qualitative (e.g., observations) information. The assessment should also be holistic and balanced—that is, it deals with a number of important areas besides substance use (e.g., vocational, social, psychological) and identifies both client strengths and limitations in the context of his or her future goals.

Assessment is the basis for planning. According to Sullivan et al. (1992), "If the assessment process is geared toward an identification of the special attributes, resources, strengths, and needs of clients, the case plan that follows will also be individually tailored" (p. 199). Rehabilitation plans should have, at a minimum, certain essential characteristics. As discussed earlier in this chapter, rehabilitation plans must be comprehensive, positive, realistic, sequential and specific, and measurable. Client involvement is the key to the development of successful rehabilitation plans because it engenders client ownership of plan. Since the client is responsible for much of the work and certainly all of the behavior change that occurs in his or her rehabilitation, it is vital that he or she embraces the plan as something important that will result in a valued improvement.

Linkage pertains to the procurement of services for clients and is a core function of case management; it should be conceptualized as an expansion of substance abuse treatment, rather than just an attempt to coordinate existing referral services (Sullivan et al., 1992). According to Crimando (1996), for referral sources to be of value, they must meet at least four criteria:

> They must be capable of providing a needed service or commodity.
>
> They must be willing to enter into a relationship in which those services and commodities can be purchased or otherwise secured.
>
> They must be located in a place that is geographically accessible.
>
> They must have attainable (to us or our clients) eligibility requirements. (p. 7)

The types of referral sources and the services utilized will vary tremendously, depending on the community, client needs, and knowledge of the case manager. Crimando and Riggar (1996), in their text *Utilizing Community Resources: An Overview of Human Services,* organized referral sources into seven groups: health and diagnostic services (e.g., home health services), social services (e.g., security income), rehabilitation services (e.g., work-hardening centers), vocational and employment services (e.g., employment security-job service), legal services and advocacy (e.g., guardianship and advocacy), education (e.g., adult education), and human services (e.g., housing and urban development). The nature and extent of services that are incorporated into a client's rehabilitation plan will depend on the strengths and limitations of the client in the context of his or her goals and the resources that exist within the community.

The monitoring and evaluation of referral services (such as job-seeking skills training, physical therapy, housing assistance, self-help support groups) require regular formal and informal communication between the case manager and the service providers. The case manager is, in fact, the central figure in the cast of service providers, monitoring client progress and ensuring that services are delivered in a timely fashion and lead to desired outcomes. In case management, evaluation consists of both process and product measures (Sullivan et al., 1992). Process measures provide information about program efficiency (e.g., were job-seeking skills training services delivered when promised?), whereas product measures determine whether the services lead to the desired results (e.g., did the client get more job interviews as a result of job seeking skills training?). Monitoring and evaluation may result in the modification of the rehabilitation because of information and experience gained from its implementation.

Finally, advocacy relates to the case manager's responsibility to identify, prevent, or combat discrimination and bias that confront clients recovering from alcohol and/or drug abuse. Advocacy means that the case manager will speak on behalf of a person or an issue in an effort to obtain entitled rights and services that other citizens enjoy. In addition to the case manager's efforts, advocacy may be enhanced through the use of human and civil rights agencies, legal aid programs, ombudsman offices, crisis intervention centers, centers of independent living, and consumer support networks. One of the strongest advocacy mechanisms for people with disabilities is the Americans with Disabilities Act (1990). It is a national mandate for eliminating discrimination against people with disabilities and provides enforceable standards against disability-based discrimination in the areas of employment, public services, accommodations, and telecommunications (there are restrictions, however, on employment discrimination against people who are currently abusing alcohol or drugs).

The implementation of case management activities is affected by a number of factors. These factors may be grouped into structural factors, such as who is responsible for case management, and service factors, such as how case management is implemented. Rapp (1996) detailed the structure and service requirements that he believed were directly related to effective case management:

Structure

1. Team structure for the purpose of creative case planning, problem-solving, sharing knowledge of resources, and support to team members.

2. Team leaders/supervisors should be experienced, mental health professionals.

3. Case managers can be paraprofessional (e.g., BA level) but need access to specialists; involvement of nurses seems particularly important.

4. Caseload sizes can vary based on client severity, geography, etc., but should never exceed 20:1. The average across-program clients should probably be 12–1 to 15–1.

5. Efforts should be made to enhance the continuity of relationship between the client and case manager.

6. Clients need 24-hour, 7 days a week access to crisis and emergency services. That service should require access to staff who have familiarity and a relationship with the client (can be and perhaps should be the case manager).

7. Pre-services, in-service, and technical assistance would be available.

8. Length of case management services should be indeterminate and expected to be on-going (although intensity at any point in time would vary).

Service

1. Case management contact with clients should be in-vivo (limit office-based contacts).

2. Frequency of in-vivo client contact will vary based on the client but should average across clients a minimum of six contacts per month. This should be supplemented by telephone and collateral contacts.

3. Case managers should deliver as much of the "help" directly as possible.

4. Referrals to traditional mental health programs (e.g., partial hospitalization, day treatment, in-office counseling, sheltered and many transitional employment programs, congregate housing, etc.) should be avoided.

5. The use of naturally occurring community resources (landlords, employers, coaches, neighbors, churches, friends, clubs, junior colleges, etc.) should be encouraged.

6. Case managers should have ultimate responsibility for client services (with the exception of medication). They retain authority even in referral situations.

7. Clients should be given equal or greater authority than case managers or other professionals in treatment and life decisions with the exception of hospitalization decisions. (pp. 29–31)

MANAGED CARE ISSUES

A case management approach to the delivery of health and human services is very consistent with newly emerging managed care programs. Managed care is rapidly becoming the dominant structure of treatment delivery and third party payment being placed upon health and human service providers by both federal/state governments (e.g., Medicaid) and private insurance companies (e.g., health maintenance organizations). These are the primary funding sources for the providers of substance abuse treatment; therefore, the very nature of

---

The Case of Wanda

Wanda has been referred to a community-based substance abuse treatment center for an evaluation because her social worker found drug paraphernalia (roach clips, pipe, and rolling papers) at a recent home visit. Wanda readily admits to smoking marijuana almost on a daily basis but states that she doesn't have a problem with pot. What she really needs help with is getting a job and getting off welfare. She tells you that even if she can get a job (which she doubts because she dropped out of school in the 11th grade and hasn't held a full-time job in her life), she'll need to find a way to get to and from work, find someone to take care of her kids while she's at work, and get help with cooking and house cleaning.

---

substance abuse treatment is being altered by the conditions being placed upon it by managed care.

Managed care is a way of organizing services that emphasizes the coordination of care among health team members; it is the organization of unit-based care, so that treatment results may be reached in a fiscally responsible time-frame while using resources that are appropriate (in amount and sequence) to the particular case type and the patient needs. Although there are variations, managed care programs usually involve insurance companies offering benefits such as prepaid financing, comprehensive service, an organized delivery system, and a predefined service population (Hale & Hunter, 1988). Hale and Hunter identified three major characteristics of managed care plans: (1) they offer a product or products that integrate both financing and management in the delivery of health care services; (2) they directly employ or contract with an organized provider network that either shares financial risk and/or has some other incentive to deliver services in a cost-efficient manner; and (3) they use an information system to monitor and evaluate patterns of financial outlays and service usage.

Case Management Under Managed Care

Managed care programs for substance abuse treatment evolved during the late 1980s and early 1990s, with case management being identified as the primary approach to promote quality, cost-effective treatment. The growth of managed care has been dramatic. By 1991 the number of managed care enrollees numbered over 36 million; further, the number of employees covered by preferred provider organizations (PPOs) grew from 0 in the late 1970s to over 37 million in 1991 (MacLeod, 1995). Anderson and Berlant (1995) recommended that case managers, under managed care systems, be frontline staff with a minimum of five to ten years of clinical experience, who have specialized training in case management techniques, and who are supplemented by easily accessible doctoral-level advisors and clearly defined systems to support the case management task. They identified the case manager's primary tasks as the following:

1. Promoting correct diagnosis and effective treatment—assisting plan members to access the best level, type, and mix of treatment; keeping alert to opportunities for enhancing the quality and efficacy of care; acting to make provider and patient aware of these opportunities (. . . case management strives to direct patients into effective forms of treatment at appropriate levels of intensity).

2. Promoting efficient use of resources—helping the patient/family access the most effective resources with the minimum depletion of family finances and finite available insurance dollars (directing patients into effective care may be the most potent cost-saving method of all).

3. Preventing recidivism—monitoring progress subsequent to intensive treatment episodes; encouraging and, if necessary, helping arrange for interepisode care to prevent recidivism.

4. Monitoring for and containing substandard care—identifying potential quality of care defects during treatment; investigating and, when needed, intervening to ensure remediation. (p. 155)

Cost Effectiveness

The hallmark of managed care is its emphasis on improving cost effectiveness while attempting to maintain quality of care. In fact, insurance or funding schemes that adopt cost-control measures are often referred to as managed care plans. Cost effectiveness has been a hotly debated issue in substance abuse treatment, as evidenced by the attention paid to it by the popular media. *Time* magazine reported in a February 5, 1996, article that the substance abuse treatment field has been criticized because the arbitrariness of the traditional month-long inpatient stays didn't make clinical sense, and frequently the treatment ended when the limit was reached on the patient's insurance coverage (Gleick, 1996). Anderson and Berlant (1995) noted that substance abuse treatment facilities created some of their own problems with the influx of private hospitals drawn into the field because of high profit margins and cheap capital investment. These programs would take advantage of the lifting of certificate of need laws and exception from diagnosis-related groups; many of them would aggressively advertise their programs, often masquerading commercials as public service announcements.

Under managed care, substance abuse rehabilitation facilities are required to offer a range of treatment alternatives, such as shorter residential stays, reduced nursing care or medical supervision, and day treatment alternatives, such as partial hospitalizations and ambulatory care programs. Anderson and Berlant (1995) indicated that many managed care plans limit coverage for inpatient detoxification and substance abuse rehabilitation. As evidence of this, Gleick (1996) reported that the average number of inpatient substance abuse treatment bed days had dropped from an average of 32 days in 1988 to 17 days in 1993.

Clearly the social and economic costs of substance abuse and dependence are extremely high. Estimates have ranged up to $115 billion per year in lost productivity, accidents, injury, medical care, and substance abuse treatment (Rice, Kelman, Miller, & Dunmeyer, 1990). Not surprisingly, studies have consistently shown that money spent on substance abuse treatment, especially for the newly identified alcoholic, is cost effective—meaning that the reductions in total health care costs are greater than the costs of the treatment itself (McKay & Maisto, 1993).

Recent research has shown, however, that more expensive treatment modalities may not be as cost effective when compared to their less expensive alternatives. One of the most extensively researched areas in substance abuse treatment has been treatment setting, specifically examining whether expensive inpatient care is more effective than less costly, nonresidential treatment options. Miller and Hester (1986) reviewed a number of studies examining inpatient versus noninpatient alcohol abuse treatment. For most alcoholics, inpatient treatment was not found to be superior to other less costly settings such as day treatment, halfway houses, or other outpatient treatment. Longabaugh (1988) found that patients who are randomly assigned to longer stays in residential treatment programs did not have better drinking outcomes than those who were assigned to shorter stays. Schene and Gersens (1986), in their review of the literature, concluded that partial hospitalization (i.e., evening treatment or weekend stays) and nonresidential treatment are viable alternatives to inpatient care. On the other hand, people with little social support or stability, more severe levels of abuse or dependence, or some degree of psychiatric comorbidity are appropriate candidates for more costly inpatient treatment (McLellan, Woody, Luborsky, O'Brien, & Druley, 1983; Miller & Hester, 1986; Nace, 1990; Orford, Oppenheimer, & Edwards, 1976). Further, people who engage in self-destructive behavior, are violent, or are suicidal will also require inpatient treatment (Miller, 1989; Nace, 1990).

Discussion Question: Does the shift to a managed care approach mean that costs/financial considerations have become more important than treatment/human considerations?

Patient–Treatment Matching

The diversity of research findings on substance abuse treatment effectiveness has led to the rise of patient-treatment matching, or the selective placement of patients into differing levels or types or treatment. Managed care embraces the concept of a "continuum of care." This concept holds that patient treatment needs change over time, often in a predictable fashion. Managed care plans typically require the use of a comprehensive program having a number of levels of care, typically detoxification (inpatient, noninpatient, residential, and outpatient), hospital rehabilitation, nonhospital residential rehabilitation, structured outpatient rehabilitation, and individual/group outpatient rehabilitation (Anderson & Berlant, 1995). Matching the proper intervention with current patient needs is hoped to lead to more effective and cost-efficient service delivery.

One comprehensive, medical-model-based patient matching system is the Cleveland Admission, Discharge, and Transfer Criteria. It uses a number of dimensions to place patients in varying levels of treatment, ranging from self-help programs up to inpatient hospital stays. Patient symptom or problem severity is evaluated on the dimensions of withdrawal severity, physical complications, psychiatric complications, life areas impairments, treatment acceptance, loss of control, and recovery environment (Hoffman, Halikas, & Mee-Lee, 1987). The logic behind the matching system is that patients with less serious problems will be referred to less intensive (and cheaper) treatment, while those with the most severe problems would receive the most intensive and expensive treatment (i.e., inpatient hospitalization). The Cleveland Criteria, however, are still in need of further refinement. McKay, McLellan, and Alterman (1992) found that some alcoholic patients treated in a day hospital met one or more criteria to be treated as inpatients (i.e., they were mismatched to day treatment), yet posttreatment follow-up found that the mismatched group was functioning at the same levels of those day hospital patients who had been properly matched.

Another patient-matching system that has been widely applied under the managed care system is published by the American Society of Addiction Medicine (ASAM). ASAM is an international specialty society of physicians from all areas of medicine who are involved with treatment, research, and education related to addiction. ASAM has published the second edition of the Patient Placement Criteria (PPC, 1996); it is the most widely used set of patient-matching criteria used in the United States. The PPC uses comprehensive national guidelines for patient placement, continued stay, and discharge of patients with alcohol and other drug problems. The PPC outlines two sets of criteria for either adults or adolescents, each with five levels of service. The levels of service for both groups are Level 0.5—Early Intervention; Level I—Outpatient Services; Level II—Intensive Outpatient/Partial Hospitalization Services; Level III—Residential/Inpatient Services; and Level IV—Medically-Managed Intensive Inpatient Services. An overview of services available for particular severities of addiction and related problems is presented at each level of care. The PPC also provides a structured description of the settings, staff, services, admission, continued service, and discharge criteria for six patient dimensions: acute intoxication/withdrawal potential; biomedical conditions and complications; emotional/behavioral conditions and complications; treatment acceptance/resistance; relapse/continued use potential; and recovery/living environment. ASAM argues that the terminology used in the criteria is consistent with the language of the DSM-IV, making it easier to use by clinicians and other treatment professionals (American Society of Addiction Medicine, available at http://asam.org under Patient Placement Criteria). Like the Cleveland Criteria, the PPC are appealing in their logic, but the criteria still require outcome validation data to support their use in improving treatment while cutting costs (Morey, 1996).

Facility Standards

In order to qualify for financial reimbursement, treatment providers must be able to meet the standards set down by the funding source or sources. Many health and human service treatment providers, including substance abuse treatment facilities, are banding together into "provider alliances" in an effort to be included in the corps of approved providers that are granted contracts and receive fee payments for services rendered. This often means that the treatment facility must "dance to the funding sources tune"; the tune comes in the form of quality assurance and treatment provider selection criteria.

Many treatment facilities, because of encouragement by managed care funding sources, are turning to brief therapy as a cost-effective alternative for substance abuse treatment. What constitutes "brief therapy" will vary markedly, depending on who is describing it. Babor (1992) outlined a number of brief therapy features in the context of substance abuse: (1) brief therapy is targeted to people with less severe dependence; (2) brief therapy may last from one to three sessions, with each session taking from 5 to 30 minutes; (3) it may take place in a variety of settings, including primary health care, outpatient com-

---

Typical Selection Criteria to Be Met by Both Substance Abuse and Mental Health Providers

Facilities
must provide a continuum of levels of care (not only acute inpatient)
average length of stay for acute inpatient cases < 10 days

Psychiatrists
accustomed to filling medication management role in conjunction with other therapists handling individual therapy
usual practice pattern involves referring patients to psychologists and social workers for individual therapy
work primarily with serious, complicated conditions

Psychologists
usual practice pattern involves referring to physician for medication evaluation when appropriate
do not routinely test all patients unless specifically indicated

Social workers
demonstrated experience in treating socio-familial issues
experienced with assessment, especially in community mental health center settings

Nurses
some general medical nursing experience
demonstrated current knowledge of psychopharmacology

All Practitioners
knowledge, experience, and training in goal-focused, brief therapy techniques
experienced in multi-disciplinary treatment approaches
routinely use peer support system to discuss difficult cases
demonstrated familiarity with community resources

SOURCE: Anderson & Berlant (1995); p. 159.

munity mental health clinics, or work settings; and (4) the goals of brief therapy are broadened to include both abstinence and moderate, nonproblematic use. Brief therapy tends to be oriented toward crisis management and employs a problem-solving, rather than personality-based, treatment orientation.

According to McKay and Maisto (1993), the research on brief therapy on substance abuse clients has some promising findings:

> First, brief interventions typically are more effective . . . than no intervention. Another result is that brief interventions also often have comparable effects to those of traditional, more intense, and longer-term programs. Furthermore, brief interventions have been shown to increase the effectiveness of later treatment. These results are surprising to many, and have significant implications for the delivery of alcohol treatment. In addition, the consistency of these findings across such diverse settings and intervention parameters lends confidence that brief therapy interventions have real effects. (p. 6)

Treatment facilities must adapt what they do to the insurance coverage if they expect reimbursement for their services. For better or worse, managed care will be a force that substance abuse treatment providers must reckon with, both in the present and the future.

SUMMARY

Treatment planning in the substance abuse field is changing. Historically, planning was the same for all clients: confrontation of the denial of substance abuse or dependence, education about the disease concept of addiction, inpatient counseling based on the 12-Step model (AA) of substance abuse, and referral to a peer support groups (e.g., Alcoholics Anonymous) follow-up or aftercare. Today, treatment planning must encompass all of the client's major needs (in addition to substance abuse), including vocational, educational, and family problems. In addition to being comprehensive, treatment plans should (1) be framed in positive terms; (2) identify goals that are realistic or attainable; (3) use specific, sequential steps that lead to goal attainment; (4) provide opportunity for the measurement of case progress.

Case management arose out of the social work and mental health fields and is being applied to substance abuse treatment. A number of different case management models have been developed, including the broker, rehabilitation, Assertive Community Treatment, and Strengths models. The characteristics of effective case management models have been identified as assessment, planning, linkage, monitoring and evaluation, and client advocacy.

Managed care has taken the health service industry by storm, and the substance abuse treatment field is no exception. Managed care plans are supportive of case management models and all managed care programs: offer products that integrate both financing and management of health care services, directly employ or contract with a provider who shares financial risks and incentives, and use an information system to monitor and evaluate patterns of costs and service usage. The major tasks of case managers under a managed care system are to promote correct diagnoses and effective treatments, efficient use of resources, prevention of relapse, and accountability by monitoring and containing care.

Managed care embraces the concept of a "continuum of care" and the proper matching of services to client needs. Patient-treatment matching in substance abuse has received a lot of attention in recent years. The American Society of Addiction Medicine (ASAM) has developed Patient Placement Criteria that have been widely applied throughout the United States. These criteria result in the placement of clients at one of five levels of service: Level 0.5—Early Intervention; Level I—Outpatient Services; Level II—Intensive Outpatient/Partial Hospitalization Services; Level III—Residential/Inpatient Services; and Level IV—Medically-Managed Intensive Inpatient Services. Many treatment facilities, in order to continue to receive financial reimbursement for their services, are implementing programs with varying levels of care and emphasizing brief therapies as an intervention strategy.

11

Special Populations

CHAPTER 11 OUTLINE

CULTURE AND ACCULTURATION

Culture binds society together and is a reflection of the manner in which that society represents itself to the world. Often, the dominant culture of a society is countered or supplemented by subcultures that reflect or reject the attributes of the dominant culture. However, culture is more than the surface representation of a group of people. It encompasses the customs, beliefs, values, knowledge, laws, norms, arts, history, language, folklore, and institutions of a group of people as a shared experience (Orlandi, 1992a). Objective, external elements (laws, institutions, and history) issues define culture, as do subjective, intangible, internal factors (norms, folklore, arts, and values).

Social norms, mores, and sanctions govern culture. Social norms are the shared rules and regulations of a group of people that define what is appropriate or inappropriate behavior. Some social norms are codified as laws and regulations by government and embrace a broad range of behaviors (jaywalking, burglary, rape, and murder). Other norms are codified by the institutions of society, particularly the religious institutions. The Ten Commandments of Judaism, the Five Pillars of Islam, and the Christian Beatitudes all represent normative systems of behavior that have influenced greatly the cultures of the world. Often religious normative systems served as the basis for the establishment of formal secular legal systems. As the world has become increasingly complex and intertwined, the clashes of religious normative systems become more apparent. Finally, norms are informally developed customs of a group of people. These informal norms may dictate social behavior (saying "please" and "thank you"), relational behavior (respect for elders, tolerating the behavior of children), and personal behavior (no belching in public). Frequently, informal norms serve to regulate drinking or drug-taking behaviors (no drinking before noon; happy hours; not drinking alone). Commonly, informal norms serve as the basis for laws and regulations, especially if they are supported widely. For example, the stricter laws governing drunk driving are a direct result of a group of informal social norms promoted by Mothers Against Drunk Driving (MADD). Informal norms may be uniform across the dominant culture, or they may reflect the beliefs of a segment of society or a distinct geopolitical element.

Discussion Question: Identify some broad societal norms about drinking and drug taking. Include both formal and informal norms. Do unique norms exist in your geographic area?

Mores represent the set of values and beliefs most cherished by a culture and with which the culture most identifies (Bellah et al., 1985). Symbols may represent mores (the flag as a symbol for patriotism) or behaviors (voting), or they may be ingrained in the lives of members of a culture (a sense of fair play). In some situations, mores evolve into formal codification such as civil rights laws or disability rights legislation.

Discussion   Identify the most important national mores in your country.
Question: Do drug and alcohol consumption mores exist? Identify and
                  discuss them.

Sanctions are the societally directed and imposed rewards and punishments
that compel people to comply with norms and mores. Some sanctions are formal, codified, and objective, including laws and regulations. In many situations,
individuals may face legal, civil, professional, and community jeopardy. For example, a rehabilitation counselor who is involved in a drunk driving accident
may face legal sanctions for violating laws against drunk driving. In addition,
the counselor may be sued in a civil action by individuals injured in the accident and may face loss of the Certified Rehabilitation Counselor Credential
for violating the Code of Ethics for Rehabilitation Counseling. Community
sanctions are usually a form of informal sanctions. The counselor may suffer
varying degrees of social disapprobation for committing an act that is inconsistent with community norms for a person of given stature or standing in the
community.

Discussion   Identify both formal and informal sanctions against drug and
Question: alcohol consumption in your community.

Not interacting with their culture is impossible for individuals. All behavior and all human experience occur within a social context, and innate human
characteristics, behavior, and the environment are in a state of dynamic interaction called reciprocal determinism. The actions of individuals determine the
actions of society, and the actions of society determine the actions of individuals. These individual–individual, individual–culture, and culture–culture interactions are both dynamic and evolutionary. They are continually changing and
evolving to differing levels of understanding and formality. For example, the
prohibitionist ideology of the 19th century evolved into the prohibitionist federal legislation of the 20th century. When prohibition failed, it was repealed as
a law, but vestiges of prohibition remain in local laws and community and individual attitudes and beliefs.

Discussion   Trace the dynamic and evolutionary processes affecting our
Question: sanctions for and against alcohol and drug consumption.

Culture is defined in many ways. One of the most basic definitions for culture is based in the old anthropological notion of race that divided the world's
peoples into three broad racial categories based on physical characteristics.
Members of the Negroid race dwelt in Sub-Saharan Africa; the Mongoloid
people included denizens of Asia and the indigenous peoples of the Ameri-
cas; and Caucasians included individuals from present-day Europe, Asia Minor, and Northern Africa. Race is also a biological classification. In truth, it is
a useful classification only if concerns exist about anatomical, structural, or

genetic differences among individuals and groups (Johnson, 1990). Race is
not very useful in the examination of cultural issues.

Ethnicity, a geopolitical, sociological term incorporating geographic ancestral place of birth, language characteristics, and political connotations has largely
supplanted *race* as a definer of an individual's cultural heritage. Occasionally ethnicity is synonymous with race; in other cases not. It achieves its importance or
its notoriety as a definer of subcultures within a larger culture. Thus, African
American designates individuals whose ancestral home was Sub-Saharan Africa
and who now reside in the United States. Euro-American is an ethnic designa-
tor for U.S. residents who are descended from individuals who resided in Europe. However, Hispanic Americans are a more heterogeneous lot, descending
from individuals whose ancestral home is Spain, but it also includes individuals
whose principal language is Spanish, who may have no Spanish blood in them.
Native American has become the term to describe individuals whose ancestors
were the indigenous people of North and South America. Yet, uncertainty and
a lack of standardization fail to define clearly who is a Native American. In
some settings an individual must be descended only from individuals of Native
American ancestry to be considered Native American. The standard established
by the Bureau of Indians Affairs (BIA) requires that an individual be one-fourth
Native American by blood in order to claim Native American heritage, although some tribes have lower standards for tribal benefits (Thomason, 1991).
Thus, in some instances, Native American heritage can be claimed when the
individual is only one-eighth (i.e., one great-grandparent is a Native American)
Native American by blood. The U.S. census recognizes Native American heritage on the basis of self-identification, without requiring further proof.

Asian Americans spring from the diverse cultural and national groups of
Asia. While Euro-Americans came from a diverse group of nations, they shared
a common Judeo-Christian religious bond and a basic root language structure.
Asian Americans are a more heterogeneous lot, coming from different political
entities, with distinct languages and several different religious traditions. The
Asian-American individual whose ancestors hailed from the jungles of Southeast Asia has little in common with the Asian American descended from the
peoples of the steppes of north-central Asia. The Filipino Asian descendant may
be considered Hispanic American, not Asian American, because the family's
principal language is Spanish. Clients from all ethnic minority groups enter rehabilitation services with different needs, beliefs, attitudes, values and experiences and significant interpersonal differences exist within each ethnic minority
(Johnson & Associates, 1984).

Discussion Questions: Think about your own ethnicity. How has it shaped your
values, attitudes and beliefs? How has your ethnicity shaped
your drinking and drug consumption patterns?

Life span development serves as a definer of culture and cultural subgroups for some individuals. Adolescents have a unique set of values, attitudes,
and beliefs, separate from the dominant culture; similarly, the elderly have

their own values, beliefs, and attitudes, shaped by their life experiences. While some life span development periods remain fixed, others are more fluid. The Baby Boom generation is a life span development period based on date of birth and represents more a life span cohort than a life span developmental period, for example.

Discussion   What are the significant issues that appear to have affected your
Questions: life span developmental group? Have you seen changes in drug
                  and alcohol laws and consumption patterns during your life-
                  time? How have those changes affected you and your peers?

Society itself serves as a definer of culture and cultural values, beliefs, and attitudes. Imposition of stigma, second class status, or stereotypic notions consign individuals with disabilities, women, and individuals with alternative sexual lifestyles to separate cultural niches. Similarly, society has defined a culture of drug dependency and alcohol dependency and assigned certain characteristics to individuals seen as representing that culture.

Discussion   Is there a drug culture? An alcohol culture? What are the
Questions: defining characteristics?

In this chapter the roles of ethnicity, life span development, and societal definition will be examined with respect to their creation of unique drug and alcohol use, abuse, dependency, and treatment issues.

CULTURAL CONCEPTS

Understanding several basic constructs is important to comprehend the impact of culture on drug and alcohol use. Ethnocentrism is a belief that a particular culture is the only culture that makes sense, espouses the correct values, and represents the right and logical way to behave. Individuals who are ethnocentric might be said to be monocultural in their orientation. Bicultural individuals identify with more than one culture simultaneously. Increasingly America has become a multicultural society, in which many differing cultures coexist. Truly America is probably one of the most, if not the most, multicultural societies in the world. On an individual level, multiculturalism is the effort to be responsive to and to relate to several different cultural groups simultaneously. Cultural pluralism is a reflection of the expanding diversity of society and the importance of preserving and maintaining the identity of differing cultural groups. Often this is accomplished through cross-culturalism and cultural relativism. The communication process that results when individuals who are members of one culture interact with members of another culture is cross-culturalism. Important factors in the process include the groups or individuals who are involved, the type and style of communication, and the political

process that occurs. The unconditional attempt to understand the diverse beliefs and behaviors of another culture is an example of cultural relativism.

Discussion   Identify and discuss the success of national and local efforts at
Question: multiculturalism and cultural pluralism.

Orlandi (1992b) raises the issue of cultural competence, suggesting this
construct incorporates a set of personal and interpersonal skills held by individuals reflecting their understanding of cultural differences and similarities
within, among, and between groups. Table 11.1 depicts Orlandi's model for
cultural competence.

According to Orlandi, the culturally competent person is someone who
completely understands cultural issues and conflicts, is committed to change,
and is skilled in needed abilities. In contrast, the culturally incompetent individual is oblivious to cultural problems and differences and is insensitive, apa-
thetic, and totally lacking important skills. The culturally sensitive individual is
aware of and sympathetic to cultural issues and problems but lacks the skills required to effect needed change. Ideally, all counselors should be culturally
competent; in reality all counselors have varying degrees of competence, sensitivity, or incompetence. However, Rubin et al. (1995) assert that counselor insensitivity to the problems and issues of individuals from minority subcultures
results in disproportionate denial of services and the provision of less effective
service. The result is poorer rehabilitation outcomes. Further, they argue, counselor insensitivity manifests itself in lower counselor empathy, greater levels of
misunderstanding and misdiagnosis, and alienation of clients leading to early
withdrawal from services.

Acculturation has two meanings. At the group level, acculturation refers to
the mutual influence of two or more different cultures in close contact. On a
personal level, acculturation reflects the tasks, struggles, and challenges faced
by an individual adapting to a new or different culture. It involves modification of values and attitudes, which may be slow, especially among adults. Additionally, acculturation includes behavioral change that is often faster and easier
to discern, but behavioral change may be more superficial. Changes in personal

Table 11.1 The Cultural Sophistication Framework

	Culturally Incompetent	Culturally Sensitive	Culturally Competent
Cognitive Dimension	Oblivious	Aware	Knowledgeable
Affective Dimension	Apathetic	Sympathetic	Committed to Change
Skills Dimension	Unskilled	Lacking Some Skills	Highly Skilled
Overall Effect	Destructive	Neutral	Constructive

SOURCE: Orlandi, M. A. (1992b). Defining cultural competence: An organizing framework. In M. A. Orlandi,
R. Weston, & L. G. Epstein (Eds.), *Cultural Competence for Evaluators: A Guide for Alcohol and Other Drug Preven-
tion Practitioners Working with Ethnic/Racial Communities.* Rockville, MD: U.S. Department of Health and Human
Services, Office for Substance Abuse Prevention.

customs, dress, language, lifestyle, and habits are among the personal adaptations resulting from acculturation. Some individuals may become fully assimilated into the dominant culture, while others may accommodate to it. Interestingly, individuals who become assimilated adopt the drinking and drug-consuming habits of the dominant culture. For example, Jews who become assimilated and who drop or reduce their participation in religious rituals display drinking practices and problems that more closely approximate the general population. The demands faced in adapting to a new or different culture may cause the development of acculturative stress. Acculturative stress follows when environmental or internal demands tax the individual's ability to cope or adapt.

Discussion Question: Consider instances when you were thrust into the position of responding to or adapting to a new or different culture. What stressors did you feel? How did you respond to those stressors?

Acculturative stress has been implicated as a cause of alcohol or drug dependence, and stress is known to cause impairment in decision making and impairment of physical health and recovery. Adaptability decreases, and problems may emerge in several life areas, including family and social functioning and occupational functioning. Furthermore, stress plays a role in acceptance of disability and may impede both the counselor-client relationship and the recovery process.

Despite recent attention given to multicultural issues, most drug and alcohol treatment and prevention resources in this country target the majority culture. A variety of reasons contribute to this reality. Since either the federal or state governments fund the most widely available treatment and prevention programs, groups with the most political power have been most successful in obtaining programs for their communities. Trimble (1995) notes that the literature describes few prevention programs targeted at minority groups, and the literature is similarly devoid of articles about treatment for minority individuals. Political power is growing in minority communities but not quickly enough to demand additional funding to respond to quickly multiplying drug and alcohol problems. Moreover, minority groups who have a self-perception that governmental programs serve to disenfranchise or limit opportunities may be suspicious of government-sponsored programs targeted at drug and alcohol problems.

Discussion Question: Consider the prevention and treatment resources in your community. Identify the political factors that mitigate for and against minority group participation in those resources.

Economics play a key role in the establishment of community-based programs, determining the distribution and targeting of resources. Wealthy communities are more likely to have sufficient treatment and prevention resources than poorer communities, and individuals of higher economic status clearly have greater access to more treatment options. Moreover, professionals may be reticent to work in poor minority communities for low salaries or poor working conditions. Historically, minority group members are employed in poorer paying jobs that offer few fringe benefits such as health care insurance. Treatment options for these individuals are limited often to publicly funded or free programs. They simply do not have the economic resources to afford costly, private treatment. Even if financial resources are available, other economic factors may surface. Minority individuals serving as the principal wage earner for large extended families may not be able to take time away from work for dependency treatment or may not be able to afford peripheral costs associated with treatment, such as transportation, family counseling, and child care.

Discussion Question: What are the economic forces/constraints that dictate treatment availability in your area?

Associational factors such as family and community often dictate drinking and drug-taking behaviors. Adolescent and adult problematic drinking behaviors are clearly related to a group of risk factors, including familial alcoholism, poor school and social performance, low levels of parental attachment and family dysfunction, early onset of conduct disorders in childhood, and greater levels of antisocial behavior in preadolescence (Trimble, 1995; Zucker, 1994). Children raised in minority families where significant levels of acculturative stress exist are vulnerable to several of these risk factors. Conversely, many minority families display important assets promoting responsible use, including large, supported extended families, a cultural tradition of abstinence or temperance, and an emphasis on school and social achievement. Similarly, a strong minority community with well-ingrained values promotes positive drinking. However, other forces may supplant the community. For many young people, gangs provide peer recognition, support, a feeling of belonging, and community cohesion not available otherwise (Padilla, Duran, & Nobles, 1995).

Overarching all other factors related to the development of culture is language. Language is the element that binds cultures together and gives it meaning, values, and a world view. It is both the informal and formal representation of a culture's belief system, sense of self-identity, and the cement that holds a culture together. No subculture exists without the undergirding of a unique language structure. For example, a graduate student protested the critical comments of her advisor, who had suggested the language used in her thesis was too rudimentary. "But I learned in Expository Writing 101 that simple language is best and that I should refrain from using big words." The advisor replied, "Academia is the one culture in which the use of big words is salutary." The cultural role of language illustrates why Ebonics is important to the African-American community, not as a substitute for standard English but as part of the African-American cultural heritage.

Discussion   Do unique language structures define your culture? Identify
Questions: some of those structures. What is the influence of geography
                  on language and culture? For example, what word is used to
                  describe carbonated beverages: soda, pop, tonic?, Coke?

COUNSELOR CULTURAL SENSITIVITY

The increasing diversity of the United States' population means that counselors will encounter individuals from other cultures on an increasing basis,
and several authors note the importance of preparing counselors to work
competently with culturally divergent groups (Armstrong & Fitzgerald, 1996;
Rubin et al., 1995; Walker, 1991). As suggested by Orlandi's work, competence
implies more than sensitivity. Competence includes the possession of sensitivity and a subjective idea, and it also includes knowledge, a sense of the relevance of cultural concepts, and the ability to recognize and be aware of per-
sonally important variables (Armstrong & Fitzgerald, 1996). Martha Lentz
Walker (1991), a rehabilitation educator of considerable renown, defines cultural competence as follows:

> The ability of individuals to see beyond the boundaries of their own
> cultural interpretations, to be able to maintain objectivity when faced
> with individuals from cultures different from their own and be able to
> interpret and understand behaviors and intentions of people from other
> cultures nonjudgmentally and without bias (p. 6).

Implicit in this definition is the ability of the counselor to bring both subjective and objective principles to the counseling relationship. There is a recognition of personal values and assumptions and recognition of the value and le-
gitimacy of differing values and judgments. Part of the counselor's objectivity
lies in the ability to understand the sociopolitical forces that influence minority culture members and to understand that counseling theories, strategies, and
techniques are not politically, morally, or culturally neutral. Every interaction
that occurs with a client from another culture is tinged with elements of cross-
cultural interaction. The culturally competent counselor recognizes this reality
and is able to interpret and understand the behaviors of individuals from other
cultures without bias or judgment. On the concrete level cross-cultural differences may be as subtle as differing gaze and attending patterns or as obvious as
differing language and dress standards. More abstractly, differences may exist in
values systems, relational hierarchical structures, and even in the perceptions of
the value and utility of counseling. Unfortunately, counselors often respond either on the basis of their stereotypes and bias, without seeking an understanding of the culturally relevant characteristics of the client. Ultimately, counseling services grounded in stereotypes and cultural bias result in unfair and
unwarranted conclusions about clients and negative service outcomes.

Avoiding problems based on cross-cultural differences may be as simple as asking the correct questions about client beliefs, values, and attitudes early in the counseling relationship. Counselors may be reticent to question clients about their values, relying instead on their own limited knowledge base. However, significant questions may be difficult to discern or may be difficult to ask. Consequently, counselors may make assumptions that are not true, rather than risking the exposure of their own lack of knowledge and information.

ETHNICITY AS A DEFINER OF CULTURE

Ethnicity, either based on racial characteristics, national heritage, or native language is probably the most common definer of a divergent culture. Unique issues and concerns arise when providing dependency counseling services to individuals from distinct ethnic cultures.

African Americans

Currently the largest minority ethnic group, African Americans, constitute approximately 13 percent of the U.S. population. As a description, African American designates a group of people descended from residents of Sub-Saharan Africa. The majority of African Americans are descended from individuals brought to this country during the slave trade prior to the mid-1800s. While African Americans represent a distinct culture, it is a cultural tapestry woven from diverse threads. The culture reflects the origins of African Americans from geographically distinct parts of Africa and from tribal groups with unique languages, cultural practices, and kinship practices. It also reflects regional differences in the United States, with the northern experience differing from the southern experience and urban experiences differing from rural experiences. Despite this inherent diversity, the African-American cultural experience has been viewed as linear and unitary, with unfortunate consequences. "The development of a valid description of the phenomenology of being African in the United States has been hindered by the tendency on the part of social scientists to view African Americans as a monolithic group, by active denial and distortion of their accomplishments, and by their tendency to focus on the limitations rather than on the strengths of their culture and community" (Grace, 1992, p. 57).

Akbar's work (cited in Butler, 1992) identifies six trends illustrative of unique African-American cultural behavior.

Language. Language is a symbolic representation of the mental processes of a group, according to Akbar. Since the African-American experience is characterized by affect and feeling, standard English may not reflect the simultaneous complexity and subtlety of the African-American communication process. Thus, Ebonics, African-American English, is best not viewed as a substandard form of English communication but rather as an alternative form, incorporating phrases, nuances, and speech patterns more reflective of the African-American culture. Among African Americans, African-American language is characterized by more extensive use of body language, including gestures, and as a "modality for maintaining rhythm in expression as well as dramatizing that which [spoken] language fails to communicate" (p. 34). Communication through spoken language is central to the counseling relationship, and yet many counselors fail to grasp the meaning and contextual elements of Ebonics and their importance in the counseling relationship (Beaman, 1994; Kottler, 1992).

Oral Patterns of Information Transmission. The predominant mode of information transmission in the United States is visual. From kindergarten on through graduate school, learning centers around reading and observation, and visual–motor activities are more highly valued than oral–motor activities and aural–motor activities. Conversely, oral forms of information transmission typify the African–American culture with antecedents reaching back to African roots and slavery when African Americans were forbidden to learn to read. Akbar suggests that the oral tradition is one reason African–American children do poorly in school. More cogently, it may serve to explain why bibliotherapy may be of little value for some African Americans and why orally or aurally expressive forms of therapy may be more powerful.

People Orientation. According to Akbar, African Americans inextricably tie the speaker to the message and the context of the message. Because of the oral tradition, it is impossible to separate these three elements of communication. Consequently, African Americans may be less likely to accept information on face value and are more likely to analyze communication in terms of the congruence of the message, messenger, and the contextual elements (relevance, environment, intention) of the message.

Interaction vs Reaction. As illustrated most vividly in the Sunday morning sermons in traditional African–American churches, African–American language includes a call and response pattern. In this interactional language paradigm, the listener is not a passive participant whose responses and reactions occur at defined moments, such as at the end of a speech. Instead, the African–American pattern emphasizes and encourages spontaneous reactions and pronouncements of encouragement, engaging the speaker and listener in an interactive dialogue, characterized by emotional content and an expressive style (Hale-Benson, 1986).

Thought Patterns. Years of exclusion from participation in formal education opportunities have evolved among African Americans a form of thinking and problem solving that relies more on intuition, internal cues, and reaction and feelings than on external information. Resulting from the influence of cultural heritage and life experiences, these thought patterns are especially suited to environmental situations in which social interactions are highly valued. These intuitively based thought patterns, however, are not without problems. The rate of HIV infection among African Americans continues to grow, and, as a group, African Americans are less likely than others to seek treatment for HIV or AIDS, with tragic consequences. For instance, McNair and Roberts (1997) reported that cultural norms and cultural mediating variables may affect the sensitivity of African–American women to HIV/AIDS risk cues, resulting in

higher rates of infection and lower rates of treatment participation. Speculation attributes developments such as these to continued reliance on intuition
and internalized thought processes instead of consideration of the empirical
public health and medical evidence about AIDS prevention and treatment.
Others have suggested that the African-American community has been victimized by past public health scientific studies, notably the Tuskegee syphilis
studies and thus is more likely to rely on intuition and personal insight than
information from government or scientific groups.

Spontaneity. The ability to be highly adaptable and flexible to environmental and social changes is another facilitative characteristic of the African-
American culture.

The extended family plays an important role in the African-American
culture and may include members who are related by blood, both proximally
(grandparents, aunts, uncles) and distantly (cousins, great-aunts and great-
uncles) and members not related by blood but by social patterns of kinship
and affiliation (neighbors, fellow church members). The extended family
provides a shield against the tensions of life, a place of refuge and haven, a
support system, and a spiritual center made possible through the family's involvement in religious and symbolic rituals (Alston & Turner, 1994). Recent
research evidence suggests that African Americans who have a strong sense
of racial identity and self esteem bolstered by cultural traditions and the family are less prone to develop drug and alcohol problems (Foulks & Pena,
1995).

Historically the African-American church has been identified as a source
of cohesiveness and support for African Americans and a major resource in
times of rage and pain. More recently some of the initiatives of the Nation of
Islam have shown promise in combating inner-city drug and alcohol problems,
although the methods of this organization remain mired in controversy. Both
organized and informal neighborhood and community groups have been
meaningful in reaching out to African Americans with drug and alcohol problems, as have African-American social and fraternal organizations.

**Discussion
Questions:**   What African-American groups have been influential in drug
and alcohol issues in your community, state, or nation? What
are some of the successes? What are some of the failures?

Ambivalence, uncertainty, and continued questions mar the data concerning
drug and alcohol use abuse and dependence within this community. The literature suggests that African Americans as a group have drinking rates equal to or
lower than the general population (Alcohol Alert, 1994; Gordon, Gordon, &
Nembhard, 1994; Wade, 1994), although others have asserted that alcohol abuse
and alcoholism rates are higher in the African-American community (Watson,
1990). Similar inconsistencies are evident in examining the data concerning
drug problems. Two things are clear, however. First, much of the research on
African-American drinking practices is flawed because of sampling and survey
difficulties, and the limited research performed with a sample of African Amer-

icans dependent on drug or alcohol is plagued by inconsistencies in data collection. Second, all of the evidence suggests that the African-American community (and especially African-American males) has suffered more severe consequences from drinking and drug taking than the general population (Gordon, Gordon, & Nembhard, 1994; Wade, 1994; Watson, 1990). Higher prevalence of alcohol-related health problems exist in this community, and the African-American community appears to suffer disproportionately from alcohol and drug-related violence. According to Wade (1994), the leading causes of death for African-American youth include drug and alcohol-related homicide, suicide, drug abuse and accidents; among white youth, cardiovascular disease and accidents were the primary causes of fatality. Employment rates for members of the African-American community lag behind rates for the general population, and when disability is factored in (including substance abuse disabilities), the gap grows significantly (Wright & Emener, 1992).

Crack cocaine has had a particularly devastating effect on the African-American community. In some studies of crack cocaine (Hoffman et al., 1996; Wallace, 1991), African Americans constituted more than 90 percent of the sample; African Americans are six times as likely to be incarcerated for crimes (Wade, 1994), and the numbers of young African-American males in correctional institutions is higher than the number of African-American males enrolled in higher education (Gordon, Gordon, & Nembhard, 1994). In part, this high rate of incarceration is attributed to stiffer penalties for crack cocaine offenses.

Finally, African Americans in the lower socioeconomic strata may have fewer treatment resources available to them, and those treatment resources may be of questionable efficacy. Treatment strategies for crack cocaine addiction are still in the developmental, evolutionary stages, and limitations imposed on treatment resources by scarce public funding reduce the availability of treatment.

Hispanic Americans

The broad umbrella minority group title of Hispanic American shelters a heterogeneous mixture of 20 million U.S. residents who belong to this group because of national heritage, principal language, or ethnic background. The federal government uses Hispanic American to describe this group. Other terms include Chicano, a sociopolitical term describing individuals of Mexican-American heritage, which has fallen into disfavor in some parts of the country, and Latino (or Latina), a term used to describe individuals from Central or South America. Interestingly, Brazilians may be included in the Latino and/or Hispanic American culture even though their native language is Portuguese.

Discussion   Are specific terms used to describe Hispanic Americans in
Questions: your part of the country? Have some terms fallen out of or
                 into favor? Whom do you regard as Hispanic American?

The largest group of Hispanic Americans (about 60 percent) are the 13 million Mexican Americans. While it is stereotypical to think of most Mexican

Americans as first- or second-generation residents of the United States, many individuals claiming Mexican-American heritage date their U.S. residency back many generations. The 1848 Treaty of Guadalupe Hidalgo ended the U.S.–Mexican war and ceded the territory encompassing the states of California, Nevada, Arizona, New Mexico, Texas, Utah, and half of Colorado to the United States. The 80,000 Mexican citizens of this territory became U.S. residents overnight. The Mexican-American population is centered in the Southwest, but it is growing in the Northwest and Great Plains as more individuals seek better employment opportunities. Many migrant farm workers are choosing to settle permanently in agricultural communities year round, rather than following the crops north.

Puerto Ricans (2.5 million) constitute the next largest group of Hispanic Americans, concentrated in the New York-New Jersey metropolitan area. The Commonwealth of Puerto Rico was given to the United States by the 1899 Treaty of Paris ending the Spanish American War, and Puerto Rican residents received U.S. citizenship in 1917. Cuban Americans number about 1.1 million individuals, principally residing in South Florida. The more recent Cuban émigrés entered the United States after the 1950s Cuban revolution and lived on Florida's east coast, mainly in the Miami-Dade County area. An older Cuban-American community exists in the Tampa, Florida environs, comprising descendants of Cubans who started the cigar industry in Tampa early in this century. Finally, the Hispanic-American group includes individuals whose national heritage is from Spain, the countries of Central and South America, and the Philippines.

It is impossible to ascribe particular cultural characteristics to this group or to individuals within the group. Racial characteristics of group members reflect African, European, Native American, and Asian descent. Many Hispanic Americans are bilingual in Spanish and English; others speak English only, and some may speak Spanish only, and as indicated earlier some may speak Portuguese as a primary or secondary language. Many are monocultural, while others may be tricultural. Their cultural beliefs and practices may reflect their nation of origin, the broader Hispanic-American culture in general and the broader U.S. culture.

Discussion Questions: Do you know individuals from various sectors of the Hispanic-American community? How are they similar? How do they differ? What do you know about their attitudes, beliefs, and practices about drugs and alcohol?

The diversity of the Hispanic-American population creates difficulty in examining group characteristics, and any assertions about a unique Hispanic-American culture must be viewed with caution and skepticism. For example, one of the major concerns about drug and alcohol consumption and use patterns and research findings is the failure of most statistics and reports to distinguish between the various Hispanic subgroups. Nevertheless, certain characteristics appear to transcend the various cultures. In particular, the broad

Hispanic–American culture is typified by strong family units, with a well-defined hierarchical system valuing respect for elders and for males. Traditionally, males have the primary leadership and financial responsibility for the family, while women are assigned traditional roles of nurturing and self-sacrifice. The family identity may be more important than personal identity, especially among Mexican Americans. Moreover, the extended family may include a broad range of aunts, uncles, cousins, and family friends. This extended family is a powerful force in treating drug and alcohol problems. Individuals with dependency problems tend to maintain close family contacts, and Hispanic–American families are willing to intervene in dependency problems and support recovery.

Personalismo takes the reliance on the family a step further to incorporate reliance on the social group, another powerful force. Role models are respected and emulated, especially for their inner qualities. Social groups and individuals practice *simpatía,* the honoring of central values and customs, and mandating a sense of respect and politeness in interactions. A sense of personal modesty and dignity is incorporated in the meaning of *simpatia* as well. Finally, *machismo* is an important transcultural value among Hispanic Americans. Correctly and traditionally interpreted, *machismo* embodies a tradition of honor, responsibility, dependability, dedication, and generosity combined with courage, assertiveness, and self-confidence. Unfortunately, in both the Euro-American and Hispanic–American cultures, *machismo* has become synonymous with arrogance, aggression, and selfish sexuality.

Drug and alcohol consumption data, although flawed, suggest some trends among the Hispanic–American population. Adolescents show early onset drug and alcohol use and have high rates of polydrug use and inhalant use. Among the high-risk factors facing adolescents are acculturative stress, high rates of poverty, high teen pregnancy rates, low school performance and success rates, and high availability of drugs and alcohol, particularly in impoverished inner-city neighborhoods. Gangs have a strong negative influence on Hispanic–American youth, too.

Hispanic–American adults who are less well assimilated into the broader culture have higher drug and alcohol consumption rates and lower rates for participation in help seeking. As a group, they have higher death rates than expected due to alcohol problems. In general, the evidence suggests that Hispanic–American males have alcohol consumption rates consistent with the general population, while Hispanic–American females consume less alcohol than the general population. Among Hispanic Americans, Mexican-American males are the heaviest alcohol consumers, whereas females from this subculture are the lightest consumers. Hispanic Americans born in this country have higher rates of consumption than immigrants.

Hispanic families immigrating to the United States experience both acculturative stress and problems related to assimilation. Since the youth in these families adapt to the new culture more quickly, including a faster rate of language acquisition, they achieve a more powerful position in the family than normally expected in the Hispanic culture. Because of language facility, adolescents become translators for the family and consequently control or broker many adult interactions with the dominant culture. More problematically, Padilla and Salgado de Snyder (1992) suggest that Hispanic adolescents develop significant drug and alcohol problems because of poverty, lack of parental attention in families where both parents work and single-parent families, and the increased availability of drugs and alcohol in a society with very different values. Hispanic men who immigrate to the United States without their families show higher patterns of drinking. These high-risk behaviors are attributed to acculturative stress resulting from distance from immediate family members, lack of a social support system, language isolation, and lack of familiarity with the dominant culture (Casas, 1992). The precipitating force catalyzing immigration and the legal or illegal nature of immigration may create stress. Historically, many Hispanic Americans immigrated to the United States for economic reasons; more recently Hispanic Americans have come to the United States to escape political oppression or to flee civil war in their native countries. Consequently, this latest immigrant group may suffer from post-traumatic stress disorder, increasing their vulnerability to psychoactive substance abuse and dependence. This vulnerability may be exacerbated by an uncertain future in this country, concern for friends and family back home, and loss of economic and social supports.

Hispanic Americans are overrepresented in the population of individuals with HIV/AIDS. Intravenous drug use practices, unsafe sex practices, limited available information, and the vocationally forced separation of males from extended and nuclear families are contributing factors.

Counselors who work with Hispanic Americans should recognize the importance of tapping into naturally occurring resources and alliances. The family is seen as a source of strength and pride, and family involvement in treatment is crucial as is an understanding of the dynamics of family life. *Personalismo* can be a powerful force in group therapy, although self-disclosure may be limited by *machismo* attitudes. Hispanic Americans may be slow to self-disclose initially, and it is important to proceed slowly, winning trust and rapport through demonstration of personal interest, correctly pronouncing names, engaging in small talk, and being sensitive to cultural issues. Finally, counselors must be cognizant of the self-perpetuating cycle of poverty that may exist, caused by limited vocational and educational opportunities, language difficulties, and cultural biases.

Native Americans

Native Americans number about 2 million U.S. citizens (.7 percent of the population), about half of whom live in urban areas. Limited consensus exists about who is a Native American, or even what tribal structures exist. Thomason (1991) suggests 505 Native American tribes have achieved recognition by the federal government, while Heinrich, Corbine, and Thomas (1990) put the number of tribes at 478. Moreover, the individual states recognize 365 tribes and bands, and approximately 150 different Native American languages are acknowledged. Consequently, great variability exists within the Native American population, and care must be taken to avoid stereotyping on the basis of general assumptions or limited information.

Despite the variability of this population, a depressing consistency exists with respect to Native American health, employment, and socioeconomic and dependency problems. As a group, Native Americans have been notoriously underserved and inappropriately served by counseling, human services, health care and vocational rehabilitation programs (Marshall, Johnson, Martin, Saravanabhavan, & Bradford, 1992; Marshall, Martin, Thomason, & Johnson, 1991). Unemployment rates range from 18 percent to 66 percent, and the median income among Native American groups is about half that of the general population. Arrest rates are ten times that of Euro-Americans and three times that of African Americans. Adolescent suicide rates have increased by 1000 percent in the past 20 years, and alcohol has been implicated as a major cause of accidental death among adolescents and adults (Smith, 1991).

Alcoholism rates are thought to be at least twice the national average among Native Americans (Heinrich, Corbine, & Thomas, 1990), and patients admitted to Indian Health Service hospitals have a 3.28 times higher likelihood of alcoholism diagnosis versus the U.S. hospital average. Among Native Americans admitted to state-federal rehabilitation services, the rate of alcohol abuse problems was 3.34 times the national average (Marshall, Martin, & Johnson, 1990). Of the ten leading causes of death among Native Americans, at least half are directly attributable to or related to alcohol. Native Americans have significantly higher rates of liver disease, fetal alcohol syndrome, diabetes, nutritionally related hypertension, and car accidents. Cirrhosis of the liver is higher among women of childbearing years than among Native American men of comparable age (Marshall, Martin, & Johnson, 1990). As many as two-thirds of Native Americans fail to complete high school, and college attendance is extremely low, particularly at the graduate level (Marshall et al., 1991). These data have particularly sad consequences. Because few Native Americans graduate from graduate-level counseling programs, there are few Native American counselors available to treat a population in desperate need of services.

Why alcohol has had such an horrific impact on Native Americans may in part be explained through cultural considerations. In 1981, Zephier asserted that Native Americans had experienced 30,000 years of sobriety and 200 years of alcohol problems. While it is likely that pre-Columbian tribes fermented alcohol-containing beverages, there is little documentation of alcohol problems and little discussion of alcohol as a food substance or as a ceremonial element. Euro-American settlers, traders, and missionaries first introduced alcohol to Native American cultures, and that early exposure was almost universally negative. Traders and settlers often used alcohol as a coercive tool to cheat Native Americans out of lands or trade goods. Missionaries sought to control Native American behavior by advocating absolute abstinence, a practice that continues today on many "dry" reservations. History makes clear that changes introduced into a culture bring about alterations in morality, values, beliefs, and attitudes and that these alterations are slow to occur. Because Native Americans have been exposed to alcohol for a relatively recent period, it may well be that

Native American cultural practices with regard to alcohol are still in an evolutionary stage. Nowhere is this clearer than on reservations where alcohol is banned. On those reservations, young people never see alcohol consumed as food or in "normal" social environments or situations. Consequently, no models exist for appropriate drinking. Alcohol enjoys the status of forbidden fruit, elevating its acquisition and consumption to an adventure-seeking, thrilling activity. On vast western reservations, tribal members drive long distances to acquire alcohol in "wet" towns surrounding the reservation. Bars and taverns are nonexistent on the reservation, and the elders or tribal authorities may frown on drinking in homes or at formal social gatherings, so drinking occurs in decidedly dangerous places—in cars and outside on the prairies. Unfortunately, it is common for individuals to become intoxicated, wander away from the group, and freeze to death on cold winter nights.

In their research, Weisner, Wibel-Orlando, and Long (1984) identified five patterns of Native American drinking, all of which are influenced by tribal affiliation, socioeconomic status, cultural identity, and demographic characteristics. Partying is a period of continuous drinking on weekends and is referred to as "serious" drinking. In urban environments, partying is typified by groups of Native Americans going from bar to bar and then to an open-air environment after closing hours. Partying has strong elements of cohesion, exclusivity, and ritualism and is viewed by some scholars as analogous to raiding and hunting parties of past eras. Native Americans on reservations may go to substantial legal and driving risk to obtain and conceal alcohol from elders and tribal police. The group context of partying contributes to high degrees of sociability and bonding and may be seen as normative behavior for young people. However, the sociable elements of partying often deteriorate as the drinking continues, resulting in violence and fights.

Individuals whose drinking style is referred to as "maintaining" exhibit a unique form of excessive but controlled drinking. These individuals have the role of maintaining sufficient control to keep social interactions going, prevent fights, and to care for others. Typically these individuals have very high tolerance levels and have learned to function in a state of continuous inebriation. Their role of community barfly may be their only legitimate role.

"Heavy drinking" is a drinking style characterized by periods of excessive drinking interspersed with periods of abstinence usually stimulated by family crises, health problems, incarceration, or treatment. As opposed to maintenance drinkers, heavy drinkers are more likely to experience significant life difficulties related to alcohol consumption and relapse readily.

The Native American drinking style called "white man's drinking" is reflective of the reality of dealing with a bicultural environment. While most Native American drinkers consume alcohol in social situations, even if they are maintainers or heavy drinkers, individuals who practice white man's drinking often are solitary drinkers without a strong social network. Recovery from alcohol dependence may be hindered by the absence of a support system within the tribe or community.

Finally, "teetotaling" Native Americans are often practitioners of lifelong abstinence. Revered as elders, these individuals have been referred to as the spiritual fabric of the tribe. Nonetheless, teetotalers seem to have limited impact on Native American drinking, largely because of the Native American philosophy of noninterference in the lives of others. Noninterference implies the right of all individuals to conduct their lives in their own fashion and to learn from their own mistakes (Fisher & Harrison, 1997). Consequently, abstinent elders may frown upon the drinking behaviors of younger tribal members but may not interfere. In the dominant culture, some may view this as codependent or enabling behavior. Within the Native American culture, noninterference is a venerable and hallowed tradition. However, according to Fisher and Harrison (1997), this "notion of allowing one to learn from mistakes may have had a significant impact upon the development of alcohol abuse and alcoholism among Native Americans throughout generations" (p. 58).

The interconnectedness of all experiences of life and all things in the world is another important Native American tradition. Many Native American cultural traditions conceptualize life as a circular or cyclical series of events and emphasize harmony, balance, and mutual support. The introduction of alcohol abuse and alcohol dependence badly skews the balance of the circle of life, and recovery must focus on restoration of that balance. Respect for and understanding of Native American cultural and spiritual traditions is vital, as is inclusion of family members and community members in the treatment process. However, balance restoration is more difficult when alcohol dependence is accompanied by crunching poverty, a history of joblessness, and severe health and physical problems. Recovery, then, becomes an all-encompassing series of events, involving total life restructuring in many ways.

SOCIETY AS A DEFINER
OF SPECIAL POPULATIONS

Ethnicity and race are obvious considerations in examining cultural influences on drug and alcohol consumption, abuse, and dependence. However, in many cases society itself defines certain populations as culturally different or distinct where drugs and alcohol are concerned.

Women

Noted alcoholism expert Sheila Blume (1988) recounts many of the ancient myths and legends about alcohol consumption and women. A 4000-year-old Persian legend tells of a woman with sick headaches who sneaked into a storeroom holding wine labeled as poison. Drinking the wine to kill herself resulted instead in a sense of joy and relief, and she continued to consume alcohol, possibly depicting the story of the first alcoholic woman. The story of the Egyptian goddess Hathor recounts the tale of Hathor destroying mankind and wading in the blood. The god Re changes the blood to red beer, which Hathor drinks, becoming intoxicated. The killing stops, and mankind is saved by the drunkenness of a woman. The biblical account of Lot reveals that his daughters conspire to get him drunk and have sex with him, as he is the only available male. Thus, the first case of alcohol-related incest is described. Samson's mother is counseled by an angel to not drink wine during pregnancy, the first example of counseling for fetal alcohol syndrome prevention.

Discussion Question: Discuss other instances concerning women and alcohol and drug consumption in legend, mythology, and religion.

Psychoactive substance use and women, however, is not just the stuff of legend. Roman laws punished wine drinking by women with death, and alcohol prohibition laws were linked to laws proscribing adultery. The Women's Christian Temperance Union (WCTU) led the fight for prohibition in the 19th and 20th centuries. Interestingly, many of the opiate addicts of the late 19th century were women, addicted either because of their use of opium-laced patent medicines or from smoking opium (Abadinsky, 1997).

Women have long been held to a stricter standard than men have when it comes to drugs and alcohol (Gomberg, 1988; McDonough & Russell, 1994). Philosopher Emanuel Kant in 1798 noted that women do not get drunk for fear of violating community standards of piety and chastity, a clear example of the stigma a woman faced then and faces now about drugs and alcohol (Blume, 1988). Stigma about women and drinking even extends to research. Nearly all of the studies of alcoholism and drug dependence have focused on male samples, and little is known about many female psychoactive substance issues.

Discussion Question: Discuss other examples of the stricter standards women face concerning psychoactive substance consumption.

Data reveal that about 60 percent of all adult women in the population drink, and 12 percent to 16 percent of women can be classified as heavy drinkers. Estimates of the number of female alcoholics range from 3 million to 7 million, depending on the source (McDonough & Russell, 1994). However, women are less likely than men to be in treatment. Women are the largest group using benzodiazepines (Ativan, librium, Valium, etc.) drugs. Over 1.875 million women have a history of taking this type of drug for a year or more. Twice as many women as men take benzodiazepines, and they are three times as likely to abuse them. Among women with eating disorders, an almost exclusively female issue, concurrent amphetamine and cocaine abuse is seen frequently. Finally, the number of women, especially of childbearing age, abusing cocaine and crack cocaine has grown dramatically. The 1990 National Household survey reported that about 500,000 women of childbearing age reported cocaine use in the month prior to the survey.

Blume (1988) argues that women who become dependent on psychoactive substances are triply stigmatized, a theme echoed by other authors. They face the stigma shared by all individuals who are dependent; they face the stigma of being a drunken or addicted woman; and they face the stigma caused by the linkage of promiscuity and alcohol or drug consumption. A high incidence of sexual trauma exists among women who enter substance abuse or dependence treatment, and the relapse rate for this group is significantly higher (Wadsworth, Spampneto, & Halbrook, 1995).

Gender differences in alcohol and drug dependency are not limited to psychological issues. Alcohol is absorbed and metabolized differently by women, resulting in higher blood alcohol levels and creating greater susceptibility to hepatic, cardiac, and cerebral damage (Urbano-Marquez et al., 1995; Nixon, 1994). Differences in blood alcohol levels are related to lower amounts of body water in female bodies and reduced activity of alcohol-metabolizing enzymes in the stomach, which allows more alcohol to pass directly from the stomach to the bloodstream (National Institute on Alcohol Abuse and Alcoholism, 1990; Frezza et al., 1990).

Identification of women with psychoactive drug problems and access to needed treatment is limited for women. Especially among the middle and upper socioeconomic classes, female drug and alcohol use is more likely to occur at home, in private. Consequently, women are less likely to be identified by traditional gatekeepers to treatment: employers and law enforcement personnel. Women in the workforce may be stigmatized or viewed with suspicion if they attempt to "drink like the boys." They face the double jeopardy of trying to fit into the power and social circles of the workplace, while enduring the continued prevalence of continuing stereotypes. Naturally this contributes to feelings of stress, devaluation, and low self-esteem that may exacerbate alcohol and drug problems.

Alcoholic women often are married to alcoholic men. In this relationship women tend to be held to higher standards of morality and influence. Society expects women to exert a positive influence upon drinking and drug-taking behavior in marriage, and again, women who are unable to do so are doubly stigmatized. The codependence literature provides some evidence that women who are raised in homes where the father is alcoholic may marry an alcoholic both to try to "fix" the alcoholic spouse and to deal with unresolved childhood issues (Beattie, 1987). In certain situations, women in alcoholic marriages may become alcoholic themselves. As a control mechanism they may drink with their husbands in an effort to regulate his drinking. Unfortunately, they may end up drinking in an alcoholic fashion themselves. Despite the gains of the women's movement, many women are still viewed in the context of their relationships. They are somebody's wife, daughter, girlfriend, or sister, and female alcohol consumption is linked strongly to their relationships (Wilsnack, Wilsnack, & Klassen, 1986). This view is more than symbolic when alcohol and drug problems eventuate. Economic and culturally dictated dependence may force many women in need of treatment to remain in negative relationships and to eschew treatment. If the male partner is the primary wage earner and insured individual, insurance coverage may not be available for treatment for the female partner. Even if the woman is employed, she may be working in a job with limited fringe benefits, including insurance and available time off (sick time or vacation time) to participate in treatment. The role of the woman in the marital/family relationship may obviate treatment participation. If a woman is seen as the family caretaker or nurturing partner, the family may overtly or covertly object to or resist her participation in treatment. They may also value her participation in treatment at a lower level than would be the case for the male partner. Motherhood presents unique treatment concerns for women. Some treatment centers may be loathe to admit women who are pregnant, particularly those in the late stages of pregnancy, and lack of child care availability is recognized as a significant barrier to treatment admission for many women (McDonough & Russell, 1994).

Victimization by domestic violence or sexual violence is an all too often occurrence related to psychoactive substance dependence among women. Kantor (1993) points out that spousal abuse is inextricably tied to alcohol and that women who are problematic alcohol consumers are more prone to be victims of violence, but this is not a simple linkage. Other factors, including cultural issues, socioeconomic status, and history of abuse in the family of origin of both spouses, contribute to the incidence of domestic violence. Glover, Janikowski, and Benshoff (1995) examined the prevalence of incest involvement among women and men admitted to treatment centers across the nation. In their sample of 732 individuals enrolled in treatment in 35 treatment centers, more than half of the women (55 percent; $n = 113/204$ female participants) reported at least one incest contact prior to treatment. The number of previous incest contacts ranged from 1 contact to 104 contacts. Significantly, incest is not a gender-specific issue. Nearly a third of the male respondents (29.4 percent) in this study reported participation in at least one incest event. As might be expected, the women in the incest group in this study were significantly less likely to report positive feelings of self-esteem, and they were more apt to be in treatment for multiple drug and alcohol problems. The authors noted that, despite its prevalence, incest victimization is not addressed in many treatment programs. They noted that many facilities declined to participate in the study, contending that incest victimization was not a problem for their clientele. Other facilities suggested that their counselors were either uninterested in incest as a problem or ill-prepared to deal with it. "Unfortunately, many counselors are not cross-trained in substance abuse and sexual abuse issues and may genuinely fear the consequences of opening an issue that they are ill-prepared for and cannot close" (p. 192). Both Widom (1993) and Glover, Janikowski, and Benshoff (1996) assert that alcoholic drinking among victims of childhood incest may be a coping mechanism to allow them to deal with their memories, emotional pain, and feelings of isolation, exploitation, and loneliness. The risk of relapse is significantly increased among incest victims if the victimization is ignored or downplayed in the substance abuse/dependence process. Indeed, the confrontational, male-oriented approach to treatment found in many facilities may be problematic in dealing with female incest victimization problems (Wadsworth, Spampneto, & Halbrook, 1995). Unfortunately, programs specializing in treating incest and violence issues may not address psychoactive substance abuse/dependence problems. Consequently, adequate treatment for women with victimization concerns usually will require collaborative networking among at least two or more specialized agencies.

Discussion   What resources exist in your area for the treatment of incest
Question: victimization or domestic violence victimization?

Just as treatment facilities may be inadequate in their ability to respond to incest issues, counselor training programs may be deficient in their preparation of counselors. Few educational programs appear to address these issues in their course offerings, and many neophyte counselors will enter practice with little or no formal training in dealing with sexual abuse or domestic abuse.

Other unique treatment considerations exist for women. Women begin drinking at a later age than men, on average, but enter treatment at about the same age. Thus, the disease processes related to alcoholism are telescoped, and adverse physical consequences develop sooner and are more severe. On average, women drink less than men, but since they are smaller and have more body fat and less muscle mass, alcohol is more concentrated in their bodies. Body fat has less water than muscle, and it is the water in the body that dilutes ingested alcohol, allowing alcohol concentrations to rise to higher levels, and leading to more dire physiological consequences. Women in treatment report a greater incidence of suicidal attempts and depression. In studies, 20 percent to 25 percent of women with alcoholism problems report a history of unipolar depression, and long-term care of that depression must be a component of the abuse/dependence treatment plan.

As illustrated by the following case example, treatment of concurrent depression and psychoactive substance abuse is fraught with pitfalls. The client, a middle-aged woman, had relapsed and called seeking admission to an inpatient treatment center. In the preadmission review, the clinical team reviewed her previous admission. She had been diagnosed with concurrent alcoholism and depression. On her initial admission she was withdrawn, teary, and exhibiting many of the classic psychological signs of long-term, unipolar depression and the physiological signs of chronic alcoholism. She completed treatment successfully following stabilization with antidepressive medication and was discharged with a treatment plan that included abstinence from alcohol, participation in mental health counseling, and continuation of her antidepressive medication. The clinical review team assumed that a depressed, withdrawn, physiologically impaired client would be seen on readmission. Instead, the client arrived at the treatment center looking very healthy and alert. She greeted staff members by name and reacted positively to her readmission. Staff members were frankly puzzled about this very different presentation. It was not until a staff member completed the initial history that the reason for the startling change in this client became apparent. She had remained abstinent from alcohol and had participated in AA meetings, but she had become dissatisfied with her mental health counseling and the side effects associated with her antidepressive medication. Taking matters into her own hands, she began to self-medicate her depression with cocaine. Her reason for seeking readmission centered on her fear of addiction to cocaine—unfortunately, a fear that was well founded. She had used cocaine the day of admission and was high upon admission. Following a short detoxification period she reverted quickly to her depressed, withdrawn state, and she and the treatment team now faced the issues related to a triple diagnosis. Discharge recommendations included follow-up counseling care in an agency specializing in dual disorders.

Many women enter treatment with a history of benzodiazepine drug use. Since these drugs are commonly prescribed and relatively safe in terms of their potential for lethality through overdose, many assume that detoxification from the benzodiazepines is simple and straightforward, akin to alcohol detoxification. Clinically, however, the picture is far different. Because of the neurotoxic effects of this class of drugs, abrupt discontinuation can result in seizures, tremor, disorientation, and hallucinations beginning two to ten days following cessation of use. Death may result. Detoxification from benzodiazepines requires a carefully monitored weaning away from the medication, preferably in an inpatient, medical setting.

Still other women enter treatment exhibiting classic signs of malnutrition characteristic of long-term alcoholism, yet their age and history of use are inconsistent with this diagnosis. They are underweight, and their body chemistry blood analysis may be abnormal. While these signs may be attributable to alcoholism, the possibility of the presence of an eating disorder must be examined. In particular women who enter treatment with a history of amphetamine abuse or cocaine abuse may have a hidden problem with anorexia or bulimia.

Wadsworth, Spampneto, and Halbrook (1995) assert that most treatment services for psychoactive substance dependence are dominated by a male-oriented philosophy and may be insensitive to the needs of women entering recovery. Many women with dependence problems are hidden users, concealing their use from family members, professionals, friends, society, and themselves. As a result they may have limited insight about the role drugs and alcohol have come to play in their lives. However, because their use is hidden and private, their ultimate reactions and their impact on others may be quite different from the reactions and actions of men. White and Chaney (1993) conceptualize this difference in terms of shame and guilt. They argue that male-oriented recovery models, such as AA, focus on guilt, yet many women experience shame rather than guilt. Guilt is "self-indictment for doing [and] self-blame for behavior" (p. 16). Conversely, shame is "internalized indictment of being [and] self-blame of one's character . . . one's very essence" (p. 16). While the Alcoholics Anonymous philosophy is geared toward dealing with guilt issues, it does little to ameliorate the feelings and perceptions of self-loathing, self-blame, and self-hatred. Recently programs have evolved exclusively for women who are dependent, notably Women for Sobriety (WFS). Described in greater detail in Chapter 8 WFS seeks to bring about a cognitive restructuring for participants, aimed at creating new, healthy self-perceptions and world views. The difference between the AA emphasis on powerlessness and dealing with guilt and the WFS emphasis on empowerment and dealing with shame is typified in the introductory statements member make at meetings. "Hello, my name is John, and I am an alcoholic" conveys a very different message from "Hello, my name is Susan, and I'm a competent woman." More often than men, women bring histories of victimization, self-destruction, and low self-esteem to treatment and characteristically may be less responsive to the confrontational strategies of conventional treatment (Farr, Bordieri, Benshoff, and Taricone, 1996). They are more apt to respond positively to mutual support and affirmation and efforts directed at overcoming societal and cultural barriers to personal growth and development (Illinois Women's Substance Abuse Coalition, 1985; Lewis, Dana, & Blevins, 1994).

Visionary programs for supporting and empowering women with dependence problems are not yet universal, however, and many women (especially in rural areas) will continue to participate in "traditional" treatment programs and attend Alcoholics Anonymous and Cocaine Anonymous meetings. Indeed, some women may prefer participation in those programs, and anecdotal and documentary evidence suggests their effectiveness for many women. Important considerations for women participating in traditional treatment include obtaining a positive female sponsor, participating in treatment that offers all-female group opportunities, and developing a network of positive female role models to emulate. No matter what the treatment setting or treatment philosophy, the multiple problems often associated with female dependency issues call for collaborative networking among multiple service providers.

The Elderly

Individuals who are elderly, usually defined as individuals 65 years of age and older, constitute about 13 percent of the U.S. population. This age cohort is one of the fastest-growing groups, as medical and lifestyle advances gradually increase life expectancies. While the cohort represents about 13 percent of society, dramatic differences are found when comparing drug and alcohol consumption rates with those of the general population. As might be expected, this group of 30+ million individuals consumes 20 percent to 25 percent of all prescription medications, and it is this consumption that presents the most significant drug problems for individuals who are elderly. Little to no data exist about the use of illegal substances by this age group, and illegal substance use is not regarded as a significant problem. About two-thirds of noninstitutionalized individuals who are elderly use one or more prescription drugs, and a similar number take one or more over-the-counter medications on a daily basis. Table 11.2 details the most frequently used drug types among individuals older than

Table 11.2 Drug Types Used Most Frequently by Individuals Who Are Elderly

Drug Type	Percentage of Elderly Using
Analgesics	67%
Cardiovascular	34%
Laxatives	31%
Vitamins	29%
Antacids	26%
Antianxiety Drugs	22%

65. Physicians write 30 percent plus of all prescriptions for Seconal, a popular sleeping medication, and Valium for individuals over the age of 60.

Alcohol use and abuse among older individuals appears to be lower than the use and abuse patterns of the general population, but this assertion is fraught with problems and ambiguities (Atchley, 1994). Clear reasons exist to support the speculation that use and abuse rates are lower. Many older individuals are living on fixed incomes, which, particularly for older single women, are at or below the poverty level. They may not have disposable income to purchase alcohol. Since many older individuals are taking one or more prescription medications, they may be reluctant to consume alcohol for fear of drug-alcohol interactions. Most individuals lose body mass and body water content, resulting in increased sensitivity to alcohol and reduced tolerance. Additionally, lifestyle changes forced by retirement and withdrawal from participation in social and recreational activities may reduce alcohol consumption rates. Finally, there may be an overall cohort effect that reduces alcohol use among this older generation, especially for women. As a group these individuals lived through the Great Depression and Prohibition during their childhood, adolescent, or young adult years. The moral messages of not spending money frivolously (i.e., for alcohol) or not drinking at all may have become well ingrained in this cohort. Different rules existed for alcohol consumption for women, especially during the early part of this century. Women were expected to drink moderately or not drink at all. Proscriptions existed about where women could drink. Taverns would have separate entrances for women to enter the dining area, and women were expected to refrain from entering the bar area.

Discussion   Name other forces that may be a limiting factor in alcohol
Question: consumption among individuals who are elderly.

Estimates of alcoholism among elderly individuals range from a low of 2 percent of this cohort to a high of 15 percent (Benshoff & Roberto, 1987), although most authorities speculate that the rate of alcoholism is less than 10 percent. One reason for low rates of alcoholism for this group may be that traditional gatekeepers to treatment do not identify them as having problems. The vast majority of older individuals who drink in a problematic fashion are hidden drinkers. Because they are retired, they are not exposed to workplace scrutiny of drinking behaviors. Many older individuals no longer drive and thus are unlikely to be arrested for driving under the influence. Ambulatory problems or sensory problems may cause individuals in this age group to drink at home rather than out in society. Finally, very few research studies on addiction or alcoholism have examined drug and alcohol problems among individuals who are elderly (Crandall, 1991).

The biggest factor creating the apparently low rates of alcoholism among the elderly may be the attitudes, beliefs, and misperceptions of family, friends, and treating professionals, however (American Medical Association, Council on Scientific Affairs, 1996; Benshoff & Roberto, 1987). Benshoff and Roberto

(1987) coined the phrase "Nice little old man (or lady) syndrome" to describe the response of professionals and society alike to drug and alcohol problems in elderly individuals. Confronted with an array of symptoms and behaviors characteristic of alcoholism or drug dependence, professionals are loathe to make a diagnosis of dependence. Instead, they respond, "He's such a nice little old man. He couldn't be an alcoholic. It must be some problem related to aging." Ataxic gait and balance problems are attributed to arthritis and joint problems rather than to alcoholism. Cognitive dysfunction is dismissed as expected problems of old age or as dementia, rather than being attributed to the effects of sedative drug consumption. As a consequence of all of the above factors, alcoholism problems and drug dependence may be greatly underdiagnosed in this age cohort, resulting in fewer treatment admissions and ultimately greater costs to the individual, families, and society.

Discussion Question: Discuss other factors that may lead to misdiagnosis or under-diagnosis of drug and alcohol problems for this age group.

Alcoholism in individuals who are elderly is subdivided into early-onset and late-onset alcoholism. Early-onset alcoholism begins prior to age 65 and continues past age 65. Late-onset alcoholism begins after age 65, usually in response to the stresses of later life. Individuals in the early-onset group are intoxicated twice as many days per month as late-onset alcoholics, have more health problems, and are more likely to drop out of treatment. There is a saying among pilots: "There are bold pilots, and there are old pilots, but there are no old-bold pilots." It is likely there are few old-bold alcoholics. Individuals who maintain their alcoholism into old age probably have learned to moderate or control their drinking in order to remain marginally functional in society. Additionally, they may have a well-developed support (or codependent) system in place to protect them from some of the ravages of later-life alcoholism. A large group of early-onset, but now abstinent, male alcoholics reside in nursing homes and suffer from Korsakoff's syndrome and other alcohol-related neurological and physiological problems.

Individuals with late-onset alcoholism are thought to develop alcohol problems as a consequence of poorly developed coping mechanisms for the problems of later life. As a group they more commonly drink at home, and their drinking is often accompanied by a situational depression related to loss. Bereavement resulting from the loss of a loved one, most often a spouse, may precipitate a drinking or drug problem (Kostyk, Lindblom, Fuchs, Tabiz, & Jacyk, 1994). Additionally, the death of a spouse may also mean the loss of a control mechanism, and some individuals may resume earlier, maladaptive drinking patterns. Other losses may catalyze drinking problems. Even though retirement is now characterized as a socially and vocationally appropriate end to a career, many individuals experience profound identity loss. Others find themselves with excess free time and have no hobbies or activities, resulting in stress. Marital conflict may ensue when a husband and wife are now forced to spend more time with each other, and the balance of power and responsibility in the home and relationship shifts. Physical loss and decline are a universal consequence of aging to which most people adapt without significant problems. Some individuals may use alcohol to self-medicate the aches and pains of old age, while others use alcohol to escape from the reality of declining physical ability and health. Unfortunately, the consequence of this behavior is nearly always exacerbation of existing pains and ailments or the creation of new ones. Alcohol potentiates the action of many medications prescribed for conditions related to aging, and combined use poses grave consequences (Peluso & Peluso, 1989).

Many of the drug and alcohol problems encountered by older individuals are rooted in physiological changes related to aging. Absorption of some drugs from the gastrointestinal tract (GI) is reduced because blood flow declines to the GI tract with aging. The older body usually has a higher concentration of body fat and a lower concentration of body water. Consequently, drug concentration levels will be higher for water-soluble drugs such as alcohol and lower for fat-soluble drugs. Other mechanisms lead to higher drug and alcohol concentration levels in the bloodstream. Slowed rates of metabolism and excretion (urinary tract, GI tract, perspiration) are related to aging and lead to higher drug and alcohol concentrations in the body. Finally, body mass is an issue. Many older adults lose body mass as they age, and for them a standard "adult" dose of a medication may be too much.

Drug concentration changes related to aging exacerbate the rates of adverse drug reactions, drug-related hospitalizations, and fatalities among individuals who are elderly. Adverse drug reactions occur three to seven times more often, and 12 percent to 17 percent of hospital admissions for acute problems are drug or alcohol related. Finally, half the drug-related fatalities in this country occur as a result of drug reactions experienced by older people.

A variety of social and psychological factors contribute to drug and alcohol problems among the elderly. Multiple chronic health problems may lead to the consumption of multiple prescription and over-the-counter drugs, increasing the risk of drug interactions and overdose. Elderly individuals often see their family physician for medical care and see a specialist for arthritis and another specialist for cardiovascular problems, for example. Each physician may be prescribing medications, unaware of other medications being prescribed or OTCs being consumed, a condition referred to as polypharmacy (Falvo, Holland, Brenner, & Benshoff, 1990).

Memory and scheduling problems may result in underconsumption or overconsumption, especially when large numbers of drugs are involved. Additionally certain drugs may cause drowsiness or confusion, exacerbating the risk of problems. Self-medication with over-the-counter medicines or alcohol to supplement the effects of prescription medication creates severe problems for many who are aging. People tend to view OTC drugs as less powerful and not apt to contribute to adverse reactions. However, body mass issues and metabolic and excretory changes may increase the power of OTC drugs and increase the risk of adverse reactions. Recently, both the popular and scientific press extolled the health virtues of small amounts of beer or wine. However, little attention has been given to the potential danger of mixing alcohol with other drugs for the elderly or to defining a "small amount."

The consequences of psychoactive drug abuse and dependence for older people include physical, neurological, and social problems. Specific identified risks include higher incidences of certain cancers, sleep disturbances, anemia, heart disease, kidney and hepatic problems, accidents (Riekse & Holstege, 1996), and osteoporosis. The combined consumption of alcohol and pain-relieving analgesics may cause gastrointestinal bleeding. Malnutrition is often seen in elderly individuals with alcoholism problems, attributable to substituting alcohol for food, forgetting to eat, eating an inadequate diet, or spending food money for alcohol. Alcohol and drug consumption may mask the symptoms of physical problems, making diagnosis and treatment more difficult (Tice & Perkins, 1996).

Alcohol and drug use may serve as a precursor to dementia (Rieske & Holstege, 1996), and chronic alcohol dependence is associated with a number of other neurological maladies most commonly seen in older individuals. Peripheral neuropathy manifests itself as muscle weakness and sensory loss in the extremities. Chronic letptomeningitis (wet brain) and chronic brain syndrome are seen often. Both of these diseases cause cognitive and ambulatory dysfunction, and both benefit from dietary improvements and abstinence from alcohol. Wernicke's disease is an organic, toxic psychosis characterized by ataxia, wide gait, disorientation, and confusion. It occurs as a consequence of thiamin deficiency resulting from inadequate diet, reduced intestinal absorption, metabolic changes, or cirrhosis of the liver (Segal & Sisson, 1985), and it is readily treatable with abstinence and proper nutrition, including vitamin therapy. Untreated, Wernicke's disease often progresses to Korsakoff's psychosis. Individuals with Korsakoff's display many of the characteristics of Wernicke's syndrome; they also suffer from memory encoding and recall problems, and display confabulation. These individuals are unable to store new memories, although their long-term memory may be intact but distorted. To accommodate for and conceal recent memory loss, Korsakoff's victims will tell long, involved, and florid stories in response to simple questions. Neophyte counselors are often impressed with the forthcoming nature of these individuals until it becomes clear that they have no recent memory at all. Individuals with Korsakoff's are unable to recall simple items such as the day of the week or the names of staff members who are working with them. At present, treatment for individuals with Korsakoff's is limited to abstinence and supportive protection. There is no viable treatment, and most of these individuals reside in long-term care environments. They are not good candidates for counseling and therapy.

The social consequences of alcohol and drug dependence center around increased isolation and social withdrawal. The denial of problems and the desire to hide drinking and drug-taking behavior may result in the individual withdrawing from normal social interactions. It is common for family members and friends to discount problems early in the emergence of abuse and dependence. Later those same family members may avoid or reject the individual out of frustration, disgust, despair, or denial (Tice & Perkins, 1996).

The treatment prospects for elderly individuals are quite good, especially for individuals with late-onset alcoholism. Ironically, this population has been and continues to be largely unserved by the dependence treatment community (Brown, 1982), with only a few specialized treatment units in existence. In part, the limited services available for older people with dependence problems reflect the attitudes of society and the professional community in general. Dependence treatment professionals may not view older people as good candidates for treatment, and questions may arise about the value of serving this population. In many treatment centers, older individuals may not "fit" well with the rest of the treatment group, and this may be viewed as problematic. Finally, older individuals may not have financial or insurance resources to pay for treatment.

Discussion   What other factors influence the decision to treat or not to
Question: treat an older individual for a dependency problem?

Treatment for this group should focus on the support system and concurrent negative emotional issues that may impact alcohol or drug dependence. Treatment providers should be aware of the physical and cognitive deficits that older individuals may experience. They may not be able to accomplish some tasks as quickly, or they may need additional explanation or support and understanding. Grief and loneliness are significant treatment issues with this group (Kostyk et al., 1994). In many cases alcoholism or drug dependence is precipitated by loss and exacerbated by poor coping skills and a limited or nonexistent social network. Traditionally, treatment centers on another loss as recovery progresses: the loss of alcohol or drugs. Failure to address loss issues and to build positive coping skills will surely lead to relapse.

Adolescents

While little attention is directed at abuse and dependence problems of older individuals, much effort has been directed at preventing and treating drug and alcohol problems at the other end of the age continuum. Nothing attracts national attention more quickly than a report that teenage drug or alcohol use is on the rise. In fact, data from the National High School Drug Use Survey suggest that drug use among adolescents reached its zenith about 1980 and remained at a steady or even declining level until the early 1990s, when an upward trend began (National Clearinghouse for Alcohol and Drug Information, 1997). The percentage of high school seniors who reported the use of any illicit drug peaked at 52.4 percent in 1979 and fell to a low of 27.1 percent in 1992 before rising to a level of 39 percent in 1995. Marijuana use reached its peak in 1979 (50.2 percent), and use declined steadily before trending upward in 1993 to a 1995 high of 34.7 percent. In contrast to the overall trends, stimulant use among high school seniors reached its high point in the mid-eighties. Cocaine use was reported by 13.1 percent of the class of 1985, and stimulant drug use peaked at 26 percent in 1982. Crack cocaine use was first examined in 1986 when 4.1 percent of high school seniors reported use. Reported crack use fell to 1.5 percent of high school seniors in 1991 and has hovered between 1.5 percent and 2.1 percent since then. As might be expected in a country where alcohol presents the greatest adult drug problem, alcohol is the chemical most frequently used by teenagers. Of the class of 1979, 88.1 percent reported at least one episode of alcohol consumption during the previous year. Alcohol consumption reports have declined steadily to a low of 76 percent in 1993, the last year for which data are available. However, the picture is less positive for indicators of alcohol abuse. In 1990 the High School Drug Survey began asking if students had been drunk in the previous year. Slightly more than half of all respondents answered affirmatively; similar responses have occurred throughout the nineties. Other data suggest that about a third of high school seniors have engaged in binge drinking (five or more drinks at one setting), increasing the likelihood of intoxication-related problems such as accidents, violence, and high risk behaviors (Ellickson, 1995).

Discussion   Discuss the trends and factors contributing to changes in
Question: adolescent drug and alcohol use over the years.

Alcohol, tobacco, and marijuana are described as "gateway" drugs, and their use is thought to exceed 90 percent for adolescents. Doweiko (1996) includes inhalants in the category of gateway drugs, asserting that it is a drug often used in adolescent experimentation. Experimentation with gateway drugs is thought to precede the use of other, more harmful drugs (Ellickson, 1995; Fisher & Harrison, 1997), a sort of domino theory of drug abuse. In reality, while the vast majority of adolescents experiment with alcohol, tobacco, or marijuana, the use of more dangerous drugs is much more limited. Several authors (Abadinsky, 1997; Doweiko, 1996; Fisher & Harrison, 1997) point out that our understanding of adolescent drug use patterns is not entirely precise. The National High School Survey collects data from about 15,000 to 19,000 students enrolled in high schools across the country. It examines student responses and fails to collect data from individuals who have dropped out of school or students who remain enrolled but who have stopped attending school. Yet, the data are clear that dropouts and students with high absentee records are at greatest risk for drug and alcohol problems. Second, while the survey provides a broad look at national patterns, it may overlook or obscure local patterns or issues of importance. For example, it fails to distinguish between urban and rural concerns, and it may understate or underestimate the impact of local or regional events. Finally, the survey examines current drugs of use and abuse, and it may be slow to pick up trends or the emergence of new drugs. Crack first appeared in the survey in 1986, and steroids first appeared in 1989, yet anecdotal and clinical evidence suggests problems were occurring prior to those dates. Abadinsky (1997) suggests that the results of the survey may be skewed by conscious or unconscious errors in information attributable to the self-report format. Some students may underreport their drug or alcohol use by responding in a socially acceptable response set manner.

Others may exaggerate their use to impress their peers; and still others may report inaccurate information out of ignorance about drugs or because of recall problems.

Discussion   Discuss your personal perceptions of changes in drug and
Question: alcohol consumption patterns during the past ten years.

Fisher and Harrison (1997) identified a variety of risk factors predisposing adolescents to use of, abuse of, or dependence on drugs or alcohol. They suggest that family consumption patterns and family attitudes and perceptions about drugs and alcohol may influence use and abuse patterns. Low levels of family bonding and communication and high levels of family conflict are also endangering factors. School problems including persistent behavior problems, academic failure, low attendance rates, high tardiness rates, and social rejection during the elementary years contribute to increased likelihood of abuse problems among teens. A childhood history of hyperactivity, learning disabilities, and conduct disorder have all been cited as possible precursors or markers for eventual substance abuse (Fishbein & Pease, 1996). Hawkins and his associates (1992) assert that peer influences, family influences, early onset of use, and alienation and rebellious characteristics are all predisposing factors. There is a long and extensive history linking adolescent drug and alcohol use and membership in gangs (Fagan, 1993). Increasingly, the co-occurrence of violence and drug-consuming behaviors is a pervasive facet of gang drug use.

From a developmental perspective, individuals who begin abusing drugs and alcohol during their teenage years are at great risk for later life problems and crises. Erikson (1968) argues that adolescence is a time when individuals learn to (1) get along with peers, authority figures (i.e., teachers), and others; (2) develop a sense of who they are in relation to other people and distinguish between the demands of self and the needs and demands of others; and (3) develop a sense of personal, individual identity. Respectively referred to as the stages of industry vs inferiority, group identity vs alienation, and individual identity vs identity confusion, these stages incorporate basic skills needed for successful adult living. Robert Havighurst, another developmental theorist, asserts that adolescents face a group of specific developmental tasks that prepare them for adult functioning as successful individuals. Both Havighurst and Erikson argue that noncompletion of adolescent developmental experiences may result in specific life difficulties. Erikson contends that identity confusion occurs when the individual fails to safely make the transition from the security of childhood status to the more ambiguous and threatening role of adult autonomy, resulting in a failure of the individual to develop a strong, clear sense of personal identity. They may take one of two paths, either withdrawing from family friends and peers into isolation or losing themselves in the crowd (Santrock, 1990). Marcia's work (as cited in Santrock, 1990 and Vinacke, 1968) expanded on Erikson's concepts, postulating four methods of identity resolution in adolescence. Some individuals experience identity diffusion, showing little interest, commitment, or affinity for particular ideological or societal roles. Identity foreclosure describes a situation in which the individual has prematurely fixed the self-identity by adopting an identity role based on the values and mores handed down by parental figures. In this situation, the adolescent has often not conducted a sufficient exploration of possible options and opportunities. The identity moratorium stage is characterized by vague commitment to the resolution of identity issues. Unlike the two previous intervals, individuals in the moratorium phase are exploring identity issues but in an unfocused fashion. The identity achievement stage is typified by a clear commitment to a series of life goals related to identity, vocation, family, and self.

Individuals with identity confusion problems are variously described as unattached, unable to find themselves, cognitively disorganized, and impulsive. They often are thought to have trouble forming warm, accepting relationships but instead have a series of superficial, sporadic relationships. Finally, their pathologically prolonged identity crisis often culminates in an inability or unwillingness to assume personal responsibility for their actions. Adherents to psychiatric models might describe these individuals as having a personality disorder or an adjustment reaction to adult life.

No matter what label is assigned or what theory is followed, the characteristics displayed by individuals unable to explore and resolve identity issues closely parallel the characteristics of individuals who experience drug and alcohol problems. Thus, the concern for drug and alcohol abuse among adolescents must extend beyond short-term, quick solutions aimed at curbing adolescent consumption.

Discussion Questions: How does the failure to achieve identity achievement manifest itself in drug and alcohol problems? Do individuals in particular phases seem more prone to drug and alcohol problems?

Developmental problems may arise in areas other than personality. Jean Piaget, the Swiss educator, developed a four-stage process to explain intellectual development. Like other developmental theorists, Piaget believed intellectual development was a function of personal development and then environment, conceptualizing the ideas of assimilation and accommodation. Assimilation refers to the process of fitting previously acquired skills and expressive qualities into the environment. Using assimilation, the young child realizes that crying will evoke a response from caregivers in the environment. Accommodation alludes to the development of new behaviors and cognitions to meet the demands of the environment. Permeating Piaget's work are the ideas that intellectual development proceeds from crude, egocentric states to a state of higher cognitive organization characterized by abstract thinking skills and greater degrees of control over self and the environment (Vinacke, 1968).

Piaget defined four stages of intellectual growth: sensorimotor stage, preoperational stage, concrete operations, and formal operations. This stage model is unvaried in its sequencing, and each stage derives from and transforms the previous stage. The first two stages occur during the first six or seven years of life and depict the movement of the child's intellect from a state of egocentric, reflexive activity to a state in which the child is able to use signs and symbols and make distinctions between objects and groups of objects. The concrete operations stage roughly is consistent with the elementary school years and marks the development of concepts of order and system as well as the ability to manipulate numbers. The formal operations stage is the highest level of intellectual development according to Piaget and is characterized by the emergence of abstract thinking and the ability to generate hypotheses (i.e., the ability to ask What if?). Not all adults achieve the abilities inherent in formal operations, and even so, abstract thinking is required for relatively few adult tasks. Because Piaget's stages occur in sequential fashion, it is evident that problems encountered in early stages will result in magnified problems in later stages. Thus, children growing up in an alcoholic home, deprived of intellectual support and stimulation during their years of intellectual development, may experience significant deficits in abstract thinking abilities. Similarly, adolescents who begin using drugs and alcohol during the early teenage years may have difficulty developing formal operational skills. In part this may be due to the negative influences on cognition of mood-altering drugs. What is more important, school tardiness, frequent absences, or dropping out are likely to limit the ability to develop abstract cognitive skills.

Donald Super, in work that spanned six decades, postulates that adolescence is a period of exploration of vocational career orientation and examining specific career directions. He argued that vocational self-concept is tied closely to overall self-concept and that subsequent vocational behavior is grounded in the total self-concept. According to Super's (1957) model, adolescents go through stages of exploration and crystallization during which they examine various career alternatives and begin to solidify their vocational preferences. Vocational choice is strongly influenced by socioeconomic status, personality characteristics, educational background, and opportunities to which the individual is exposed (Power, 1991). Clearly drug or alcohol abuse is included in the influencing factors with respect to both identity and vocational choices among adolescents. Vocational role is a fundamental indicator, component, and definer of adult status. One of the primary icebreaker questions used by individuals in new encounters is "What do you do for a living?" The response to that question serves as a definer of status and standing within the culture. Consequently, and importantly, the failure of adolescents to develop a sense of vocational identity may have long-lasting vocational, socioeconomic, and social implications for later life.

Sexual Orientation

The 3.7 million gay men and lesbians are thought to have significantly higher risk factors for the development of drug and alcohol problems. Various commentaries suggest that as many as 30 percent of gays experience drug and alcohol problems, compared to about 10 percent of the general population. However, very limited research centers on the drug and alcohol problems of this group, and research design and methodology questions are abundant (Jung, 1994).

One of the most commonly cited risk factors for gays is the gay bar scene (Stevens-Smith & Smith, 1998). For many gay individuals, the gay bar is the only place to meet new friends, socialize, and recreate, free from the stigma and prejudices of a largely homophobic society. While recreation and leisure choices have expanded in recent years with the advent of gay bookstores, coffee shops, church groups (e.g., the Metropolitan Community Church), and other social venues, the gay bar remains a dominant force in the gay culture. Since the bar is a dominant force, many speculate that alcohol-related risk factors increase proportionately for gays because alcohol is so intimately and ubiquitously tied to socialization. Traditionally alcoholism research in the gay community has focused on gay bar patrons, largely because they represented a sample of convenience. Gay bars are the one place where large numbers of gay individuals can be located and approached about drug and alcohol use issues. However, the use of a bar or tavern as a sampling site may spuriously increase estimates of drinking and drug-taking behaviors by examining a sample from a setting where one would expect higher levels of alcohol consumption behaviors. Researchers who have examined alcohol and drug use behaviors in more representative gay populations (Paul, Stall, & Bloomfield, 1991; McKirnan & Peterson, 1989) assert that drug and alcohol problems exist at a higher rate in the gay community. They note that this phenomenon is true across genders. Both homosexual men and women are thought to have higher use rates and risk factors for problem development than their heterosexual counterparts. Wojakowski (1997) suggests that as many as 35 percent of lesbians have a history of excessive drinking, compared to 5 percent of heterosexual women, for example.

Discussion Question: Discuss strategies to collect more accurate drug and alcohol use/abuse/dependence data within the gay community.

A number of more abstract concerns, however, probably exceed the drug and alcohol risk factors imposed by the gay bar scene. Many gay and lesbian individuals demonstrate fears and anxieties about rejection from friends, families, and society. For many these fears and anxieties are born of actual, devastating experiences. Society virtually demands that gay men and women conceal their sexual identity from friends, family, peers, coworkers, and colleagues, and "coming out" often results in rejection and alienation (Finnegan & McNally, 1989). Unfortunately many individuals who do not have a well-developed repertoire of coping mechanisms may turn to drugs and alcohol to relieve their emotional pain.

Many gay individuals are unwilling to disclose their sexual orientation, opting to remain "in the closet" for fear of retribution, rejection, or oppression (Pohl, 1991). Their inability or unwillingness to resolve self-identity, self-worth, and self-acceptance issues often leads to feelings of low self-esteem, self-hatred, depression, despair, and alienation (Wojakowski, 1997). Just as in the general population, these feelings and self-perceptions are inextricably tied to substance abuse and dependence.

While members of the gay and lesbian community may be at higher risk for drug and alcohol problems, treatment resources sensitive to gay and lesbian concerns are in scarce supply, and many gay and lesbian individuals are reluctant to enter treatment. For some gay or lesbian individuals, acknowledgment of a drug or alcohol problem is doubly stigmatizing. Failure to acknowledge either or both issues sets up an endless cycle of denial, repression, substance abuse, and continued problems. Individuals who do seek treatment may be faced with homophobic attitudes in treatment centers. Often facilities will not address sexual orientation issues in the intake or assessment process and will actively discourage the discussion of sexual orientation concerns during treatment. As recently as 1973 homosexuality was considered a mental disorder by the American Psychiatric Association. According to Stevens-Smith and Smith (1998) the research evidence concerning the attitudes, perceptions, and behaviors of counselors is contradictory. Some research suggests that counselors tend to have more positive attitudes toward gays and lesbians; other studies indicate that heterosexual counselors have heterosexist attitudes and stereotypic beliefs about homosexuality. They may incorrectly attribute drug and alcohol dependence behaviors to sexual orientation problems or assume that all gay and lesbian individuals have similar concerns, lifestyles, and behaviors. A greater concern for individuals may be the reactions of fellow treatment participants. Gay and lesbian individuals may be reluctant to disclose their sexual orientation in group for fear of encountering the same types of homophobic behaviors as in the rest of society. This is a problem faced in ongoing recovery, too. The ability to openly discuss sexual orientation problems in treatment and recovery is essential, yet many Alcoholics Anonymous groups exhibit stereotypes and value systems inconsistent with inclusion and full participation of gays and lesbians. Dr. Melvin Pohl suggests that the religious language and seeming religious orientation of many peer self-help groups may deter many gay and lesbian individuals in recovery from participating (1991). As Pohl notes, homosexual behaviors or open admission of homosexual status is inconsistent with the ideology of nearly all mainstream religious groups. Commonly many individuals have trouble coping with the religious language inherent in peer self-help fellowships; gays and lesbians may have problems beyond the general population. Recent years have seen an explosion in membership in gay- and lesbian-specific AA groups and in the emergence of other self-help groups serving the gay and lesbian population. These groups include recovery clubs such as Lambda, Live and Let Live, Alcoholics Together, and others. Unfortunately, many peer self-help groups specifically for gay and lesbian individuals are found only in urban environments.

Specialized treatment is available for gay men and women at Pride Institute in Minnesota, CleanStart in Chicago, and at scattered other sites around the United States. As a group characteristic, gay men and women tend to be better educated, have higher incomes, and better health insurance than the general population. However, many gay individuals may be reluctant to enter

treatment, fearing either job loss, higher insurance rates or insurance cancellation, and double stigmatization. The potential for insurance cancellation or
coverage reduction is especially troublesome for gay males, who may feel coverage is needed to deal with the potential acquisition of AIDS. At one time gay
males were the group at greatest risk for contracting AIDS. However, IV drug
users now have about three times the risk of gay males for contracting AIDS,
and gay males who use IV drugs comprise the subgroup at greatest risk. Moreover, the specter of AIDS contraction remains very real in the gay community,
caused mainly by unsafe sex practices often linked to the disinhibiting effects
of alcohol or drug consumption. Thanks to aggressive AIDS prevention and
education programs, infection rates have fallen dramatically in recent years.
Many AIDS patients are living much longer as a result of improved health care
practices and expanded medication options.

While the gay and lesbian communities have higher risk factors for drug
and alcohol problems, little literature exists that details specific gay/lesbian consumption patterns or practices. Some gay men have been reputed to use amyl
nitrite to enhance sexual pleasure. Available over the counter prior to 1980,
amyl nitrite is a liquid that dilates blood vessels and speed up the heart rate and
causes the user to feel stimulated and euphoric. The drug is packaged in glass
ampules that are snapped, producing a popping sound and conferring the street
name "poppers." The volatile vapors are inhaled by the user. After amyl nitrite
was reclassified as a prescription drug, some users turned to butyl nitrite to get
high, and others continued to obtain amyl nitrite, often illegally diverted from
hospital supplies. Anecdotal evidence suggests that cocaine use among gay males
is popular to enhance sexual pleasure and to alter consciousness.

Recently great concern has emerged about the use of methamphetamines
as a sexual aphrodisiac and mood altering drug in the gay male community
(Gorman, 1996). Known on the street as speed, methamphetamine is easily and
cheaply synthesized and can be ingested by smoking, eating or drinking, intravenous injection, or absorption through the mucous membranes. The form of
methamphetamine that is smoked is known as ice on the street. According to
Gorman, compelling evidence exists linking AIDS and speed use (1996). A
number of methamphetamine epidemics have occurred, including one in the
1950s characterized by abuse of benzedrine inhalers, followed by a 1960s epidemic tied to the 1960s drug scene and most recently the methamphetamine
epidemic of the 1990s.

Amphetamines and methamphetamine have declined in popularity for traditional medical uses, supplanted by safer, more effective pharmaceuticals, and
today the only accepted use of amphetamines is the treatment of children
with attention deficit hyperactivity disorder (ADHD). Nearly the entire available supply of methamphetamine is illicitly produced, and production is
driven by user demand. Geographically, methamphetamine abuse centers in the
western United States, especially in areas with a large gay population. Other
identified user groups include bikers, truckers, and some construction workers, according to Gorman. Because speed is typically manufactured in small,
clandestine labs that seem to pop up at random, it is difficult to track its use

and availability, and little is known about the drug, its history of use/abuse, and appropriate treatment protocols. Ecstasy is a methamphetamine analogue (3–4 methylenedioxymethamphetamine) that gained great popularity in the late 1980s as the love drug among the heterosexual and homosexual communities, particularly among afficionados of rave dance parties and techno rock music (Palfai & Jankiewicz, 1997). Formally referred to as MDMA, the drug is also known as XTC, essence, clarity, and a number of other colloquial terms. Typically ingested in tablet form, the drug produces mind-altering stimulant effects and hallucinations.

Gorman argues that the use of speed in the gay population is linked to increased rates of HIV infection. Intravenous use clearly heightens the disease contraction danger, but the real increase in infection rates centers around unsafe sexual practices caused by speed's disinhibiting effects. Additionally, evidence is mounting that some individuals with AIDS may be using speed to self-medicate AIDS-related symptoms or to treat AIDS-related depression. The violence and social isolation associated with speed use contradict its use among individuals whose immune systems require all possible physical and psychological support.

Discussion Question: Discuss the short- and long-term consequences of speed use for individuals who are HIV positive.

Treatment concerns about working with gay and lesbian individuals do not center around specific drug use types but more on the ability and sensitivity of the treatment provider to serve individuals whose life experience may be significantly different from that of the counselor. Sexual orientation must be discussed openly, honestly, and nonjudgmentally in counseling sessions. Counselors must not fall prey to the stereotypic notion that all gay and lesbian individuals have sexual orientation problems. Some will have worked through these issues and are ready, willing, and interested in drug and alcohol recovery as their first priority. Others will have significant personal issues that must be addressed and resolved as part of the recovery process. Demonstrating a willingness to examine and discuss specific sexual orientation concerns is the first step in the process of serving gay and lesbian clients. Too many counselors and facilities fail to include questions about sexual orientation in the intake and assessment process, unwittingly giving the impression that this is not an important concern. Others may intentionally omit questions about sexual orientation because they feel ill-prepared to consider sexual orientation issues or because they do not want to deal with those issues. Normalizing sexual orientation issues by including sensitively phrased and appropriately timed questions sends a message to gay and lesbian clients, to heterosexual clients, and to staff that issues related to sexual orientation are an important and standard part of the treatment process. Counselors should not forget that many clients will have unresolved sexual issues according to the research of Glover, Janikowski, and Benshoff (1995). Consequently, normalizing sexual orientation and other sexual issues will create benefits for all clients.

Discussion   Discuss strategies to "normalize" and promote the thoughtful
Question: analysis of sexual orientation concerns in counseling. Analyze
the impact of this concept on clients, staff, and other groups.

SUMMARY

Culture includes the beliefs, values, mores, knowledge and skills shared by a
population or group. It is often defined by race, however more useful definers
of culture are ethnicity, life span development or societally generated definitions. Cultural issues presuppose interaction of individuals with each other and
with surrounding cultures. These interactions are both dynamic and evolutionary. Acculturation has a dual meaning: it includes the struggle individuals face
in adapting to a new culture and it refers to the interaction of two cultures in
close proximity.

The syntax of cultural concepts is broad and varied. Ethnocentrism refers
to a belief system that an individual's own culture is preeminent; conversely,
multi-cultural and culturally pluralistic persons recognize and value the contributions of multiple cultures. Culture is influenced by language, politics, family, economics, and many other factors. The increasing diversity of society
requires counselors to go beyond mere cultural sensitivity to cultural
competence. Competence incorporates understanding and sensitivity with a
commitment to continued knowledge acquisition and change. The culturally
competent counselor is aware of and understands personal cultural values, attitudes and beliefs and simultaneously understands the social forces affecting the
client, while retaining the ability to be supportive and objective.

Ethnicity is the most prevalent definer of culture. African Americans constitute the largest ethnic group in the U.S. and it is far from a monolithic
group, reflecting substantial diversity. Akbar has identified six cultural characteristics central to African Americans: Language, oral patterns of information
transmission, people orientation, interaction vs. reaction, distinct thought patterns, and spontaneity. The extended family, the church, and other African
American groups play a significant role in this culture. The data suggests that
African Americans have drinking rates similar to the general population, but
that the consequences of drinking may be more severe. The impact of crack
cocaine has been especially devastating to the African American community,
and fewer treatment resources for this problem are available.

The heterogenous group referred to as Hispanic American includes individuals because of shared national heritage, principal language or ethnic background. Many Hispanic Americans date their residency in the United States
back hundreds of years, while others are newly arrived, and still others move
back and forth between this country and their home nation. The broad range
of this culture makes it difficult to ascribe particular group-wide characteristics with certainty. Generally this culture values extended families, a strong
family hierarchy, and traditional roles for men and women. Unique concepts

like *personalismo, simpatia,* and *machismo* are reflective of important Hispanic American values. Drug and alcohol data for this population are flawed, but reflect early onset of adolescent consumption behaviors, and higher consumption rates for less well-assimilated adults. Hispanic Americans have a higher than expected rate of HIV/AIDS.

Native Americans number about 2 million Americans affiliated with a variety of tribes, bands, and clans. As a group, Native Americans are confronted with significant health, unemployment and socioeconomic problems, often related to alcohol consumption. Half of the ten leading causes of death in this group are attributable to alcohol, including high rates of cirrhosis, diabetes, fetal alcohol syndrome, and car accidents. Some scholars trace the development of these alcohol problems to the mostly negative history of alcohol distribution and use among Native Americans. Five patterns of Native American drinking have been identified: partying, maintaining, heavy drinking, white man's drinking and teetotaling. Native American cultural practices including the importance of the extended family and life balance can play a significant role in the recovery process.

Society defines some groups as culturally distinct where drugs and alcohol are concerned. Women, elderly individuals, adolescents and gay and lesbian individuals represent four such groups. Women face the increased stigma around drug and alcohol consumption because of societal attitudes about gender roles and drugs and alcohol. Other factors facing women include high rates of incest, sexual abuse, and domestic violence related trauma, limitations in treatment, and physiological issues that make treatment different. Women with alcohol problems are often seen in relationships with men with alcohol or drug problems and are often victimized sexually. Despite high rates of victimization, many treatment facilities are ill-equipped to deal with traumatic problems. Women are more likely to suffer concurrent depression, and to abuse benzodiazepines. Many women who use stimulant medications (e.g., methamphetamines, cocaine) suffer from eating disorders. Treatment services are male oriented and male dominated, but a number of groups, notably Woman for Sobriety, are emerging as treatment resources or treatment adjuncts.

Individuals who are elderly constitute the largest growing age cohort in the country. They are frequent users of both prescription and over-the-counter medications, however alcohol consumption patterns appear to be lower than the general population. Economic, physiological, and attitudinal factors serve to depress rates of alcohol use. Elderly individuals with abuse problems are divided typically into late-onset and early-onset groups. Late-onset alcoholics begin drinking later in life, usually in response to specific stresses or losses. Early-onset alcoholics begin their problem drinking earlier in life and continue to abuse alcohol after age 65. This group is more difficult to treat. Older individuals face many unique problems, often related to the physiology of aging, or changes in socioeconomic status. Many elderly individuals do well in treatment, however treatment agencies have largely ignored this group.

Adolescent drug and alcohol use is a topic of continuing national concern and the subject of much data collection and research. The gateway drugs (alcohol, tobacco, and marijuana) and crack cocaine are the principal drugs of concern with this population. Several risk factors seem to predispose adolescents to drug and alcohol use, including family issues, school problems, peer influences, childhood hyperactivity problems, and early onset of use. Many of the problems related to adolescent alcohol and drug use can be seen in developmental problems. Consequently, solutions to teenage drug and alcohol problems do not lie in short-term solutions. Psychological, educational and vocational issues must be addressed.

Gay men and lesbians seem to have significantly higher risk rates for drug and alcohol problems. The gay bar scene is thought to contribute to increased consumption. Other more potent factors seem to include anxieties and fears related to sexual identity, possible rejection by family and friends, and issues related to the resolution of self-identity and self-esteem. Specific treatment resources for this population are limited, and many traditional treatment providers espouse homophobic attitudes and beliefs. Some specialized treatment programs have been developed, along with gay and lesbian-specific 12-Step groups. Analysis of consumption patterns reveals a high rate of stimulant drug abuse, often tied to sexual behavior. Successful treatment is linked to abandonment of homophobic attitudes, and a willingness to openly examine and discuss sexual orientation issues as part of the treatment process.

12

Substance Abuse as a Coexisting Disability

CHAPTER 12 OUTLINE

Nearly one-fifth (49 million+) of all Americans have some form of disability (Rehabilitation Research and Training Center on Drugs and Disability, 1996). While a variety of formal definitions of disability exist, the term itself is generally thought to imply a "condition that impairs or imposes restrictions on a person's ability to function at normal or expected levels of mental or physical activity" (Nagler & Wilson, 1995, p. 257). The concept of disability has evolved from an original, post–World War I concept of disability encompassing only physical impairments or sensory loss. The first individuals who served in the newly created state-federal rehabilitation system were WWI veterans who had suffered war-related injuries. Later, in the 1940s, disability came to incorporate mental retardation and mental illness. Learning disabilities joined the roster of disabilities via educational disciplines in the late seventies. More recently, diseases such as Acquired Immune Deficiency Syndrome (AIDS), cancer, and other progressive disorders and diseases have been included in the disability paradigm. On a formal basis, substance abuse and substance dependence have traditionally been regarded outside the disability framework until the passage of the Americans with Disabilities Act (ADA), although some states, notably South Carolina, have offered vocational rehabilitation services to individuals with substance abuse problems for many years. Title I of the ADA offers an individual with a history of alcohol or drug abuse protections as a qualified person with a disability. The law does distinguish between drug users and alcohol users. Individuals who are using illegal drugs are excluded from protection. They must be abstinent from drug use and participating in or be a graduate of a rehabilitation program. The law is somewhat more flexible with respect to alcohol use, recognizing as a person with a disability an individual who is currently using alcohol. For clinical purposes, the ADA clearly intends to protect individuals with a documented history of substance abuse/dependence who are making or have made personal rehabilitative efforts.

Prior to the passage of the ADA, a limited number of individuals with drug or alcohol dependence problems were served within the state-federal rehabilitation system. These services tended to be offered by progressive state rehabilitation agencies, individual counselors, or agency offices with a particular interest in or motivation to serve clients with drug and alcohol problems. Frequently offices or state systems would (and still do) establish arbitrary guidelines for eligibility for services. Establishing minimum lengths of sobriety prior to eligibility is a common requirement; other requirements include attending a specified number of Alcoholics Anonymous meetings prior to acceptance for services or completing an inpatient treatment program. Many counselors routinely include continued participation in AA as part of the Individualized Written Rehabilitation Program (IWRP). In most situations arbitrary guidelines such as these have served to include compliant, cooperative clients and to exclude most individuals with drug and alcohol problems from the state-federal system. The experiences of Sydney illustrate the problems encountered by alcohol- and drug-dependent individuals in the state-federal vocational rehabilitation system.

The Case of Sydney

Sydney had a history of drug and alcohol dependence dating back five years. He began attending AA and Narcotics Anonymous and enrolled in a local college where his admissions and financial aid counselor suggested he might qualify for department of rehabilitation services support for his education. Syd went to the local state rehabilitation office and applied for services, only to be told that he would have to demonstrate a year of sobriety before he would be eligible for rehabilitation services. After completing a year of college with an *A* average and the requisite year of sobriety, Syd reapplied for rehabilitation services. This time the counselor reviewed his progress and decided that he did not have a disability. He was no longer drinking and using drugs and was functioning well as a member of society. He was declared ineligible for services.

Discussion Question: Does your state or local rehabilitation system have regulations concerning the eligibility of individuals with drug or alcohol abuse and dependence problems?

Individuals with drug and alcohol problems have had difficulty accessing the rehabilitation system, and, correspondingly, individuals with traditional disabilities have been underserved by the substance abuse treatment network. Prior to and even subsequent to the passage of the Americans with Disabilities Act many substance dependence treatment facilities were not accessible to individuals with ambulatory disabilities (i.e., individuals who use wheelchairs). The nature of therapy and a shortage of qualified interpreters was thought to preclude participation by deaf individuals. The abstract nature of many substance abuse concepts was perceived to limit participation by individuals who had developmental disabilities, and transportation and access problems and the extensive use of bibliotherapy ruled out therapy participation by individuals with visual problems. Few people with "traditional" disabilities sought treatment, and fewer still were served. The passage of ADA required all facilities, including substance abuse treatment services, to be fully accessible to everyone. More importantly a grassroots movement of disability advocates emerged in the early nineties, promoting the inclusion of individuals with disabilities in all needed and required services, including substance abuse treatment. Along with this advocacy came growing recognition that individuals with traditional disabilities were often at greater risk for the development of substance abuse and dependence treatment services. The research carried out by Dr. Dennis Moore of the Substance Abuse Resources and Disability Issues (SARDI) program of the School of Medicine at Wright State University has consistently revealed that individuals with traditional disabilities are at greater risk for substance abuse problems and are less likely to have services available to them (Moore & Li, 1994). Even when professional services are available and accessible, people with traditional disabilities face problems accessing aftercare and peer self-help programs. Many AA and NA meeting are held in church basements or similar settings with architectural barriers because the ADA does not require most nonprofit groups to achieve accessibility standards. Individuals who need interpretive services for the deaf must provide their own at a cost burden that may be extravagant. Some meetings are held in places inaccessible by public transportation, ruling out participation by individuals who do not or cannot drive. This is not just a disability-specific issue, although it occurs more often and more specifically with some disabilities. Obviously individuals who are blind cannot drive. What is more important, many individuals with disabilities live in poverty and cannot afford a car, no matter their disability.

Discussion Questions: Are your local substance abuse treatment centers accessible to people with disabilities? Are AA and NA meetings accessible?

This chapter will examine the coexistence of substance abuse and dependence disabilities with traditional disabilities. It will review demographic data, outline unique concerns related to traditional and substance abuse disabilities, and offer guidelines for service provision.

SUBSTANCE ABUSE/DEPENDENCE COEXISTING WITH PHYSICAL DISABILITIES

Traumatic Brain Injury

Of all the disability classifications, traumatic brain injury is the disability most commonly associated with coexisting substance abuse or dependence. Annually an estimated 50,000 to 70,000 Americans experience head injuries resulting in significant, enduring neurological impairments, and a total of more than a million Americans suffer ongoing neurological problems or loss (National Institute on Disability and Rehabilitation Research, 1994). Alcohol is implicated in at least half of all automotive (the leading cause of head injury) and bicycle accidents and is even more commonly associated with head injuries caused by violence (Naugle, 1990). Data have not revealed the number of head injuries attributed to drug-related violence, but clearly this is another very high-risk area.

Traumatic brain injury occurs when a blow or outside force is applied to the head. The blow may be direct—for example, when the head strikes the steering wheel in a car accident—or it may be indirect, as when the brain rebounds within the cranium as the result of an outside force. Football players often suffer concussions (i.e., loss of consciousness without any lasting neurological effects) as the result of a violent tackle. The head, well shielded by a helmet, may not be contacted, but the jarring effect of the tackle may cause the brain to rebound in the skull, resulting in contusions to the brain or occasionally the formation of hematomas. Traumatic brain injury may be the result of an open injury in which the brain is exposed and damaged as a consequence of trauma-related penetration of the skull and direct damage to the brain. A closed head injury occurs when the brain is damaged by a blow or rebound force but no actual skull penetration is evident. Most traumatic brain injury is the result of closed head injury, although violence-related head injury may be the result of a bullet wound or other penetrating injury.

Brain damage may eventuate following a cerebrovascular accident (stroke) or as a result of anoxia caused by a cardiovascular accident (heart attack). Generally this brain damage is not the result of direct, outside trauma or force, but it clearly results in trauma to the brain. Most strokes and heart attacks happen among older individuals as a consequence of normal age-related events, but drug and alcohol use has been implicated in both stroke and heart attack in younger individuals.

As might be expected, males in their late adolescent and early adulthood years are at greatest risk for traumatic brain injury (Naugle, 1990). Nonwhites (African Americans and Hispanic Americans) are 49 percent more likely to experience traumatic brain injury (Jagger et al., 1984). Traumatic brain injuries occur most frequently during evening and nighttime hours and on weekends when individuals are engaged in leisure activities, driving, or drinking. They take place most often in the warm weather months, according to Naugle. Interestingly he points out that fewer accident-related head injuries transpire during cold weather, despite more hazardous road conditions. He speculates that drivers may be more cautious and more likely to wear seat belts during winter driving conditions.

Not all alcohol- and drug-related head injuries happen to individuals who are drug or alcohol dependent. Many individuals suffer injury as a result of acute intoxication or drug use, and some individuals have accidents as a sequella of hangovers or withdrawal. Still others are victims of drunk or drug-impaired drivers. Whatever the use/abuse/dependence circumstance, the data are clear that drugs and alcohol are closely linked to the etiology of traumatic brain injury. Yet, evidence is equally clear that trauma center personnel often fail to evaluate or identify alcohol or drug use or abuse as a precipitating event and fail to make appropriate referrals for drug and alcohol evaluations and treatment (Shipley, Taylor, & Falvo, 1990).

Many individuals suffer physical problems secondary to traumatic brain injury. They may experience paralysis or hemiparesis, gait or balance disturbances, reduced motor and ambulatory speed, and loss of coordination (Collum, Kuck, & Ruff, 1990). While these physical losses can result in severe impairments from a physical rehabilitation standpoint, the emotional, cognitive, language, and sensory deficits resulting from traumatic brain injury pose more serious rehabilitation challenges.

Many individuals with traumatic brain injury suffer memory problems and especially short-term memory loss. Treatment of drug and alcohol problems may be limited by the client's inability to follow directions, recall instructions, or understand even concrete counseling suggestions. Individuals with short-term memory loss may confabulate to conceal their memory deficits, a phenomenon also seen in chronic alcoholics who have Korsakoff's syndrome. They may invent stories or events to fill in memory gaps. Unfortunately, confabulations may be interpreted as denial, deception, or lack of treatment compliance rather than a true, neurologically imposed problem.

Decreased self-awareness and insight are often seen in clients. Impaired cognitive functioning may result in an inability to make connections between behaviors and their consequences. Often TBI clients were risk takers before suffering their injury and often suffered their injury as a result of high-risk behavior. Their impaired judgment and insight may lead them to continue high-risk activities and limit their ability to ascertain the added risks of mixing drugs, alcohol, and high-risk situations. Situations or activities requiring abstract reasoning may be especially difficult also because of cognitive losses. Some individuals lose the ability to integrate and analyze information, and they may have great difficulty comprehending even the most simple concepts such as "one day at a time." William Peterman (National Head Injury Foundation, 1988), recognizing the difficulty many traumatic brain injury survivors have with abstract concepts, has rewritten the 12 Steps in more concrete and understandable language.

1. Admit that if you drink and/or use drugs your life will be out of control. Admit that the use of substance after having had a traumatic brain injury will make your life unmanageable.

2. You start to believe that someone can help you put your life in order. This someone could be God, an AA group, counselor, sponsor, etc.

3. You decide to get help from other or God. You open yourself up.

4. You will make a complete list of the negative behaviors in your past and current behavior problems. You will also make a list of your positive behaviors.

5. Meet with someone you trust and discuss what you wrote in step 4.

6. Become ready to sincerely try to change your negative behaviors.

7. Ask God for the strength to be a responsible person with responsible behaviors.

8. Make a list of people your negative behaviors have affected. Be ready to apologize or make things right with them.

9. Contact these people. Apologize or make things right.

10. Continue to check yourself and your behaviors daily. Correct negative behaviors and improve them. If you hurt another person, apologize and make corrections.

11. Stop and think about how you are behaving several times each day. Are my behaviors positive? Am I being responsible? If not, ask for help. Reward yourself when you are able to behave in a positive and responsible fashion.

12. If you try to work these steps you will start to feel much better about yourself. Now it's your turn to help others do the same. Helping others will make you feel even better. Continue to work these steps on a daily basis. (Reprinted with permission of the Brain Injury Association.)

Some individuals with traumatic brain injury may experience problems related to attention span deficits or concentration skills. They may be unable to focus on a task, or may have difficulty following the sequences required to complete a task, or may be easily distracted. In part, these deficits may be related to long-term memory loss. Skills acquired by individuals as children, referred to as old learning, may be extinguished from the memory banks, making new learning experiences tedious, slow, and frustrating (Telzrow, 1990). That frustration can lead to anger and socially inappropriate outbursts, and many individuals with TBI must work on anger management and coping skills and on the use and practice of appropriate social skills (Rehabilitation Institute of Chicago, 1991). Because they act and behave differently, individuals with TBI may be wrongly labeled and stigmatized as mentally retarded or mentally ill, especially by the lay public. This can present particular problems for participating in peer self-help recovery groups such as AA and NA.

Discussion Question: What are some of the issues individuals with TBI might encounter while attending AA meetings?

Instead of acting out problems, some individuals who have experienced traumatic brain injury may become flat in affect or blunted in expression, appearing withdrawn and isolated. These characteristics may be attributable to the head injury, or they may be a side effect of medication the individual may be taking to control seizures or other neurological problems. Unfortunately, depression is quite common after head injury (McGuire & Sylvester, 1990), so identifying the etiology of affective blunting may be difficult for the practitioner. Some individuals have very labile emotions, exhibiting broad emotional swings, further compounding assessment and treatment issues.

Language and communication deficits occur very often following traumatic brain injury and range from difficulties in formulating and comprehending language and communication patterns to performing the actual biomechanics of speech (Marquardt, Stoll, & Sussman, 1990). Open head injury caused by penetration typically results in focal damage in which a particular skill or ability is lost, while closed head injury usually results in more diffuse language and communication problems. The broad generic term used to describe difficulties in understanding or using written or verbal communication or in expressing thought is *aphasia*. The inability to understand what is communicated by others is referred to as *receptive* aphasia. Receptive aphasia can affect several modalities of communication or can be limited to a single modality. Some individuals may be able to understand written material but are not able to understand verbal communication. *Expressive* aphasia similarly may encompass single or multiple modalities and is the loss of the ability to express thoughts, desires, or needs. Individuals who have expressive aphasia may have difficulty with word order, recalling the names of particular objects, or forming speech into coherent patterns. Misarticulations and labored speech are also seen in expressive aphasia. Spontaneous recovery of some or all aphasic problems may occur during the recovery process, but many individuals never recover complete return of function.

Depending on the site of brain damage, some individuals may experience sensory deficits. Loss of visual acuity, hearing loss, and loss of the senses of taste and smell are sometimes seen in individuals who have experienced traumatic brain injury.

Vocational and educational problems are often seen in individuals who have experienced traumatic brain injury. Younger individuals with TBI often have not established a vocational identity and may have difficulty developing a career or even getting a job if they have severe impairments. Individuals with an established career may not be able to return to their previous jobs and may have problems with new jobs. Even if head injury–related impairments are not severe, individuals with TBI may fatigue more quickly or may have less tolerance for stress.

Most individuals with TBI return to the community and to their homes. Unfortunately a high incidence of divorce exists among this population, and family members report high levels of stress, somatic complaints, and depression. Isolation from peers, community social life, vocational experiences, and the loss of support systems can result in depression and suicide.

Treatment efforts with individuals with traumatic brain injury should emphasize slow, deliberate, well-planned strategies. Most existing treatment programs are too fast paced and rely too heavily on cognitively loaded materials. Lengthy reading and writing assignments are usually not appropriate, and TBI clients need more time to process verbal and written information and to conceptualize, formulate, and deliver verbal messages. Treatment may need to be time limited to allow for fatigue factors and multiple admissions tolerated as the TBI recovery process continues. Finally because traumatic brain injury is so closely linked to substance abuse and dependence, staff from both the substance abuse and brain injury disciplines should be cross-trained.

Mobility Disabilities

Many disabilities cause functional impairments in the realm of mobility. Typically these include spinal cord injuries, arthritis, muscular dystrophy, cerebral palsy, and other related or similar disorders. Approximately 1 percent of the U.S. population has a mobility disability (2.5 million+ people) and about 1 million of those individuals use wheelchairs as their principal means of mobility. Most of the attention about drug and alcohol concerns has been focused on spinal cord injuries, although increasing examination of drug and alcohol issues with other mobility issues is occurring. In part, this is attributable to the success of the independent living movement, growing disability advocacy efforts, improved community accessibility, and advances in both acute and chronic medical care technologies. For many years individuals with severe mobility impairments were isolated from society by the severity of their disabilities or by accessibility barriers. Individuals who were formerly warehoused in institutions are now living, working, and socializing in the community. Technological advances have resulted in many individuals surviving severe trauma and returning to home and family. Consequently the numbers of individuals who have mobility impairments will probably increase in coming years, and the increase will occur across the life span. Many individuals today are surviving congenital problems that might have been fatal 20 years ago, and individuals with certain other disabilities are surviving far longer than before. For example, individuals with spina bifida frequently expired as a consequence of a fluid buildup in the cerebrum or severe infection prior to reaching their adulthood. Advanced surgical techniques, improved care modalities, and new antibiotics now mean that most individuals with spina bifida live well into adulthood and function in the mainstream of society (Heller et al., 1996; National Information Center for Children and Youth with Disabilities, 1994), and they experience greater risk for drug and alcohol problems.

Arthritis is usually thought of as an ailment that afflicts older members of the population, although juvenile arthritis affects younger individuals. New medicines and new technologies have improved the lives and community participation of individuals with arthritis and other similar problems of old age. From a drug and alcohol perspective, the greatest concern with this group may be alcohol-drug and drug-drug interactions. The standard treatment course for both juvenile and adult-onset arthritis includes analgesic or anti-inflammatory medications whose effects may be potentiated by alcohol or illicit drug consumption. Alcohol is used to self-medicate pain or to supplement medication. Often multiple prescriptions for pain relief medications may be obtained from multiple physicians, a practice referred to as polypharmacy (Falvo et al., 1990). The threat in this instance involves dependence on multiple pain medications.

Spinal cord injury (SCI) occurs in 25 to 35 Americans per million citizens each year, with young males who engage in high-risk behaviors (i.e., driving too fast, diving, rock climbing, etc.) (Heller et al., 1996) comprising the greatest prevalence group. Typically the site of injury to the spinal cord determines the extent of residual loss and impairment. Spinal cord injuries occurring in the cervical region usually result in paralysis to all four extremities (quadriplegia), while an injury at or below the first vertebra in the thoracic spine eventuates in paralysis to the lower extremities (paraplegia). In addition to mobility problems, individuals with spinal cord injuries will have bowel and bladder problems and sexual dysfunction concerns, again highly dependent on the level of the injury.

While the data vary greatly from study to study, alcohol and drug use are thought to be related to spinal cord injury from 25 percent to 75 percent of the time (Helwig & Holicky, 1994; Tate, 1994). Furthermore, evidence suggests that higher levels of drug and alcohol use occur post-injury among individuals with SCI.

Following injury, a number of factors combine to increase the risk of drug or alcohol abuse and dependence problems. Increased isolation from friends, family, and the community and natural controls on drinking and drug-consuming behaviors often occur. In the general population many individuals with drug and alcohol problems are identified and referred to treatment by a regulatory, gatekeeping function of society. For example, drinking and drug problems often surface on the job, and employers frequently refer individuals

---

The Case of Vinnie

Vinnie was a 25-year-old white male who was completing his bachelor's degree at the local state university. He lived in accessible housing on campus and used a manual wheelchair for mobility. Every Friday and Saturday night, and often other nights of the week, he would wheel himself down to a local student bar, where he always got intoxicated. The bartenders served Vinnie even after he was visibly intoxicated, and the other patrons tolerated his rude and obnoxious behavior after he got drunk. After closing hours on many nights, he would be found passed out in his chair out in the parking lot, and on more than one occasion he was discovered lying in the parking lot or adjoining alley next to his tipped-over chair. On these occasions the campus police or city police invariably picked him up and transported him home but never arrested him. When questioned, bartenders, patrons, and the police all commented that drinking was the one normal social outlet Vinnie experienced, and all voiced their concern and sorrow about his paralyzed condition. Nobody expressed any concern about a possible alcoholism problem.

---

to treatment. Being arrested for driving under the influence is another gatekeeping/referral mechanism. Many individuals with spinal cord injury are unemployed or do not drive and thus are effectively shielded from treatment referral and intervention. However, as the preceding case study illustrates, the attitudes and perceptions of society often serve to enable drug- or alcohol-dependent behavior among individuals with spinal cord injuries.

Discussion Question: Discuss the multiple dangers Vinnie was facing because of his drinking style.

Medication interaction is a common problem for individuals who experience spinal cord injuries. Muscular spasticity is often seen post–SCI, and muscle relaxants from either the benzodiazepine family or the barbiturate family of drugs are often prescribed to control muscle spasms and reduce pain, potentiating a synergistic effect between the drugs and ingested alcohol. When alcohol and benzodiazepines are ingested simultaneously, the liver concentrates on metabolizing the alcohol, and the benzodiazepines remain in the bloodstream for a longer period of time and in a higher concentration. Barbiturate and concurrent alcohol use has a potentially lethal effect, as alcohol potentiates the central nervous system depressant effects of the barbiturates. Lethality aside, barbiturates are dependence-causing drugs, and cross-tolerance with other barbiturate drugs or alcohol will result from long-term barbiturate use.

Some individuals with spinal cord injury impairments are unable to tolerate even low doses of hallucinogenic drugs. In other individuals, delayed metabolic or excretory rates may result in retention of drugs in the body for an extended period of time and at higher dosage levels than normal. Gastric problems may develop in individuals who take aspirin or cortisone-based medication for inflammation and drink alcohol. Using acetaminophens for their anti-inflammatory properties bypasses the gastric inflammation problems of other analgesics and anti-inflammatories but may result in liver damage and an impaired ability to metabolize alcohol.

Marijuana is ingested by some individuals to control muscle spasticity, but long-term marijuana use may be related to the development of pulmonary problems and depressed immune system functioning. People who are quadriplegics with a high level of impairment have reduced pulmonary function, and they more easily contract pneumonia.

The disinhibitory effects of depressant or mood-altering medications are especially problematic for many individuals who have sustained spinal cord injury. The failure to maintain a standard schedule of bladder control and hygiene may result in the development of severe, incapacitating bladder or kidney infections. Individuals with reduced sensation will develop decubitus ulcers (bedsores) if they fail to shift positions in their wheelchairs every so often. Finally, individuals who participated in high-risk behaviors prior to spinal cord injury may continue to participate in those behaviors after injury and particularly while high or intoxicated.

Polypharmacy is a problem among individuals with spinal cord injuries, too. Frequently SCI patients are seeing multiple physicians for multiple problems and may be receiving multiple medications, resulting in increased risk for dependence or overdose. Some individuals use their medicine access and supply as a social mediator. They purposefully obtain mood-altering medications to share with or sell to their friends and peers.

Secondary gain is another risk factor for individuals with spinal cord injuries. Secondary gain refers to unintended benefits that happen as a result of participation in a rehabilitation program. Many SCI patients receive Social Security Disability benefits, or, if they were injured on the job, workers' compensation benefits. These benefits are intended to provide a satisfactory standard of living until the individual is able to return to gainful employment, but they may also provide sufficient income to support a drug or alcohol dependence, particularly when the individual is also consuming no-cost medication. Ultimately many individuals become comfortable with the leisure, drinking, and drug-taking time afforded by benefit programs and lose all motivation to return to work or more functional participation in society. Moreover, society permits them to continue in this dysfunctional, disabled role through its paternalistic views of disability and people with disability (Rubin & Roessler, 1995). Secondary gains, isolation imposed by disability status, and the limitations imposed by disability combine to create feelings of worthlessness, hopelessness, and helplessness, and turning to drug and alcohol abuse is a frequent coping mechanism for dealing with these feelings. Some feel that life cannot get any worse and that drugs and alcohol offer respite from their situation. Others may use drugs and alcohol for relaxation, to socialize, or to fit into the culture of society. *J. R.'s Story: The Disability of Chemical Dependency* depicts graphically the multiple problems associated with coexisting spinal cord injury and substance abuse/dependence.

**Discussion
Question:** Discuss societal views and perceptions of disability that may lead to increased use of drugs and alcohol among people with spinal cord injuries.

Individuals with spinal cord injuries face a variety of barriers to treatment. Prior to the passage of the Americans with Disabilities Act many treatment centers were not accessible to individuals with mobility limitations or who used wheelchairs, and some may be inaccessible still. If the individual with a spinal cord injury is able to gain access to the facility, other, more subtle barriers may prevent participation in treatment. Most inpatient treatment facilities have rigorous, jam-packed schedules. Often clients must be awake, dressed, and at breakfast or a morning therapy group by 7:00 or 8:00 A.M. Individuals with severe spinal cord disabilities may require a long time period for dressing, personal care activities, and eating, and many facilities are unwilling to accommodate those needs. Economic barriers may limit access to treatment. Individuals who are unemployed may not have private or public in-surance coverage for drug and alcohol treatment and may be relegated to publicly funded, often overcrowded programs with long waiting lists, and a continuum of care may not exist. Finally, many treatment centers and counselors may not understand the importance of taking certain medications such as benzodiazepines to control muscle spasms.

The Case of Julie

Julie is a 40-year-old female who suffered a severe spinal cord injury at the C4 level as a result of an especially antagonistic viral infection at age 20. As an individual with quadriplegia, Julie requires an electric wheelchair for mobility and needs considerable assistance with dressing, personal care, and eating. She can use a manual wheelchair for short distances, but she fatigues easily. She is employed as a computer programmer. Recently Julie was diagnosed with alcohol and benzodiazepine dependence as a result of job-related difficulties. Her insurance carrier agreed to pay for ten days of intensive inpatient drug and alcohol treatment, and Julie was admitted to the treatment program accompanied by her personal care attendant and her support dog. Agency rules did not allow Julie to bring her laptop computer to treatment. Despite the avail- ability of assistance, Julie was often late for morning groups and had to eat breakfast in her room because of time constraints. She missed some afternoon groups because of her personal care needs and was unable to turn in some written therapy assignments in a timely fashion because of her slow writing speed. Upon discharge the treatment review team assessed Julie as minimally in touch with her issues of dependence, and it was noted that she did not seem fully committed to the treatment process and the peer recovery model used by the facility. Several individuals on the team noted that her support dog was a distraction to the treatment process. Her prognosis was listed as guarded, and she was referred to participation in Alcoholics Anonymous and outpatient counseling following discharge.

Discussion   Discuss the accommodations required for full participation
Question: in drug and alcohol treatment programs for individuals with
                 severe spinal cord injuries.

Sensory Disabilities

Visual Impairments   About 4.25 million Americans have severe visual impairment (i.e., are unable to read ordinary newsprint with glasses or contact
lenses), and the vast majority of them are over 55 years of age (Dickerson,
Smith, & Moore, 1997). While no agreed-upon definitions of blindness and visual impairment exist, for practical purposes *blindness* is usually thought of as
the inability to perceive light, while *visual impairment* implies a loss of function
as a result of visual limitations (Moore, 1997). Very limited data exist about the
prevalence of substance abuse as a coexisting disability, but existing studies suggest that individuals with visual impairments have drug and alcohol problems
at significantly higher rates than the general population (Sacks, Barrett, & Orlansky, 1997) and that this is an underserved population in drug and alcohol
treatment.

One of the reasons for the failure to serve this population may be its relative
isolation and separation from many of the normal gatekeeping and marketing
awareness functions of the drug and alcohol treatment industry. As nondrivers,
individuals with visual disabilities do not get arrested for driving under the influence (DUI) and are not referred to treatment through this process. Many individuals with visual impairments are employed in homebound settings or in
independent businesses set up under the provisions of the Randolph-Shepherd
Act, and they lack employer recognition and referral for job-related drug and
alcohol problems. Finally, many drug and alcohol treatment and prevention services market their availability through visual media—newspapers, posters, flyers,
and magazines—effectively making those marketing efforts inaccessible to individuals with visual disabilities.

If individuals are identified for treatment, problems exist with typical treatment modalities, often because many treatment centers rely heavily on treatment activities and materials requiring visual skills, for example, bibliotherapy.
Clients are expected to read AA or other treatment literature and are often required to write journals and/or accounts of their drinking and drugging experiences. Videos are another popular treatment tool that may have limited
utility with this population. While most treatment materials are available in
large print or Braille, the ability of individuals to use either format is widely
variable. Lectures about recovery topics should include a verbal explanation of
handouts, overhead transparencies, and any material written on a chalkboard
or displayed on a bulletin board.

Most individuals with severe visual impairments have well-developed mobility skills, usually either through independent travel, white cane use, or guide
dog use, but exposure to a new, unfamiliar environment may create anxieties
and concerns. The first phases of treatment often must be devoted to orienting
the person to the new environment. Sighted individuals are usually able to

---

The Case of Mike

Mike is a 35-year-old male who became blind following an industrial accident. He received a large financial settlement and is financially independent. Diagnosed with alcohol dependence, he was referred to 12 days of inpatient treatment. Anticipating his arrival, the treatment center had Braille copies of all of their treatment materials completed, at considerable expense. Mike arrived for treatment on the appointed day, carrying his tape recorder, which he used as his principal communication medium. The staff proudly presented him with several large boxes of Brailled materials and were profoundly dismayed to learn that he could not read Braille.

---

make an instant assessment of new surroundings and begin to establish their comfort level in their new surroundings. While many individuals with visual impairments accommodate rapidly to new environments, others may need more time and more support. Accommodation needs are as diverse as identifying and learning the best route of travel from the bedroom to treatment rooms and office to learning and recognizing staff and peers solely without reliance on typical visual cues. Clients with visual impairments can't just go down the hall, turn left at the third door, and talk to the counselor wearing the red dress in the group room with the blue door. Clients in outpatient programs usually have fewer facility-specific accommodation issues, but they may have more difficulty getting to appointments because public transportation or paratransportation (special transportation services for people with disabilities) services are limited. Facilities that have strict regulations about missed appointments or late appointments may need to examine their policies to accommodate the ability of the client to get to treatment.

Discussion Questions: Identify the transportation alternatives available to clients with visual disabilities and clients with other disabilities in your immediate area. Can clients who do not drive get to drug and alcohol treatment facilities? What are the advantages and disadvantages of each option?

Discussion Questions: Discuss the possible media alternatives that might be needed for clients with visual impairments. Discuss the advantages and disadvantages of each alternative. Are some alternatives useful with individuals with other disabilities or problems?

Other problems may arise for individuals with visual difficulties because of the extensive use of group therapy in drug and alcohol treatment. They may have difficulty tracking the flow of the group dialogue, especially until they learn to distinguish different voices, and they risk missing many of the visual clues that are an important and rich component of group therapy. It is especially important to supplement group therapy with extensive individual therapy specifically geared at determining if the client is developing a full understanding of the recovery process.

One of the vital considerations in providing drug and alcohol treatment to individuals who are visually impaired is the order of the onset of the substance abuse and visual impairment disability. Individuals who suffer severe visual impairment require a period of adaptation, adjustment, and acceptance to their disability. In part, this adaptation and adjustment centers around the acquisition of new mobility skills and life organization skills, and the replacement of visual styles and forms of communication (i.e., reading and writing) with other styles and forms of communication. Mobility training is widely available through state agencies for the blind and visually impaired, as are life organization skills. These skills center on personal hygiene skills, appropriate clothing identification and selection skills, and activities of daily living. Many of the things sighted individuals take for granted are often lost to individuals with visual impairment. Women must learn to apply makeup without visual cues; men must learn to shave with no mirror image for guidance. Both genders must develop new strategies for selecting matching clothing. Another facet of visual impairment centers on selection of a new medium for communication. While many individuals who are blind use Braille, not all individuals who experience visual impairment as adults are able to learn to use Braille. As a communication medium, Braille has several disadvantages. Creating Brailled materials usually involves time and expense, and Brailled materials are significantly more bulky than visually oriented reading materials. Braille writing and Braille embossing (i.e., Braille typing) are noisy and potentially distracting in education and treatment settings. Tape recorders are used for communication purposes by many individuals, including individuals with visual impairments. Their great utility lies in recording lectures for later playback and to record in verbal form the material that sighted clients may be recording in written journals or diaries. It is a reasonable accommodation to allow individuals with visual impairment to use recorders in lieu of completing written assignments. Much treatment literature is already available on tape, and that which is not can be easily and quickly recorded for client use. It may be preferable to provide two tape recorders for client use so that the client can use one recorder to listen to treatment tapes and use the other recorder for making personal notes or recording reactions and thoughts for later review with the counselor.

Some clients with residual vision may be able to utilize printed materials, either in the form of large-print books or through magnification of standard print. Computers loaded with word processing software capable of font enlargement may be helpful in many situations. In addition to print or magnification considerations, other factors include the stability and range of the client's vision, environmental factors including lighting and glare, and the ability of the client to distinguish colors (Luxton et al., 1997).

Regardless of the communication medium selected, counselors should expect reading speed and reading comprehension to be lower. Individuals who use Braille, large-print, or magnified materials fatigue more quickly and may need more time to complete and assimilate learning materials. In addition, review of complex materials is usually more daunting with alternative media formats. Substance abuse counselors and agencies can receive technical assistance on appropriate assistive devices from the American Foundation for the Blind (AFB) from their state rehabilitation agency serving individuals with blindness and visual impairment. Large-print, Braille, and recorded materials are available from the American Printing House for the Blind (APH).

Hearing Loss and Deafness Hearing loss is a common impairment, afflicting 20 million Americans, especially when they reach their forties. Such people are referred to as hard of hearing. Additionally, another 2 million Americans have no functional hearing and are considered to be deaf. Research data suggest that the prevalence of drug and alcohol problems among deaf and hard-of-hearing individuals at least approximates if not exceeds the rates of drug and alcohol problems in the general population (Guthman, Lybarger, & Sandberg, 1993; Rendon, 1992). Several reasons may account for higher levels of drug and alcohol problems within the deaf community. In many locales a separate Deaf (with a capital D) community exists apart from the general society. Deaf individuals may socialize together, worship together, and participate in separate social events. A well-established Deaf culture exists with a shared history, shared goals and values, and a shared sense of purpose and direction. Unlike many other disability groups who encourage the use of person first language (i.e., person with a disability), members of the Deaf culture prefer to be referred to deaf individuals and promote the continuation of a Deaf culture. The common bond is American Sign language (ASL) (Guthman & Sandberg, 1997).

American Sign Language is a language with its own syntax, grammar rules, and idioms that is difficult to acquire. Fluency in ASL is regarded as essential for effective communication for deaf people, but that very fluency sets the deaf apart from verbal speech users, often resulting in isolation, stress, or paranoia. Not all deaf individuals are able to learn ASL, so they rely on lipreading as their principal communication mode, but data suggest that only about 26 percent of language content is understood by lip readers. Still other individuals rely on self-taught strategies of note sharing and gestures to communicate.

The ability to form and use abstract communication concepts is closely related to the age of onset of deafness. Individuals with prelingual hearing loss lose their hearing at birth or shortly thereafter. They usually have limited or no spoken English abilities or concepts and often have difficulties with abstract thought formation, an especially important consideration for success in alcohol and drug abuse/dependence treatment. Postlingual deafness occurs after the individual has acquired language skills and usually results in the retention of spoken language skills and abstract thought concepts. Obviously the age of the onset of deafness and the established proficiency of language skills will vary from person to person. Late-deafened adults are a growing group of individuals who lose their hearing in adulthood as the result of trauma, disease, or genetic problems. While these individuals have well-developed language and abstract thought skills, they often experience problems in vocational, social, and family areas.

The Case of Ray

Ray is a 50-year-old college professor who had normal hearing until he suffered a head injury in a rock-climbing accident, leaving him with complete bilateral hearing loss. A vital and dynamic teacher, Ray discovered that he could no longer communicate with his students in the classroom. He tried to learn American Sign Language, but he became frustrated easily because of his lack of fine motor skills. In any case, he did not enjoy communicating through an interpreter. His university reassigned him to a research and service position, but Ray had never enjoyed either research or administration and quickly became bored and fearful of losing his job altogether.

An outdoorsman, Ray attempted to resume rock climbing and rappeling but experienced difficulties when he could no longer hear the important verbal safety commands essential to those pursuits.

Ray's family included his wife and three teenage sons who tried to be supportive of his disability-related problems, but Ray began to feel increasingly excluded from family activities. Eventually he spent his evenings browsing on the Internet, ignoring normal family events such as concerts, football games, and shopping trips. Formerly active in a number of professional organizations and community boards, he resigned his memberships.

Ray developed back pain as a consequence of spending long hours at his computer and began taking pain relief medication. When the medication failed to alleviate his pain, he augmented it with alcohol. On-the-job drinking soon followed. Fortunately Ray's university had a first-rate employee assistance program, and when he experienced job-related alcohol and drug problems he was referred to treatment. The initial treatment assessment revealed that he had obtained pain medication prescriptions from three different physicians and was drinking over a pint of vodka each day. Because of the isolation imposed by his deafness, neither his friends, family, nor colleagues were aware of the extent of his substance abuse.

Discussion Question: Discuss the treatment issues Ray and the agency staff will encounter in the treatment process.

The Sign for Drugs

The professor was lecturing about substance abuse to a class of graduate students that included a deaf student. As the professor began discussing illegal drugs, he noticed that the ASL interpreter was using a specific gesture to refer to illegal drugs and used that same gesture for all illegal drugs. The interpreter signed with a motion mimicking the injection of intravenous drugs into the forearm. Concerned that the interpreter was not making the distinction between IV drugs and drugs administered through other means, the professor stopped the lecture and asked the interpreter about the signs and if the lecture was unclear or ambiguous with regard to differing drugs and their mode of administration. The interpreter responded that the sign in question was the appropriate idiomatic sign for *all* illegal drugs.

The substance abuse attitudes of the Deaf community present barriers to treatment. Within the Deaf community, substance abuse is very stigmatizing and seen as a sign of moral failure or weakness. Drunkenness is a sin to be avoided at all costs and certainly not to be displayed in public. Even the signs and idioms used in American Sign Language may have a pejorative tone about drugs.

Discussion Question:	Discuss the implications of a single sign being used to convey information about different drugs with different modes of administration.

Guthman and Sandberg (1997) assert that the few deaf individuals seen in alcohol and drug treatment are markedly disproportionate to their actual numbers in society and estimates of the numbers of deaf individuals who require treatment. The obvious communication barrier presented by deafness, however, is only one barrier. Attempts to establish deaf-specific drug and alcohol treatment programs have sometimes been met with denial, anger, and hostility by the Deaf community. Some members of the Deaf community, already feeling stigmatized and isolated from the general population by deafness, are unwilling to assume the added burden of the label of alcohol or substance abuser. The fear of being stamped with a double deviance has prevented many deaf individuals from seeking treatment and has hindered the establishment of much-needed programming.

Prior to educational mainstreaming, many deaf children were raised in residential schools, separated from family and community. Consequently there is some feeling that as adults these individuals are at greater risk for developing drug and alcohol problems as a result of the isolation imposed by a segregated, residential educational system. Many individuals learn their normal and abnormal drinking and drug-consuming practices from cues in the home and community. They observe parental drinking practices, eat in restaurants where alcohol is served, interact with peers who use drugs and alcohol, and usually can observe typical alcohol and drug consumption in the general population. Conversely, children attending residential schools are exposed to fewer models of appropriate (or inappropriate) substance consumption and often are exposed to stricter regulations concerning drugs and alcohol. Drug and alcohol prevention programs are of varying intensity and quality, and residential school students may learn more from their often ill-informed peers than from prevention efforts. As is the case in the broader society, peer-transmitted information may be erroneous, underinformed, and sensational. Consequently deaf adult alumni of residential schools often have limited knowledge about the drugs and alcohol and their impact and have fewer skills to deal with adverse situations.

Providing treatment to deaf adults is fraught with many difficulties. In the literature often alcoholism is referred to as the lonely disease; interestingly, deafness is also called the lonely disease, and the impact of this dual loneliness can be overwhelming. Deafness isolates individuals from participation in the societal mainstream, perhaps more so than any other disability. For many deaf people, drugs and alcohol become coping strategies to deal with isolation and separation. Unfortunately they may be supported and reinforced in substance abuse practices by deaf peers and socialization opportunities in deaf bars and social events and may be reluctant to give up both abusing behaviors and a peer group. Often individuals in recovery are admonished to, in the words of the treatment vernacular, find new playmates and new playpens. This is a difficult task for nearly everyone in recovery and may seem to be a difficult task for deaf individuals who cannot easily develop new social experiences and new colleagues because of communication barriers.

Communication serves as a barrier to treatment for many deaf and hard-of-hearing individuals and especially for individuals who are totally deaf. Talk-oriented models of individual and group therapy can be translated for clients who are fluent in American Sign Language, but qualified ASL translators are often in short supply, and hourly rates for translation may be prohibitive. The use of unqualified translators should be avoided at all costs. Inaccurate or fragmentary information may be communicated, or unqualified translators may editorialize in their translation. Even if substance abuse treatment facilities can provide translation for formal treatment activities, the lack of available translation for informal interactions (meals, social and recreation activities, etc.) will continue to isolate the deaf client from full program participation. Many videos are now available in closed caption format, but restocking an existing video collection with captioned videos is costly as well, and captions may be distracting to hearing clients. Aftercare resources may be even more limited. Larger urban areas host Alcoholics Anonymous and Narcotics Anonymous groups, either solely for or translated for the deaf, but deaf individuals in smaller, rural communities may be shut out of peer self-help group participation. Individual counseling can be a meaningful therapeutic experience for hard-of-hearing individuals who use hearing aids, and they can often participate in group therapy, but they may have more difficulty tracking the conversation or filtering out extraneous sound and noise. Similarly, individuals may work well in individual counseling but may be less effective in a therapy group where the lipreader must attempt to follow the conversations from several different speakers with varying speaking styles. Finally, the high-pitched or nasal speaking tones of early deafened individuals may present comprehension problems for fellow group members.

Discussion Question: Discuss strategies that might be used to maximize group therapy participation for hard-of-hearing people or lip readers.

Many deaf individuals who were born deaf or became deaf at a very young age demonstrate very low reading comprehension abilities, often at or about the fourth-grade level. These deficits may reduce their ability to participate in bibliotherapy activities or to complete required forms and paperwork. Special care must be taken to ensure that accurate information is provided on written intake and assessment forms and that informed consent is truly informed consent.

Deaf individuals are less likely to have strong support systems, or even interaction with their families. Some individuals may be isolated from their birth families as a result of being educated in a residential school, and other individuals may be isolated from the rest of the family by communication barriers. Occasionally families develop idiosyncratic communication systems employing a combination of standard and nonstandard signs, gestures, lip reading, and note writing, just as all families develop unique family communication styles. Unfortunately, that which works in the family setting usually does not translate well to the larger society.

Mental Illness

No single coexisting substance abuse and disability issue has received more attention than mental illness and substance abuse in the professional literature and in the development of specialized programming. Variously referred to as Mental Illness-Chemical Abuse (MICA), Mental Illness-Substance Abuse (MISA), Substance Abuse-Mental Illness (SAMI) programs, and commonly known as dual-diagnosis programs, they developed in response to an increasing number of dually diagnosed individuals seeking help. The demand and need for services have grown in recent years for a variety of reasons. Many individuals with the dual diagnosis of substance abuse and mental illness formerly were institutionalized in state-operated facilities for the mentally ill, but the development of new psychotropic medications and the continuing movement toward deinstitutionalization resulted in more community-based care. Individuals with severe mental illness problems now reside in small, community-based group homes or in supervised or unsupervised apartments. In the past alcohol and illicit drug consumption was proscribed and controlled by the rules and regulations of the inpatient facility. Community-based facilities have far fewer control mechanisms and, indeed, are not legally able to limit alcohol consumption by their clients. The control burden has shifted from an absolute control model made possible by institutional rules and regulations to a model dependent on education about the problems related to alcohol and drug use, with limited external controls.

A substantial number of the individuals diagnosed with concurrent substance abuse and mental illness problems are homeless or live in marginal housing situations, with little consistent contact with either substance abuse or mental health service providers and with treatment regimens that may be dictated more by economic factors, crisis situations, or legal sanctions. Marginalized by society, these individuals have few treatment options, often limited to overcrowded public programs with diminished resources. In 1990 Aliesan and Firth described a comprehensive program offering phased day treatment services on a five-day-a-week basis to individuals with concurrent substance abuse and mental illness problems. Today, funding cuts and shifts to a managed care treatment philosophy have reduced dramatically the hours of program availability and the scope of treatment services, with corresponding reductions in treatment success.

Both chronic mental illness and substance abuse are relapsing conditions with frequent exacerbations, and individuals with dual disorders are seen as more challenging to treat and as having poorer outcome prognoses than individuals with single disorders (Kelley & Benshoff, 1997). Often treatment problems occur as a result of a treatment system compartmentalized into substance abuse services and mental health services with few or no connections. Frequently treatment personnel are not cross-trained, come from different disciplines, and have differing treatment and outcome philosophies. The dominance of the abstinence model in substance abuse treatment may be perceived as conflicting with medication-based care prominent in mental health treatment, and the provision of substance abuse services by staff credentialed through their own recovery may result in turf or professionalism conflicts or problems with insurance or other third-party payer institutions.

Clinically, individuals with coexisting disabilities of substance abuse and mental illness (usually referred to in the literature as dual diagnosis) are apt to fall into broad categories. Most individuals (Regier, Farmer, & Rae, 1990; White, 1993) have the DSM-IV Axis I diagnosis of schizophrenia in addition to a psychoactive drug dependence disorder. Other significant DSM-IV mental illness diagnoses related to coexisting disabilities include bipolar and depressive disorders, conduct disorders of adolescence, antisocial personality disorders of adulthood, and anxiety disorders. Data and anecdotal evidence suggest a close linkage between acting out, conduct disorders, and psychoactive substance use among teenagers who join gangs, act out sexually or violently, or have relationship development difficulties (Fishbein & Pease, 1996; Hanson & Venturelli, 1995). Anxiety disorders and antisocial personality disorders are the adult counterparts of adolescent conduct disorders and are frequently seen in the cohort of Vietnam era and Gulf War era veterans who present for treatment. In the past, a relationship was thought to exist between conduct disorders and antisocial personality disorders and opiate dependence; this relationship may be seen today among individuals dependent on crack cocaine. Individuals with bipolar disorders are seven times more likely to develop alcoholism problems (Knowlton, 1995), and clinical evidence reveals that some individuals with bipolar or unipolar depression disorders may use cocaine or crack cocaine in a dependent fashion for self-medication.

It is important to consider the interactive role of psychoactive substance dependence and mental illness, along with the order of the onset of symptoms and the etiology of symptoms. From a clinical perspective, some individuals have an identifiable psychoactive substance dependence disorder that preceded mental illness disabilities. Individuals in this group may have psychiatric disorders stemming directly from their substance dependence, such as cocaine- or LSD-induced psychosis or organic brain damage precipitated by long-term chronic alcoholism. Other situations may involve bipolar and unipolar depressive disorders, schizophrenia, and other anxiety or panic disorders resulting from long-term cocaine use (Estroff, 1987). Indeed, Estroff notes that otherwise mentally healthy individuals may suffer acute psychiatric problems if too much cocaine is ingested, ranging in order of likelihood and severity from a mania-mimicking euphoria, dysphoria resembling depression, cocaine hallucinosis, and cocaine psychosis. Exogenous depression is closely linked to long-term alcohol consumption and chronic marijuana use (Buelow & Herbert, 1995). Some individuals may develop mental illness–related functional limitations as a result of long-term psychoactive substance dependency. They may, for example, become depressed as a result of familial, social, or vocational losses experienced as a result of chronic alcohol or drug dependence (White, 1993). The view of psychoactive substance dependence preceding the acquisition of mental illness is consistent with the perceptions of the dominant treatment model, which suggests that treatment of the dependence issues should come first and that mental illness disabilities can be treated only after dependence issues are resolved (Benshoff & Riggar, 1990; Kelley & Benshoff, 1997). The corollary to this position is that failure to treat the dependence issues will automatically doom any attempt to treat mental illness concerns. Adherents to this position would argue that the disinhibitory and sensorium clouding effects of drugs and alcohol make it unlikely that dually diagnosed individuals would benefit from, or realistically participate in, therapy while they were still getting high.

The second etiological position is that some individuals have a preexisting mental illness preceding the onset of psychoactive substance dependence. Typically adherents to this position regard psychoactive substance abuse or dependence as a symptom or behavioral pattern of the mental illness, as a mechanism to hide or mask the mental illness, or as attempts to self-medicate the mental illness.

The Case of Phyllis

Phyllis was being readmitted to the chemical dependency treatment program. Her previous admission, for alcoholism treatment, was characterized by limited involvement in program activities. Staff viewed her as unmotivated and despondent over numerous life failures, including termination from her job as a sales executive, dissolution of her 20-year marriage, and estrangement from her two teenage children. News of her readmission was greeted with a groan in the morning staff meeting, and dire predictions were forthcoming about her affect and behavior upon readmission.

Much to everyone's surprise, Phyllis appeared for her intake interview in exceptionally good spirits and recounted a number of positive events in her life during the two years since her last involvement with the program. She had begun to rebuild her vocational and social life, although she was still estranged from her family. Staff were at a loss to explain this change in behavior until the precipitating event for readmission was discovered. Phyllis was arrested for cocaine possession while on a business trip and was remanded to treatment in lieu of criminal prosecution. She admitted that she had failed to keep referrals for psychiatric evaluation for depression and had discovered that cocaine use lifted her spirits and outlook considerably. It became apparent that she had continued using cocaine right up to and possibly including the day of admission. She was placed in the cocaine detoxification unit, where she detoxed without incident. However, upon transfer to the inpatient treatment unit, she was sullen and despondent, with flat affect and a teary disposition.

Discussion Question: Discuss possible strategies for supporting Phyllis in her path to recovery. How could the agency have been more helpful or supportive following her previous admission?

Individuals with psychiatric problems may use alcohol or sedative drugs to augment or supplement prescribed psychotropic medications, especially if cost is an issue. This is a phenomenon often seen among individuals with long-term, chronic, intractable mental illnesses such as schizophrenia. Because of job placement problems related to frequent symptom recurrence, these individuals may have limited economic supports. Their only income may be Social Security Disability Insurance (SSDI), a system often assailed for encouraging and fostering dependence (National Alliance for the Mentally Ill, 1997), and their only resource for medication may be public systems. Even if cost is not an issue, individuals with chronic mental illness are very likely to demonstrate co-occurring alcohol abuse problems. Unfortunately, the behaviors related to chronic mental illness (i.e., verbal acting out, poor personal hygiene skills, episodic exacerbation of symptoms and behaviors, etc.) results in these individuals being seen as "poor" clients with very guarded prognoses, and peer self-help groups may be antagonistic to their participation. Historically individuals with chronic mental illness have experienced difficulty in peer self-help groups because of their consumption of prescribed psychoactive, mood-altering medications. Many individual members of AA, for example, cling to the belief that recovery in AA includes abstinence from all mood- and mind-altering drugs, including appropriately prescribed medications, although this is not and never has been the official position of AA. Nonetheless, the implicit and occasionally explicit message conveyed by individual AA members may be to forswear all psychoactive drugs, leading inevitably to symptom exacerbation and psychiatric as well as drug- or alcohol-related relapse (Aleisan & Firth, 1990; Kelley & Benshoff, 1997).

The Case of Linda

Linda was admitted for outpatient treatment for alcoholism. Treatment progressed well, and Linda was in the final stages of a vocational counseling sequence. In the midst of a discussion about her vocational aspirations to enter nursing, she was asked when she first thought she might like to become a nurse. Calmly and matter of factly, she stated, "At about age 12. I remember it so well because that's when my father began molesting me."

Linda never discussed this issue in either individual or group therapy.

Apparently she had become comfortable with and trusting of her vocational counselor and felt that she could broach the subject. Referred back to her individual therapist, it soon became clear that Linda had used alcohol to cope with the terrible feelings of depression, low self-esteem, and guilt. She related that she often felt like killing herself, but that drinking and occasional drug use blunted these feelings.

Other individuals may use drugs or alcohol to cope with mental health problems instead of seeking psychiatric care. Glover, Janikowski, and Benshoff (1995) studied rates of incest among individuals admitted for psychoactive substance abuse treatment. They discovered a very high rate of incest involvement among both men and women and postulated that many incest victims were using drugs and alcohol as a means to cope with painful memories or to cope with continuing assaults.

It is likely that many perpetrators of incest use drugs and alcohol as coping mechanisms to deal with their impulse-control problems, deviant sexual acting-out urges and behaviors, and the feelings of guilt, shame, or rage that may accompany those feelings.

The literature and clinical evidence are quite clear that violent behaviors are often related to drug and alcohol consumption and/or a history of abusive drinking and drug-consuming behaviors (Martin, 1993; Wesner, Patel, & Allen, 1991). In these situations drug or alcohol use exacerbates preexisting psychiatric disabilities such as antisocial personality disorder or impulse control disorders.

Individuals with depressive disorders may use cocaine or marijuana, as in the case of Phyllis, to self-medicate. Interestingly, some individuals may use the sedative-hypnotic drug alcohol to self-medicate depression, with often tragic consequences. Individuals affected by anxiety disorders often "discover at one time or another that alcohol is a powerful sedative hypnotic anxiolytic, even if it is effective only over the short run. Unfortunately, like the majority of anxiolytic sedative hypnotics (benzodiazepines, for example) alcohol is addictive and causes rebound hyperexcitability when it is abruptly discontinued" (Buelow & Herbert, 1995, p. 46).

The mental illness as a preceding disability model suggests that treatment of the mental illness must take precedence and that successful recovery from psychoactive substance abuse or dependence can occur only after the mental illness is resolved or goes into remission. Unfortunately, the continued ingestion of psychoactive drugs comes into play with this model.

The third position on these coexisting disorders is that the symptoms, etiology, and onset of the disorders are indistinguishable, as conceptualized by Tracy, Josiassen, and Bellack (1995). These researchers argue that dual diagnosis may emerge from a shared or common vulnerability to a new psychiatric disorder or disorders yet unclassified. Thus, the view is not that the individual has dual disorders but that the individual is viewed as having a unique, unitary disorder that includes a range of substance abuse and psychiatric symptoms.

Clinical evidence intimates that some individuals with long-term chronic mental illness and psychoactive substance dependence may never achieve total abstinence, and the use of harm-reduction strategies has been recommended. Rather than insisting that people with dual diagnoses continuously exhibit good mental health and abstinence, a difficult achievement, the most appropriate and realistic goal might be the demonstration of positive minimal mental health behaviors, reduced or less frequent psychiatric hospitalizations, and a concurrent reduction in the severity, frequency, or number of psychoactive substance abuse events. Adherents to this position argue that the doubly relapsing nature of the two disabilities along with the usually long-term chronology of the disabilities augurs unfavorably for total, abstinence-based recovery. Successful harm-reduction strategies that break the episodic cycle of relapse and remission are viewed as more beneficial to the individual client and society instead of repeated, catastrophic relapses. This is an issue of great philosophic and clinical debate. Insistence on abstinence as the only acceptable outcome for psychoactive substance dependence may doom individuals with dual diagnosis to repeated failure and what Marlatt refers to as Abstinence Violation Effect (AVE) (Lewis, Dana, & Blevins, 1994). When a client experiences Abstinence Violation Effect, the client fails to see or to reframe a relapse or a slip from sobriety as a manageable, correctable learning experience. Instead, the relapse, especially for individuals with dual diagnosis, is seen as another failure in a life already filled with failure. The shift from an abstinence model to a harm-reduction model in which the individual is taught to monitor and control the type, frequency, and quantity of psychoactive substance that is consumed may place less of an onus on the ability to remain abstinent. Abstinence is a certainty model construct: If the individual is able to remain abstinent, it is certain that problems related to psychoactive substance will be avoided.

Because of the nature of dual diagnoses and accompanying behaviors, a third physical diagnosis often emerges. Diabetes, AIDS, cirrhosis of the liver, gastrointestinal disorders, respiratory problems, and disorders such as tardive dyskinesia are related to dual-diagnosis characteristics and behavior patterns (Kelley & Benshoff, 1997), and rehabilitation efforts are triply difficult.

The traditional outcome sought for both mental illness and substance abuse is entrance into and maintenance of recovery status. For individuals with substance abuse problems this has traditionally meant abstinence from psychoactive substances and resumption of successful functioning in family, community, and vocational spheres, usually supported by participation in peer self-help groups (i.e., Alcoholics Anonymous). Recovery from chronic mental illness is usually conceptualized as successful functioning in the community, avoidance or reduction in inpatient hospitalization episodes, and participation in pharmacologic treatment, supported by outpatient counseling or case management services. Individuals recovering from dual diagnosis are best treated through an approach that combines the best elements of both recovery strategies. Individual or group counseling or pharmacologic medication alone is significantly less effective than approaches that combine counseling, medication, education, and psychosocial interventions based on a variety of community supports and services (Kelley & Benshoff, 1997). Studies reveal that individuals who receive a variety of substance abuse education and psychosocial community support services do significantly better than individuals who receive little or nothing in the way of education and support (Crump & Milling, 1996; Jerrell, 1996). Carey (1996) advocates a heuristic model combining medical, behavioral, and cognitive approaches. She points out that clinicians and clients alike must regard recovery from dual diagnosis as a chronologically long process that is conducted in a longitudinal process. Recovery is not an event but a developmental process characterized by trust and alliance building, slow but steady change, and acceptance of the reality of relapse and rehospitalization as learning events.

EMPOWERMENT AS A STRATEGY FOR CHANGE

Empowerment, the shift from dependence to independence, is a basic rehabilitation premise, implying the existence of opportunity and the ability to move toward that opportunity. It is a developmental, sequential process, focused on independence, that for individuals with coexisting disabilities requires a double shift away from psychoactive substance dependence *and* away from the dependency-creating roles inherent in disability (Rehabilitation Research and Training Center on Drugs and Disability, 1996).

Despite the obvious reference to powerlessness over alcohol or drugs, for many individuals peer self-help groups such as Alcoholics Anonymous and Narcotics Anonymous are influential empowerment resources (Rehabilitation Research and Training Center on Drugs and Disability, 1996). They empower individuals by requiring that the person focus on what can be controlled (i.e., personal behavior and responsibility) and by promoting realization and acceptance that drug and alcohol use cannot be controlled. The mutual support system inherent in peer self-help groups provides an important resource for most people. Recovery from any disability, including both substance dependence disabilities and "traditional" disabilities, is a very lonely process. After the flurry of the initial disabling event, or the initial recovery steps, most people are left to their own resources as the people around them get on with their lives. Often individuals with substance abuse problems have alienated family and friends, and the evidence is clear that many severe disabilities result in significant family and social network changes. Suddenly the individual who was the center of much attention is the recipient of little or no attention, and it becomes too easy to succumb to feelings of despondency and loneliness. Peer self-help groups, by their very nature, create a source of mutual support, focused on recovery. They allow individuals with coexisting disabilities to move away from learned or acquired helplessness to a position of responsibility for personal behavior. Women for Sobriety programs recognize the inherent, not empowered, roles of women with substance abuse problems in their literature and philosophy. They assert, with clarity, the reality that women with substance abuse problems are doubly stigmatized and truly lacking in empowerment. That analogy holds true for individuals with coexisting disabilities. In recovery, powerlessness is not the problem—but lack of empowerment opportunities and responsibilities are.

The Independent Living Model developed in the past 25 years emphasizes personal control over life, based on having an acceptable choice of life options and minimal reliance on other people in making decisions and performing life activities (Nosek, 1992). This model is based on the premise that handicaps and stigmas are created by the social, physical, or vocational environment and are not intrinsic to impairments or disabilities. While this model is most often conceptualized in terms of "traditional" disabilities, it has great relevance for psychoactive substance dependence as well. Three principles undergird independent living. The Consumer Sovereignty Principle (DeJong, cited in Nosek, 1992) asserts that people with disabilities are in the best position to make judgments and decisions concerning their own interests and welfare. For many years decisions for and about the lives of individuals with disabilities were made by others: family, teachers, professionals, etc. Substance abuse treatment and rehabilitation facilities have long imposed rules, regulations, and policies to direct, often inappropriately, the lives of individuals with psychoactive substance abuse problems. Rules requiring attendance at "90 meetings in 90 days" or requiring every client to participate in every group creates a one-size-fits-all mentality that devalues and deemphasizes individual self-awareness, judgment, and initiative. Regulations requiring client participation in treatment planning and treatment implementation, first articulated in the Rehabilitation Act of 1973, have grown in strength and number, and consumer sovereignty is a universally recognized (if not always followed) right in rehabilitation circles. Within substance abuse agencies the importance and value of enlightened client self-awareness have been slower to develop. Historically many agencies crafted regulations designed to control client behavior and to minimize opportunities to return to substance use. However, at times these regulations are carried beyond reason or violate client civil rights.

The Case of Sean

Sean, diagnosed with cocaine dependence, was admitted for inpatient treatment. The treatment center had a firm rule: No outside phone calls were permitted during the first three days of treatment. The rule had been implemented for very sound clinical and administrative reasons and applied to all clients without exception. Sean approached his counselor, asking to make a phone call. Without listening to Sean's reasons for wanting to make a call, the counselor rejected Sean's request and took the opportunity to berate Sean for failing to "get with the program." Other counselors he approached took the same, unswerving stances. Undeterred, Sean took his request to the program director, who took the time to listen to and ultimately grant Sean's request. It turned out that Sean was not trying to avoid treatment compliance or to launch some nefarious scheme to acquire drugs or subvert the treatment process. Sean was employed as an international securities broker and was responsible for millions of dollars of client financial assets. He needed to call another broker to transfer his accounts during the time he was in treatment. Failure to transfer management of the accounts could have resulted in financial ruin for both his clients and himself.

Discussion Can inpatient treatment facilities deny the right to make
Questions: contact with individuals outside the facility by telephone?
Do special circumstances apply for individuals in treatment
for drug and alcohol problems? Is the restriction of telephone
privileges a denial of civil rights? Can agencies restrict phone
contacts for clinical reasons?

The Self-Reliance Principle contends that individuals with disabilities
must learn to rely "primarily on their own resources and ingenuity to obtain
the rights and benefits to which they are entitled" (Dejong, cited in Nosek,
1992, p. 109). Advocates of this principle argue that rehabilitation agencies and
bureaucracies have fostered dependence and reliance on the "system" rather
than encouraging and promoting self-reliance. They argue that the person who
can best do advocacy and who can best determine needs, wants, and desires is
the individual with a disability and that individuals with disabilities must develop self-advocacy skills, a rallying cry of the independent living movement.
However, some might argue, is it possible for individuals with substance
abuse/dependence-related disabilities to perform the same self-advocacy skills?
Individuals with impaired cognition, judgment, or impulse control may not
have self-advocacy skills that are oriented to recovery. Then again, individuals
with traditional disabilities are not somehow nobler, brighter, wiser, or more
skillful in decision making than are members of the general population. Self-
reliance advocates for individuals with psychoactive substance abuse and dependence problems have a powerful resource in peer self-help groups, all of
which call for personal responsibility. Conversely, they have a powerful enemy
in the attitudes and beliefs of the general population, especially with regard to
drug (i.e., cocaine and heroin, etc.) dependence. For years society has conceptualized the need to reduce drug dependence as a war on drugs. Unfortunately
the wars on drugs have translated to battle with the people who buy, sell, and
use drugs (Statman, 1993), placing them in a role of dubious self-advocacy and
self-reliance ability. Independent living champions argue that societal attitudes
and beliefs must change significantly if individuals with "traditional" disabilities are to become truly self-reliant; the task is more than doubly difficult for
individuals with coexisting disabilities.

Discussion Discuss the role of peer self-help groups as advocacy
Question: organizations for individuals with psychoactive substance
abuse/dependence disabilities. Can this role be strengthened?

The third principle, Guaranteed Political and Economic Rights, asserts that
individuals with disabilities have a right to full participation in the political,
economic, and social life of the community (DeJong, cited in Nosek, 1992).
Usually interpreted as the right to unencumbered participation in the community and vocational spheres of life, great strides occurred in this arena for
individuals with "traditional" disabilities following passage of the Americans

with Disabilities Act in 1990. However, fewer strides, and even some regression, are evident in the societal treatment of individuals with psychoactive substance disabilities. Many of the laws created by the various states in the nineties restrict the jobs that individuals with a history of substance abuse problems can perform or even restrict the freedom to participate in society. In Illinois, for example, all applicants for positions in publicly funded human service agencies must undergo a criminal background check, and individuals with certain drug-related felony convictions, no matter how recent or ancient, are disqualified from working with children and adolescents. Merely the possibility of the revelation of a drug-related problem in the past may keep some individuals from applying for jobs for the fear of public exposure. Many "three strikes and you're out" laws incarcerate individuals with three drug- or alcohol-related convictions for life, with no hope of release and no hope of rehabilitation. Indeed, the woeful state of drug rehabilitation programs in the correctional system prevents many individuals incarcerated for drug- and alcohol-related crimes from developing job skills, dealing with their dependence problems, or resolving other issues. Often society conceptualizes individuals convicted of drug- and alcohol-related crimes as wanton, heinous, terrible individuals. To be sure, some are. In reality, however, many are not, and they need and can benefit from well-conceptualized and properly implemented rehabilitation programs. Sentencing disparity, especially with regard to powder cocaine and crack cocaine, presents a significant issue for concern. Typically state and federal laws call for stiffer sentences and mandatory imposition of longer terms of incarceration for individuals convicted of crack cocaine offenses. Because crack cocaine is more often the drug of choice for urban-poor minority individuals (often African Americans), prisons have become overpopulated with young African-American males incarcerated for longer sentences with limited hope of early release. Unfortunately, these same individuals are more likely to have coexisting disabilities related to their environment, poor school systems, or gang violence.

The underlying and undergirding goal of the independent living movement, as espoused by the above three principles, is to assist people with disabilities to become as physically, psychologically, intellectually, socially, and economically independent as possible (Nosek, 1992). The presence of coexisting difficulties often more than compounds the task of creating the empowerment required for true independence.

Denial is not a defense mechanism whose use is limited to individuals with substance abuse problems, and for many individuals the first step toward empowerment is seeking treatment. The very act of seeking treatment reflects two vital considerations. The individual consciously admits the existence of a problem and takes action to deal with the problem. Prochaska, DiClemente, and Norcross (1992) point out that a willingness to take action—that is, demonstrating motivation to change—is an important precondition for participation in treatment for dependency but that action does not equate change. Consequently, becoming empowered takes more than wanting to change and seeking help. Individuals must learn an entire set of recovery skills incorporating self-reliance, self-advocacy, and self-control. Many individuals with coexisting disabilities demonstrate limited impulse control and limited abilities to delay gratification at the very core of their drug-seeking and drug-taking behaviors. These individuals typically use crack cocaine, with its nearly instantaneous euphoria, as their drug of choice.

Other individuals with long-term disabilities find themselves socialized into a lifestyle of dependency and receiving care. They grow accustomed to having their needs met by others and have little incentive to change their behavior partially because of the influences and style of a paternalistic state-federal rehabilitation system. Clients who have suffered traumatic brain injury resulting in cognitive problems represent another group of clients for whom gratification and impulse control are difficult, and this may be the most difficult, if not impossible, group to change. Recovery means moving beyond exploitation and manipulation of systems and people to an open, honest style aimed at securing and maintaining basic, entitled rights. It includes learning self-advocacy, self-control, and fundamental assertiveness skills.

Empowered recovery encompasses the development of new relationships, too. Often individuals with substance abuse and dependence problems are engaged in problematic relationships. They hail from dysfunctional families or from relationships with other individuals who abuse substances. Individuals with "traditional" disabilities often have limited relationships or relationships that are disability centered or victimization centered. Empowered recovery implies the adoption of new relationship skills, but people with coexisting disabilities have the issue of double stigma with which to deal, as well as the double burden of interacting with multiple treatment and rehabilitation systems simultaneously with frequently conflicting messages.

The Case of Bill

Bill, a 35-year-old with a significant hearing-loss problem, was admitted for treatment for his alcohol dependency. During the intake he related that he had been referred to treatment by his company employee assistance program, noting that he had a record of frequent absenteeism, shoddy job performance, friction with coworkers, and problems with his immediate supervisor. Nevertheless, he stated that he anticipated a timely return to work following his ten-day inpatient treatment experience. His company was maintaining him on sick leave status during the course of his inpatient treatment, with full salary and benefits. Proudly he noted he was captain of the company bowling team, the Tuesday Night Keggers.

Review of the intake evaluation revealed the following notation in the treatment plan under the "Vocational Issues" heading: "No apparent problems; employer's EAP is supportive, and Bill can return to work following treatment." Similarly, while addressing a number of physical problems related to his alcoholism, the "Physical Health Issues" section of the plan noted, "Bill wears bilateral hearing aids and appears able to track conversations in one-to-one settings. No intervention is required during or after treatment."

Empowerment in recovery is not limited to actions of clients. Both the rehabilitation system (including the state-federal system, the workers' compensation system, and private proprietary and nonprofit agencies) and the substance abuse and dependency treatment systems need to examine their values, attitudes, beliefs, and expectations for clients. Positive counselor attitudes and beliefs must be developed across systems and disciplines. Substance abuse counselors have a very limited awareness of disability issues and vocational rehabilitation services. Experience demonstrates time and time again that substance abuse counselors and agencies do a wonderful job with issues that are viewed as integral to the recovery process from a drug and alcohol perspective. Conversely, those same agencies do not do a very good job with issues related to traditional disabilities and to the world of work.

Discussion Questions: Does Bill have vocational issues to be dealt with in treatment? Do some issues present possible relapse problems or triggers? Will Bill's hearing problems affect his treatment potential and his outcome potential?

Many substance abuse counselors enter the field and are credentialed based on their own recovery experiences and consequently do not possess academic training in vocational and disability issues. Others enter the field through academic training in human service disciplines that do not stress disability or vocational issues. Because of crammed curricula and specific training requirements imposed by substance abuse credentialing and licensing bodies, many counselors trained at the bachelor's and master's levels do not develop skills in vocational and disability concerns. It is ironic that significant national and state policies are calling for the elimination of welfare and the establishment of vocational readiness and placement programs, yet many counselors do not have vocational readiness and placement skills.

The other side of the spectrum differs little: Vocational rehabilitation counselors have limited knowledge about substance abuse problems and in some cases may hold unequivocally negative attitudes about substance abuse and individuals identified as substance abusers.

A Conference Presentation

Two rehabilitation educators were invited to present a paper on the rehabilitation of individuals with substance abuse problems. As they stood up to begin their discussion of the disability of substance abuse, a woman sitting in the back became obviously discomfited. Finally, she rose to her feet and proclaimed to the speakers, "Sit down and shut up! We don't want to hear about people who caused their own problems through their own negative, immoral, and irresponsible behavior. We came to this conference to learn about people with real disabilities."

A Case Where Ignorance Was Not Bliss

The rehabilitation counselor confided to her supervisor that her client was not doing well in his job-training program and that she was truly mystified by his lack of motivation and success. He reported to work late, took long lunch hours, and often smelled of alcohol. The review of the case file revealed that the client had been convicted of driving under the influence of alcohol and that he had acquired his spinal cord injury when he dove into a hotel fountain after a night of partying and drinking. The Individual- ized Written Rehabilitation Program (IWRP) contained no reference to his past drinking problems. When the supervisor inquired about the need for alcoholism treatment, the counselor replied that she thought the client was past that "phase in his life" and that he had "obviously learned his lesson." The counselor expressed no need for alcoholism treatment or evaluation for her client and only grudgingly agreed to suggest that AA might be a possible option.

Discussion Questions: What strategies might be utilized to confront the professional behaviors noted in the last three boxes? How can disciplines cooperate better?

The dual nature of treatment and rehabilitation for individuals with co-existing disabilities creates a fertile environment for manipulation, falling through the cracks, miscommunication, and avoidance of responsibility by both clients and counselors. It becomes too easy to assume that the "other counselor" or "other agency" is taking care of things and that the client is getting and receiving consistent messages. Second, counselors must recognize the multiple functional limitations inherent with individual coexisting diagnosis situations and the multiple functional capacities. Too frequently counselors get tunnel vision, responding only to those limitations within the scope of their discipline. Can a client with coexisting disabilities succeed in a vocational rehabilitation program while actively abusing drugs or alcohol? Can a client succeed in substance abuse treatment if the vocational rehabilitation counselor fails to support treatment? Most importantly, can a client be successful in either or both systems without a sense of empowered recovery?

SUMMARY

Concepts and definitions of disability have evolved from a conceptualization of disability limited to physical loss to a paradigm of disability embracing a wide range of impairments, including dug and alcohol abuse and dependence. The Americans with Disabilities Act explicitly offers protections to individuals with drug and alcohol problems, although the protections differ between the two groups. Services within the state-federal system are highly variable, with some states providing excellent service; other states, however, have established regulations setting recovery standards or program participation criteria for service eligibility. In turn, many substance abuse treatment facilities have neglected the treatment needs of individuals with traditional disabilities.

Traumatic brain injury (TBI) is commonly associated with alcohol or drug use and often occurs as a result of high-risk behavior associated with drugs or alcohol. Individuals with TBI often suffer significant cognitive losses, including memory loss, diminished executive and judgment skills, and reduced communication skills. These losses create unique treatment needs, often necessitating a more concrete treatment approach. The 12 Steps for Individuals with TBI represents an effort to convey abstract material in a more understandable fashion. Individuals with mobility disabilities and substance dependence problems face concerns about medication interaction, polypharmacy, and secondary gain and may encounter physical access, time constraints, economic factors, and medication issues.

Individuals with sensory disabilities often face unique concerns with respect to isolation, communication barriers, onset of disability issues, and the use of assistive devices. Individuals who are blind or visually impaired, for example, may have significant treatment problems related to the use of treatment materials requiring visual skills (i.e., bibliotherapy, videotapes), while individuals with hearing problems are challenged by communication barriers. Participation in peer self-help meetings may be difficult. The culture and morality of the Deaf community and the paramount role of American Sign Language raise challenges idiosyncratic to deafness.

Coexisting mental illness and substance problems are perhaps the most common and most troublesome coexisting disabilities. Some attribute the prevalence of this condition to deinstitutionalization, homelessness, and limitations imposed by managed care. Treatment concerns center around the dually relapsing nature of both substance dependence and mental illness, and questions often arise concerning etiological onset issues. Medication use and drinking or using illegal drugs (medicine augmentation) are concerns, as well as the attitudes of peer self-help group members toward medication usage. Other concerns include the use of alcohol or drugs to cope with a history of childhood sexual or physical abuse by individuals suffering from depression. Recovery is a process rather than an event for this group, and some have advocated the use of harm-reduction strategies rather than a strict abstinence approach.

Empowerment, a basic rehabilitation philosophy, can be a successful strategy for change for individuals with coexisting disabilities, and peer self-help groups can serve an empowering purpose. The Independent Living Model has contributed a number of principles and ideas for empowerment: the Consumer Sovereignty Principle, the Self-Reliance Principle, and the need for Guaranteed Political and Economic Rights. Empowerment for individuals with coexisting disabilities includes seeking treatment, learning recovery skills, and developing new relationships. Positive counselor attitudes and beliefs can make a significant contribution to the empowerment process.

13

Alcohol, Drugs, and Work

Traditional substance abuse treatment paid little attention to the vocational functioning of clients; rather, treatment focused exclusively on alcohol or drug use behaviors and the importance of becoming and staying abstinent. The rationale for this approach was based on the notion that once the ingestion of alcohol or psychoactive drugs was stopped, the rest of the client's problems would become manageable. Unfortunately, many clients (if not most) found out that they continued to have difficulty functioning in major life areas (including employment) even after successful substance abuse treatment. Today, substance abuse treatment is beginning to recognize the value of a more holistic approach when working with clients. One of the major additions to the treatment field has been the inclusion of vocational programming. This chapter will address the following subject matter: the importance of work, impact of substance abuse/dependence on vocational behaviors, and vocational counseling and job placement issues of clients with substance abuse problems.

THE IMPORTANCE OF WORK

The study of work and providing clients with vocational counseling may seem only tangentially related to substance abuse treatment. The ability to seek, obtain, and maintain employment is, however, one of life's major tasks and an ubiquitous concern for people in treatment. The ability to work is indicative of overall psychological adjustment, as evidenced by its centrality to the *Diagnostic and Statistical Manual-IV* Global Assessment of Functioning (DSM-IV, 1994). The study of work and proper vocational counseling is important to everyone because the choice of an occupation will influence almost every other aspect of the person's life, including where one's family will live, where the children go to school, and with whom he or she will associate; even the worker's physical health and well-being may be affected by the type of work performed (Hoppock, 1976). Further, there is ample evidence that certain kinds of jobs can contribute to the development of drinking and drug-taking problems. Jobs such as registered nurse, physician, and dentist have higher than average rates of prescription drug abuse because of the access that these professions have to otherwise inaccessible drugs. Parker and Brody (1982) found that craftsmen, operators, and salesmen have the highest rates of alcohol-related problems. Similarly, a study by Harford and Brooks (1992) reported that the highest mortality rates due to cirrhosis of the liver were found among blue-collar jobs (construction workers and machinists) or in jobs where alcohol was easily accessible (bartenders and waitresses).

DEFINITION OF WORK

Hence, the type of work one does for a living has a significant effect on the rest of his or her life. What is *work* exactly? The answer may seem obvious, but work is a multifaceted concept that often is used interchangeably with such related terms as *employment, career,* and *job.* The most basic definition of work is that it is purposeful activity that produces something of economic value such as goods, services, or some other product (Rothman, 1987). The nature of work is varied, and it may include either physical (e.g., laying bricks), mental (e.g., designing a house), or a combination of physical and mental activities (e.g., building a house). Paid or not, hard or easy, work is effort toward a specific end or finished product. Leisure activity, in contrast, may be stimulating or relaxing, but it is free of required effort. Leisure is intrinsically satisfying with the reward in the doing, not in some end product.

Work is the most fundamental aspect of all societies and cultures. The determinant of everything that cultures do, work is at the root of a society's products, religion, politics, literature, and art (Neff, 1977). Some historians have argued that the various kinds of work performed and the distribution of what is produced constitute the essence of human history. Karl Marx took the position that the human worker was the prominent actor on the social stage. Sigmund Freud underscored the importance of work as well. When asked about the meaning of life, Freud reportedly responded that life's purpose was to "love and to work." Dreikurs (1981) believed that occupation was one of the three major life tasks (the others being friendship and love) and that the inability to work may be regarded as a serious illness.

PSYCHOLOGICAL BENEFITS OF WORK

There are a number of obvious material benefits for an individual who works in our society. Work provides the means to provide food, shelter, and security for the worker and his or her family. There are also a number of equally important psychological benefits gained from working that need to be noted as well. Work (1) contributes to the development of one's self-concept, (2) helps maintain self-esteem, (3) provides a sense of connectedness to the rest of society, and (4) gives an objective structure to one's life.

The development of one's self-concept (one's sense of self, including attributes and abilities) is a critical component to the maturation process. Work provides a significant contribution to one's personal identity. "Who you are" is largely determined to "what you do." Jobs such as priest, teacher, accountant, scientist, and dancer all have implicit personality connotations. In fact, Holland (1959, 1987) based his theory of vocational choice on the notion that people express their personalities through the choice of their occupation and that, to a lesser extent, occupations modify the workers' personalities to conform with "characteristic interpersonal environments" of the work. For instance, the job of banker requires the individual to dress conservatively and to act in a stable and responsible manner, while it is typical for an artist to be nonconventional, emotional, and creative. Holland (1987) characterized people and jobs as fitting into six corresponding personality and environmental types: realistic (e.g., mechanic), investigative (e.g., scientist), artistic (e.g., actor), social (e.g., counselor), enterprising (e.g., car salesperson), and conventional (e.g., office clerk). According to Holland's model, what you do for a living will reveal a lot about your personality. To underscore this point, note that when meeting someone for the first time, it is customary to ask, "What do you do for a living?" In reality, this is a socially acceptable way of asking, "Who are you; what are you like?"

In our society, self-esteem or a positive self-concept is intimately linked to being productive, and the clearest evidence of one's productivity in our society is having a job. At a very basic level, our cultural values of independence, competence, and contributing to society are all intimately linked to working for a living. Society values those who make a contribution to the greater good and sends messages to those individuals that they are important and worthy. These messages are internalized and result in the person's sense of self-esteem or feeling that "I'm okay" (Harris, 1969). Conversely, those who do not work are less valued by others, which is also internalized and leads to lowered levels of self-esteem and the feeling that "I'm *not* okay." Indeed people may become depressed or develop other forms of emotional problems if they become unemployed or not engaged in some form of productive activity.

People are social animals and have a basic need to fit in and be like others. All behavior, work included, may have social meaning or the objective of "wanting to belong" (Dinkmeyer, Pew, & Dinkmeyer, 1979). Work, therefore, provides a ubiquitous connection with the rest of society and helps provide a sense of belongingness. Invariably, people who experience prolonged periods of unemployment or unproductivity experience a sense of "disconnectedness" or the feeling that life is going on without them.

Work makes one conform with objective reality and gives structure to our daily lives. One's ability to successfully hold down a job is a criterion used in assessing overall psychological adjustment. The *Diagnostic and Statistical Manual-IV* (1994) uses occupational functioning as part of its Axis V assessment in estimating a person's Global Assessment of Functioning (GAF) that reflects the person's ability to cope with the environment as a psychologically healthy individual.

Despite all of the basic needs that are met by working, there are negative aspects associated with it as well. Work can be a source of problems, especially when there is an improper person–job fit. When work is boring or unfulfilling, it will result in depression, anxiety, or stress. Work may cause unhealthy competition and result in aggression, anger, or feelings of failure. Further, all work puts limits on one's freedom, placing the worker in a subordinate role that may be frustrating or demeaning. As indicated earlier, some jobs may place the worker at risk for the development of substance abuse problems. The social pressures placed on salesmen to entertain clients with alcohol may account for the comparatively high alcohol-related problems found in this occupation (Parker & Brody, 1982). Jobs such as bartending and waitressing expose the worker to alcohol on the job, and, not surprisingly, these occupations have comparatively higher rates of alcohol-related health problems (Harford & Brooks, 1992). Johnson and White (1995) found that work satisfaction in men was important in predicting alcohol quantity and alcohol-related problems (their data, however, provided evidence that generalized stress overshadows work-related stress in predicting changes in drug use in young adults). These work-related problems may be avoided or addressed by proper vocational counseling, job restructure, or finding other, more appropriate employment. Despite some of its inherent disadvantages, work is considered to be a basic, vital aspect of human existence that is necessary for both the health of society and the individual.

Discussion   Have you ever been unemployed for an extended length of
Questions: time? How do you think others viewed you? How did you
feel about yourself? Did your drinking or drug-taking patterns
change during this time?

SUBSTANCE ABUSE AND
WORK-RELATED BEHAVIORS

The notion that the alcoholic or drug addict will be an unemployed, homeless person is incorrect. Although severe alcoholism or addiction will result in unemployability, the majority of alcohol or drug abusers are employable and holding down jobs. A study by the National Institute on Drug Abuse (NIDA) found that 70 percent of illicit drug users were employed (NIDA, 1990). Cook (1989) surveyed employed adults and found that 18 percent used marijuana and 6 percent used cocaine within the last year. The estimates of alcohol and drug abuse among employees varies depending on the age, gender, income level, and occupation of the group being studied. Normand, Lempert, & O'Brien (1994) reported that illicit drug use and heavy drinking levels have declined in recent years, but they are still serious problems. They found that for all ages, about 8 percent of employed males and 6 percent of employed females reported illicit drug use in the last month, and almost 10 percent of working males and 2 percent of working females reported heavy use of alcohol.

Employees who abuse drugs come from the entire spectrum of occupations, from blue collar to white collar, from unskilled day laborers to highly skilled professionals. The economic costs to business and industry associated with substance abuse are extremely high; some estimates have been as high as $99 billion annually (Scanlon, 1991).

Banta and Tennent (1989) found that employees involved with drug use are extremely costly to employers and a detriment to the national economy. Substance abusers

- have twice as many lengthy absences than other employees.
- use more than double their sick days and benefits.
- are tardy three times more frequently.
- are five times more likely to file workers' compensation claims.

- are much more likely to be involved in accidents.

- are more inclined to steal property belonging to the employer or other employees.

- work at approximately 75 percent of their productive capability. (p. 23)

Clearly, substance abuse has a widespread impact on one's ability to meet the demands of employment, with many individuals being unable to hold a steady job because of their problems with alcohol, drug abuse, or dependence. Less than 33 percent of clients in substance abuse treatment programs are employed, and about 50 percent have less than a high school education (Craddock, Hubbard, Bray, Cavanaugh, & Rachal, 1982). Similarly, research by Platt and Metzger (1987) found that only 26 percent of people receiving methadone treatment were typically or consistently employed, while 74 percent were inconsistently employed, typically unemployed, or consistently unemployed.

Because of the myriad of occupationally relevant problems presented by substance abuse, vocational rehabilitation interventions should be an important part of most substance abuse treatment programs. Indeed, employment is typically viewed as both a positive outcome and important element to substance abuse treatment (Deren & Randell, 1990; Platt, 1995; Project MATCH Research Group, 1997). Further, retention and completion rates of substance abuse treatment are higher among those clients who are employed (DeLeon, 1984). Craig (1980) found that 31 percent of clients entering methadone treatment were employed, but those who remained in treatment for at least 12 months had a 61 percent employment rate. Platt (1995) in his excellent review of the literature on the vocational rehabilitation of substance abusers concluded that there is "an increasing awareness of the important role employment and employment-related interventions play in the treatment of and recovery from drug abuse" (p. 416). Clearly, successful substance abuse treatment has a positive relationship with successful employment.

Critical Vocational Behaviors

Substance abuse or dependence affect a wide range of human behaviors, occupational behavior being no exception. In general, there are two areas of

---

The Case of Larry

Larry is a highly skilled, talented advertising executive. He works long hours and has won awards for the creativity used in his ad campaigns. Larry attributes his ability to be competitive and highly productive to his use of cocaine. He believes that the added energy and excitement that he gets from this drug help him stay at the top of his profession. Without it he thinks he wouldn't last a week.

work-related behavior necessary for successful job retention. The first relates to the worker's ability to successfully perform essential job functions or tasks. Essential job tasks are usually listed on the employee's job description and are the worker's primary activities necessary for completing work assignments and being productive. Depending on the nature of the work, essential job functions may include answering the telephone to take messages, safely operating a backhoe, performing surgery, conducting counseling sessions, washing dishes, operating a cash register, and so on. Obviously, substance use, abuse, or dependence has a variable effect on the ability of the worker to perform essential job functions. Some jobs may be adequately performed even if the worker is recovering from recent drug use (e.g., hungover) or even under the influence while at work. Simple, concrete, repetitive job tasks may be adequately performed by a worker even when under the influence or when recovering from recent drug overuse. Such tasks can be simple assembly, hand packaging, cleaning, tending, or monitoring. Jobs that require higher cognitive functions such as problem solving, judgment, attention to detail, or discrimination/decision making will be much more difficult to complete if the worker is impaired. Unskilled jobs that require controlled physical functioning such as fine-finger dexterity, eye-hand-foot coordination, rapidity of movement, or balance, even though they may be simple, can be significantly affected by drug use. Obviously jobs that involve being exposed to unprotected heights, moving machinery, and other hazardous conditions will put the substance-abusing worker and his or her co-workers at considerable risk for injury, disability, or even death. Generally, workers who are able to avoid close contact with other people are better able to hide their substance abuse problems than are those whose jobs require significant interaction with coworkers, supervisors, or the public. Those in prestigious professions (e.g., physician, attorney, university professor, corporate executive), however, exercise a great deal of authority, autonomy, and control over their work environment and therefore are able to abuse alcohol or drugs and remain employed, despite their close job-related contacts with others.

The second area of work-related behaviors necessary for job retention is not directly related to essential job tasks but is still necessary to maintain employment. These behaviors may be referred to as Critical Vocational Behaviors (Krantz, 1971) and are important for maintaining employment in any job. These job-keeping behaviors include such things as attendance, punctuality, grooming, response to coworkers, and response to supervision. Behavioral expectations in these areas vary from job to job and employer to employer, yet each job and each employer will have established some minimum standards that must be met. Regarding attendance, most employers will allow up to 12 missed days per year (Krantz, 1971) and will fire employees who are absent more often. What constitutes promptness depends on employer practices; some jobs do not require the employee to show up until almost the beginning of the work shift, while other jobs require that the worker be at the work site and ready to go before the start of the shift. Grooming expectations vary on a continuum from requiring only minimal levels of personal cleanliness or hygiene (e.g., landscape laborer) to wearing a clean uniform (e.g., police officer) to conservative business attire (e.g., accountant). The social interaction behaviors required on the job vary from very simple (such as a punch press operator who will only rarely interact with coworkers) to very demanding (such as a car salesman who must be able to verbally communicate the features and benefits of his products to the public to make a sale). At a minimum, the employee's behavior toward coworkers must be such that he or she does not irritate, distract, or otherwise bother them, nor should he or she be victimized or taken advantage of by others (creating an administrative burden for the employer). The employee must also interact with supervisors in such a way as to show acceptance of a subordinate role but still be able to function independently so as not to require excessive time or attention from the supervisor (Krantz, 1971). Critical vocational behaviors such as attendance and response to supervision, rather than the ability to do the job, are primary causes of job separation (i.e., being fired or deciding to quit) for people with substance abuse problems.

Not surprisingly, the worker's inability or unwillingness to demonstrate these critical vocational behaviors because of a substance abuse problem will result in impaired work performance, being placed on probation, underemployment (working at jobs below the worker's capabilities), frequent termination of jobs, resulting in a "spotty" work record, or chronic long-term unemployment. People who abuse or are dependent on drugs may neglect critical vocational behaviors because their vocational needs are overshadowed by drug dependency needs. Needs typically satisfied from successful employment include such things as ability utilization, advancement, authority, compensation (pay), creativity, independence, and social status (Loftquist & Dawis, 1978). Drug abuse or addiction relegates these needs to a low level of importance and places drug use at the forefront of need-driven behaviors. Because so many drug abusers are underemployed or unemployed, they suffer from a stunted vocational development or underdeveloped vocational maturity. For example, a middle-aged substance abuser will, instead of moving up the career ladder, be relegated to working in entry-level, unskilled jobs with no retirement plan, limited health insurance, and little hope for advancement as a result of having several jobs within a short period.

As indicated earlier, however, many individuals who are considered alcoholic or drug addicted are able to maintain employment. Their ability to keep a job depends on two primary factors: the nature of their substance use and the demands of the job. The nature of the substance use pertains to the patterns of use. Do they drink only after work? Before work? During work? How much of the drug is ingested, and what is their level of tolerance for the drug? It is also important to consider if the job requires coordination, attention to detail, rapidity of movement, balance, judgment, or significant interaction with coworkers or supervisors. Therefore, the most important issues in determining if substance abuse is vocationally disabling are (1) loss of voluntary control of drinking or using drugs, and (2) the worker's ability to meet employer expectations in the face of their drinking or using drugs.

Discussion   What is your work ethic? How does this concept vary when
Questions: contrasting men versus women, high versus low educational attainment, high versus low socioeconomic class, majority versus
minority status?

VOCATIONAL COUNSELING

Approaches

Good counseling practices stem from a grounding in counseling theory because theory provides guidance and structure for the counseling professional.
There are a number of theories of vocational counseling that in turn should
determine how vocational counseling is done. The theories vary based on a
number of factors, but in general they differ in the emphasis that they place on
needs (e.g., Roe's Theory of Career Choice), personality (e.g., Holland's Career Typology), development (e.g., Super's Self-Concept Theory), worker traits
and job factors (e.g., Theory of Work Adjustment), or social factors (e.g., Social Systems Theory). None of these theories were designed specifically for
people with disabilities or substance abuse problems, but all vocational counseling concepts may be helpful in working with special needs clients such as
substance abusers.

Vocational counseling traces its roots back to the turn of the century and
to a time when work was becoming more varied and complex due to the
changes brought on by the industrial revolution. The earliest theorists in this
newly emerging field were Parsons (1909), Hull (1928), and Kitson (1925), all
of whom advocated for a trait-factor approach to vocational counseling. This
logical, commonsense approach essentially entails an explicit matching of the
client's abilities (i.e., traits) with the demands of various work environments
(i.e., factors). The vocational testing movement (that flourished in the United
States during the 1950s, 1960s, and 1970s) grew out of the trait-factor vocational counseling approach (Osipow, 1983). Other theories of vocational
choice have evolved since the early 1900s and have been placed into categories described as sociological, developmental, personality traits, and behavioral
(Osipow, 1983).

The sociological approach emphasizes the roles that the environment and
chance play in vocational selection and success. The major researchers associated with the sociological approach are Hollingshead (1949), Miller and Form
(1951), and Sewell and Hauser (1975). Because of the emphasis on societal circumstances beyond the control of the individual, such as the socioeconomic
status of one's family, these approaches do not lend themselves well to vocational counseling other than encouraging people to cope as best they can with
environmental circumstances.

Developmental approaches have grown out of the work of Buehler (1933),
with the major vocational counseling theorists being Super (1957), Ginzberg

(1952), and Tiedeman (1961). Osipow (1983) believed that the developmental approaches had three elements in common:

> (1) individuals develop more clearly defined self-concepts as they grow older, although these vary to conform with the changes in one's view of reality as correlated with aging; (2) people develop images of the occupational world which they compare with their self-image in trying to make career decisions; and (3) the adequacy of the eventual career decision is based on the similarity between an individual's self-concept and the vocational concept of the career eventually chosen. (p. 10)

Some vocational counseling theories emphasize the role that personality and the individual's needs play in vocational choice; the primary theorists in this approach are Roe (1957) and Holland (1959). These theories focus on personality traits or characteristics as being instrumental in the selection of work that is consistent with or allows for the expression of personality because it helps people to meet their needs. For example, people who have creative personalities would be drawn to artistic work (e.g., actor, graphic artist, dancer), while people who prefer concrete, structured activities would prefer realistic work (e.g., welder, engineer, bricklayer). According to Holland (1959), the exposure to the demands and environment of a particular job actually modifies the personalities of workers, so their personality better matches others who are employed in the same job or field (e.g., once employed as a banker, the individual acquires more conservative orientations in dress, behavior, and values).

Finally, behavioral approaches to understanding vocational choice emphasize the interaction between the person and the environment and the role that social learning plays in career decision making. Representative theorists in this area are Mitchell, Jones, and Krumboltz (1979), who discussed the importance of modeling or vicarious learning in the acquisition of vocational goals and behaviors. The basic assumption is that important people in the person's life (e.g., parents, siblings, peers, teachers) served as models of vocational behavior and will have a determinant effect on the individual's eventual career choice.

None of the above theories or approaches to vocational choice were developed with substance abuse or chemically dependent clients in mind. Nonetheless, they all have some relevance in counseling such clients, and it is a good idea to become familiar with the theories that underpin vocational counseling. All of the vocational theories seem to agree on a number of basic concepts (with the exception of social systems approaches that emphasize circumstances beyond the control of the individual):

1. People are different in a number of vocationally relevant areas, such as abilities, interests, needs, education, training, and life experiences.

2. Similarly, occupations differ in both their job requirements and their job reinforcers, or what they offer workers.

3. Occupational choice is important, and the choice made may either facilitate or obstruct both job success and satisfaction. In other words, occupa-

tional choices may either be realistic and result in satisfaction and success or unrealistic and result in dissatisfaction and failure. Still other choices may be somewhere in between and result in only partial success and satisfaction.

4. Occupational choices are affected by a variety of factors, most notably the individual's needs, abilities, and potential employment opportunities in the individual's environment.

5. Most people will gravitate to work that is appropriate for them, but they will make a number of occupational choices before committing them- selves to any one occupation. The work life of many individuals is com- prised of a number of different jobs taken when new occupational choices are made.

6. Vocational counseling and increased self-awareness will facilitate the occu- pational decision-making process, helping the individual to be more effec- tive and efficient and make better occupational choices.

Discussion Questions: Did you ever get help with finding a job, selecting an aca- demic major, or choosing a career? What experiences were most helpful to you and why? What might have happened if you hadn't received the help?

Vocational Counseling with Substance Abusers

From a vocational counseling standpoint, substance abuse clients may be roughly placed into one of two categories: (1) those with an underdeveloped vocational identity because of a substance abuse problem, or (2) those who have developed a vocational identity despite having a substance abuse prob- lem. A vocational identity is more than just seeing oneself as someone who has a job; it is a developmental process that results in a self-concept linked to what one does for a living. Having a vocational identity also translates into a work ethic and the ability to consistently demonstrate the following critical voca- tional behaviors (Krantz, 1971): regular attendance, acceptable punctuality, ini- tiating work activities without prodding, appropriate appearance (grooming and dress), getting along with coworkers (interpersonal skills), working well with others (cooperation), meeting quality and quantity standards (productiv- ity), following work rules and policies, being flexible in response to changes in job demands, improving job performance over time, and willingness to accept supervision or constructive criticism.

Those clients who have underdeveloped vocational identities typically be- gan abusing alcohol or drugs at an early age, and that abuse prevented them from developing work-related skills, behaviors, and a solid work history. Be- cause their substance abuse needs superseded vocational needs, they never in- vested sufficient time or energy into working. Such people are likely to have a number of common problems confronting them after they have begun the re- covery process and are planning on becoming productive. Regardless of age, be it early, middle or late adulthood, they are likely to have poor, inadequate, or unrealistic concepts of what work is and who they are as workers (RRTCDD, 1996). Often, these people have grown up in substance–abusing homes or have left stable home environments to live in situations condoning substance abuse. Therefore, the individual has not been exposed to worker-role models. Knowing how to successfully function in a work environment is a mystery to them. These problems will often result in unrealistic expectations and fearfulness about the demands of life in the world of work. Compounding these issues may be additional problems of limited education, poor reading abilities, poor math skills, and no high school diploma. Further, substance abuse needs have precluded many of life's other learning experiences, such as developing interpersonal coping skills, the ability to learn from mistakes, and limited awareness of personal values, interests, and abilities (RRTCDD, 1996).

The second category of clients includes those people who developed substance abuse problems either before or after entering the workforce but were able to seek, obtain, and maintain employment and develop vocational identities. This category includes many thousands of clients and potential clients, given the estimates that around 10 percent of the current workforce may be classified as substance abusers (Normand, Lempert, & O'Brien, 1994). Vocationally related problems that may threaten these clients include the loss of social status, home, income, and even family because of substance abuse. Having worked and invested themselves in productive activity also places them at

---

Vocational Counseling Gone Awry

Client: I've been out of treatment for nine months now and have been going to AA regularly all this time. I'm clean, I'm sober, and I'm anxious to find a job.

Counselor: That's great. I've looked at your file and note that you've held a C average in high school and have taken a number of shop classes where you consistently received As.

Client: Yeah, shop was always easy for me, and I'm good with my hands. I know how to use hand tools and most power tools and have even helped out building houses and stuff for some of my relatives.

Counselor: I can't believe how lucky this is. I've just found out about a non-union construction job. The work is as a construction laborer on a subdivision of houses that A-1 Reality is building. They're looking for construction laborers, and I know their contractor. Would you like to give it a try?

Client: You bet! This is just the kind of thing I've been looking for.

Two weeks later, the counselor found out that her client had relapsed, lost his job, and was waiting to be admitted into treatment again. Apparently, most of the construction workers at the new development ended each workday by having a few beers at the work site. The temptation was just too much.

greater risk for feelings of embarrassment and shame related to uncovered substance abuse. According to researchers with the Rehabilitation Research and Training Center on Drugs and Disability (1996), a number of on-the-job-related problems may arise, such as lack of focus on a career path, a history of errors in performance and judgment, a record of disciplinary action for poor work performance, injury to self or others, and lost money and possessions. When engaging substance abuse clients in vocational counseling, it will be important to be sensitive to all of the above issues while helping clients enter or reenter the labor force. The vocational counseling process can be a series of sequential steps, specifically exploration (of the self and world of work), identification of a vocational goal and development of a job placement plan, implementation of the job placement plan, and job placement follow-up.

VOCATIONAL PLANNING
AND JOB PLACEMENT

Exploration

The exploration stage typically takes place early in the vocational counseling and guidance process. Clients are encouraged to gather information about themselves and about the demands and rewards of various occupations and then integrate these two areas of information in an effort to help them decide where they would best fit into an occupation. Wolffe (1997) stated that both vocational and self-exploration should take place as soon as possible so that clients can work on both areas simultaneously.

Self-Exploration Self-exploration should lead to increased self-awareness in such vocationally relevant areas as interests, abilities, and values (Wolffe, 1997). Interests relate to what the individual enjoys or how he or she spends time. Super (1957) described how a counselor may go about obtaining interest-related information, categorizing interests as (1) expressed, or discovered through client verbal statements; (2) manifest, or interests shown through behavior or action; (3) inventoried, or interests estimated by client responses to sets of questions concerning likes and dislikes, and (4) tested, or interests revealed under controlled circumstances where the client is given a forced choice between engaging in one of two vocational activities (this may occur in vocational evaluations or situational assessments). Of these four approaches, interest inventories are probably the most popular method because of their psychometric properties, relation to the world of work, and widespread availability (Aiken, 1976). The use of interest inventories, relative to other types of tests, has increased dramatically in the past 40 or 50 years (Zytowski & Warman, 1982). Probably the premier interest inventory is the Strong Interest Inventory (Hansen & Campbell, 1992) that traces its roots back to the Strong Vocational Interest Blank (1927). If the client has reading difficulties, he or she can use nonreading inventories, such as the Revised Reading-Free Vocational Interest Inventory (Becker, 1981).

Similar to interests, information about client abilities may be gathered from a variety of sources such as hobbies, work history, educational background, and/or formal testing. Formal testing of abilities usually incorporates both aptitude testing and achievement testing. Tests of client aptitude tend to focus on a person's innate abilities or capacity for profiting from instruction, while achievement testing focuses on the degree to which the person has profited from prior instruction (Aiken, 1976). Aptitudes may include sensory or motor, clerical, mechanical, spatial, numerical, verbal, artistic, musical, or other creative abilities. There are several individual aptitude tests available, but for the sake of efficiency, the counselor may wish to use an aptitude test battery such as the Comprehensive Vocational Evaluation System (Dial, Mezger, Gray, Massey, Chan, & Hull, 1992) that incorporates a number of vocationally relevant aptitudes into one instrument. Achievement tests tend to focus on content taught in school, such as reading, math, language, and spelling, and are often interpreted using grade equivalents. These types of tests are also available in battery form, such as the Tests of Adult Basic Education (TABE) that produce scores in reading, mathematics, and language (CTB/McGraw-Hill, 1976).

Finally, the exploration of client values relates to the usefulness, importance, or worth that clients attach to particular activities or objects and are closely related to interests and attitudes (Aiken, 1976). Values-related information may also be gathered from directly asking clients (expressed) about what is important to them and also by observing how they spend their time and energies (manifest). Formal testing of values is less developed than interest or ability testing and is often placed in the realm of personality testing. Probably the test most closely associated with work values is Super's Work Values Inventory that measures 15 values that are thought to be important to determining vocational satisfaction and success (Aiken, 1996). In addition, there are values clarification exercises that may be applied to vocational self-exploration (Simon, Howe, and Kirschenbaum, 1995).

Self-exploration aimed at vocational development needs to take place early on, certainly prior to the completion of treatment for the substance abuse client. This type of self-exploration should be approached by both the counselor and client as a hopeful, exciting, forward-looking part of substance abuse treatment. Continued exploration after completing treatment will serve to occupy the client's time and provide needed structure to a changing lifestyle. The RRTCDD (1996) recommended that, in addition to the normal areas of self- and vocational exploration, substance-abusing clients should carefully explore the following indicators of job readiness: motivation, view of work, and self-concept. Motivation may be examined by not only what the client says but what he or she does. For instance, is the client missing appointments? Is the client punctual? How much time and effort is spent on exploration activities such as obtaining and reading labor market materials? What attitude is assumed when taking tests or completing other structured self-exploration activities? The person's view of work should be examined by addressing such

questions as: Does the person understand the meaning of work and the significance of a career? How does the person view superiors, units, schedules associated with work? Is he or she communicating effectively and dressing and
interacting appropriately? Regarding self-concept, an important question is:
Does the person's bravado and grandiosity serve to mask poor self-esteem and
low levels of self-confidence? The person's competence and ability to take
control of his or her life is an important area of exploration and will determine
if and when the person is prepared to initiate a job search.

Other important issues or challenges for counselors to explore with substance abuse clients who are in the process of career planning include "maintaining sobriety and drug-free status; management of impulses, anger, frustration;
handling confrontation; taking on new roles; time management; appropriate
dress, walk, talk; assertiveness, learning something new; dealing with authority;
changes in family relationships" (RRTCDD, p. 6.15). Another potential vocational obstacle that substance abuse counselors and clients must be aware of is
the impact that a criminal record has on job opportunities in such fields as law
enforcement, nursing, and human services. Many employers are required to do
background checks and even fingerprinting of job applicants in order to comply
with state regulations designed to protect the public.

Exploration of the World of Work   The exploration of the world of work
may take place at two levels. The first focuses on general information about the
different kinds of jobs, occupations, and careers found in the work environment. The second level is more focused on factors related to specific positions
at particular employers. The terms *job, occupation, career,* and *position* are often
used interchangeably but have important distinctions. Shartle (1959) defined a
position as a collection of tasks performed by one person that constitute the total work assignment of a particular person with a particular employer. There
are as many positions as there are workers. *Job* is defined as a group of similar
positions that are identical with respect to their major tasks and are sufficiently
alike to be grouped together and found in a particular establishment or employer. For example, a particular retailer may have a job of customer service
specialist with several people filling each position. An *occupation* is defined as a
group of similar jobs that exists in several establishments or employers. For example the occupation of dishwasher is found at almost all restaurants. Finally, a
career has been defined most broadly as "the totality of work one does in
his/her lifetime" (Sears, 1982; p. 139).

The broadest level of exploration takes place when the client examines different jobs, occupations, and career tracks. This is a very challenging task, given
the ever-evolving U.S. labor market, with new jobs and occupations being created and old ones being eliminated on a continual basis. Isaacson (1986) compared the world of work to a living organism:

> As in any complex organism, old cells die and are sloughed off, new cells
> replicate existing ones and replace them, other new cells develop as slight
> modifications of existing cells, and some new cells are totally different from

any previously existing units and take on new functions. Thus the world of work continuously and simultaneously is involved in the processes of rejuvenation, homeostasis, and evolution. (p. 161)

The U.S. labor market is very large, having over 35,000 differing occupations (National Occupational Information Coordinating Committee, 1986). To assist both counselors and clients in exploring the world of work, the U.S. Department of Labor has categorized occupational information in three important reference books: *Dictionary of Occupational Titles* (DOT; U.S. Department of Labor, 1991), *Guide for Occupational Exploration* (GOE; U.S. Department of Labor, 1979), and the *Occupational Outlook Handbook* (OOH; U.S. Department of Labor, 1996).

The DOT is now in its fourth edition, having first been published in 1939 and is "a vital part of the USES [United States Employment Service] commitment to collect and disseminate occupational data that is comprehensive, up-to-date, and economically useful" (U.S. Department of Labor, 1991; p. vii). The latest edition of the DOT provides job descriptions for over 12,000 occupations, using a standardized coding system that classifies occupations into nine categories (e.g., professional, technical, and managerial; machine trades; clerical and sales). These broad occupational categories are further divided into occupational divisions that are subdivided into occupational groups. The coding system used by the DOT not only categorizes jobs by occupation but by their level of involvement with data, people, and things. The DOT is an excellent reference source for counselors, but it tends to be too technical and limited for client use.

The GOE is much easier for counselors to use with clients than the DOT because clients are allowed to match their interests and abilities with those required of various occupations (Patterson, 1996). Occupations listed in the GOE are referenced by their DOT code, but more importantly they are categorized according to occupational interest areas such as artistic, scientific, plants and animals, protective. In addition to occupations being keyed to the DOT, occupations listed in the GOE are also described in terms of their aptitude requirements (such as verbal ability, form perception, manual dexterity) as measured by the General Aptitude Test Battery (GATB; U.S. Department of Labor, 1970).

Finally, the OOH categorizes occupations using the DOT system, but the descriptions are much more detailed, making it an ideal reference tool to be used directly by clients. Although the OOH describes a much smaller number of occupations (about 250), it provides very detailed information. In addition to the DOT job description, the OOH provides information on the nature of the work; working conditions; employment locations; training, other qualifications, and advancement; job outlook; earnings; related occupations; and sources of additional information (U.S. Department of Labor, 1996). The excellent information provided by the OOH and its ease of use make it an essential part of any vocational counselor's library of resources. Another advantage of the OOH is that it is updated about every two years and has a companion *OOH Quarterly* that provides easy-to-read articles about occupations that are useful to both counselors and clients.

In addition to exploring the different kinds of occupations and their relationships to interests and abilities, counselors working with substance abuse clients should spend time dealing with occupationally based triggers for relapse. The obtainment of a steady, full-time job in and of itself may act as a trigger for relapse. The now-employed client is removed from the treatment ex-perience/environment and may believe "If I can hold down a job, I'm not disabled by past substance dependence." Social activities (holiday parties, after work get togethers) may involve the use of alcohol or drugs by supervisors or coworkers. Seeing others using with no apparent negative effects may tempt the individual to start using again. Job-related stress, pressure, anxiety, and dealing with authority may tax the individual's coping skills, and he or she may resort to old, dysfunctional coping strategies that relied on getting high to feel better. Finally, just getting a paycheck may act as a relapse trigger if, in the past, all money was used to buy drugs. Additionally, having a stable income may result in impulsive spending, poor money management, or overspending, all of which could have an adverse effect on the person's recovery.

GOAL IDENTIFICATION AND PLACEMENT PLANNING

The selection of a particular vocational goal or set of goals for a client will obviously be a function of the client's abilities, interests, and vocational needs, in conjunction with the labor market in which he or she is looking for work. England (1991) explored the importance of 11 work goals that relate to why people select the particular work goals that they do. In the United States, the rank order of these work goals were the following:

1. Good pay
2. Interesting work
3. Good job security
4. Opportunity to learn
5. Good interpersonal relations
6. A lot of variety
7. A good match between the worker and the job
8. Good opportunity for upgrading or promotion
9. Job autonomy
10. Convenient work hours
11. Good physical working conditions.

Obviously, these rankings will vary depending on the client preference and should be explored at length when finalizing a vocational goal. Activities that facilitate the selection of a vocational goal include field trips to the local library, career center, and other community organizations, which have information about employment in the area; attendance at job fairs or career days at post-secondary schools or colleges, which will provide an opportunity to observe how employers and other applicants interact when seeking employment; and visits to potential employers to take informational tours that will help the job seeker learn about the realities of the workplace and the basic prerequisites for employment (RRTCDD, 1996).

Vocational goals and their concomitant plans should be individualized and must be "owned" by the client. Even the most sound job placement plan will fail if the client feels that something was forced upon him/her by the counselor or some other outside agency. It is important to keep in mind that the majority of the activities identified in the plan must be carried out by the client. Therefore, in order to ensure client motivation and effort in its implementation, all job placement plans should be developed with the client's full cooperation and active participation.

The job placement plan should also be developed separately—that is, the plan should not be included as part of the overall rehabilitation or substance abuse plan. The reason for this is that the use of a separate, individualized placement plan results in increased time in job search efforts and a more productive relationship or partnership between the rehabilitation counselor and the client (Hanson, 1983). This may be due to the fact that individualized job placement plans help clients to more clearly conceptualize their efforts toward obtaining employment and result in action-oriented, goal-directed behavior. The contents of the placement plan may vary widely, depending on the needs of the individual and the skills and resources of the counselor (hence, they are individualized); however, placement plans do have some common elements. At a minimum, all placement plans should (1) identify the primary and secondary job targets, (2) set the geographical boundaries of the job search, (3) detail reasonable salary/wage expectations, (4) specify the counselor/job developer responsibilities, and (5) specify the client's responsibilities. Figure 13.1 shows an example of a typical job placement plan outline.

CLIENT: _____

COUNSELOR: _____

CURRENT DATE: _____

EFFECTIVE DATE OF PLAN (when job placement activities began): _____

PRIMARY JOB TARGET: _____

D.O.T. six-digit code: _____

Estimated beginning salary: _____

Client strengths related to secondary job target: _____

SECONDARY JOB TARGET: _____

D.O.T. six-digit code: _____

Estimated beginning salary: _____

Client strengths related to secondary job target: _____

continued

FIGURE 13.1 Placement Plan

SECONDARY JOB TARGET: _____

D.O.T. six-digit code: _____

Estimated beginning salary: _____

Client strengths related to secondary job target: _____

Specify areas to be addressed by Job Seeking Skills instruction: _____

Specify problems related to job seeking (transportation, day care, job engineering or restructuring, etc.) and plans to improve specific problems:

_____

_____

List of potential employers, starting with those who are most likely to have appropriate openings:

Employer	Address	Telephone

Primary job sources to be investigated by the client (check all that apply):

_____ Family and friends   _____ Yellow pages

_____ Unions   _____ Want ads

_____ Former employers   _____ Job service

_____ School or training facility place-   _____ Private employment agency
      ment office   _____ Other (specify): _____

_____ Cold contacts (going directly to
      companies whether or not they
      are advertising openings)

Primary counselor responsibilities related to the job search (e.g., provision of job leads, provision of job-seeking skills instruction, resume preparation, labor market surveys, job analyses, job modification, monitor client progress, estimated number of leads each week to be provided by counselor, etc.):

_____

_____

Primary client responsibilities related to the job search (e.g., number of employers to be contacted weekly, number of job applications to be completed weekly, prompt follow-up on job leads, open communication with the counselor, etc.).

_____

_____

Timetable for placement plan:

   When is placement expected? _____

   If necessary, when will the plan be reevaluated?_____

By signing, the client agrees that he/she helped develop above plan and will actively participate toward carrying it out. He/she further understands that the plan is not a legally binding contract but a workable plan of action meant to result in an appropriate job for the client.

Client Signature: _____

Counselor Signature: _____

JOB PLACEMENT

There are a number of job placement challenges presented to substance abuse counselors and their clients. When substance abuse or dependence has prevented or disrupted a client's work history, the client will be forced to deal with such issues as a spotty work history characterized by successive short-term jobs; underemployment (working at entry-level jobs with no history of advancement); inability to return to prior employers because of past failures; long periods of unemployment that create gaps in the work history; a lack of acceptable references; the stigma of being labeled alcoholic or addict; restricted education or training; inadvisability of work environments that present relapse triggers; possible history of arrest or incarceration; and the decision whether to disclose a history of substance abuse or dependence (RRTCDD, 1996).

The starting point of job placement will vary depending on the client's job readiness, education, and work history. For clients with more limited backgrounds, job placement should begin more slowly, with modest goals that are easily achieved in order to build experiences and a sense of success. Volunteer positions, temporary jobs, internships, supported employment, and other worklike activities may be the most appropriate (RRTCDD, 1996). All of these activities provide experience and confidence so the client may progress on to more structured, competitive employment. Clients with more intermediate backgrounds or who have potential but lack credentials may wish to launch their job search by completing a short-term training program that results in a particular certificate or credential that qualifies them for employment (e.g., welder, truck driver, typist/word processing, nurse's aide).

Job-Seeking Skills

Most clients will benefit from formalized job-seeking skills instruction. Job-seeking skills are those behaviors that increase the probability of getting an interview and a job offer by presenting the job applicant in the most favorable light possible. It is important to note here, however, that the best job-seeking skills will be useless if the client's job goal is inappropriate. Job placement activities always flow from sound vocational counseling and goal selection. With that caution in mine, job-seeking skills typically include how to identify and use various sources of job leads; complete an application form completely, accurately, and without emphasizing any negative aspects of the applicant; develop a resume that combines both chronological and functional features crafted to emphasize the client's most desirable characteristics; write letters of application; line up good references; and positively present oneself in a job interview (Salomone, 1996).

The identification and use of job leads require clients to vigilantly read classified ads in newspapers; visit the local employment agency; make cold calls to employers (i.e., visiting employers who aren't advertising an opening but have positions closely related to the client's job goal); use informal sources such as relatives, friends, and acquaintances; and (given today's job market) search the Internet. Some clients will benefit from joining (for a fee) a job club, which is an organized group that provides such services as group counseling/support, a buddy system that pairs job club members to provide encouragement and individualized advice, and other resources such as telephone banks, photocopiers, fax machines, mailing addresses, and so on (Salomone, 1996). Research has found that the job club tends to be the most effective method of various job placement approaches (Azrin, Philip, Thienes-Hontos, & Besalel, 1980).

Completion of job applications, although usually straightforward, requires close attention. Misspelled words, missing information, or a sloppy appearance will quickly eliminate the client from the applicant pool. It is advisable to have the client complete a blank application form and take it along whenever applying for jobs. That way the completed form may be used as a reference for details that are often forgotten, such as the addresses and phone numbers of references, the exact chronology of the work history, and names of former supervisors. Invariably, clients will be asked on an application if they have any conditions (e.g., disabilities) that would prevent them from successfully fulfilling the job requirements. At this juncture the client/job applicant must make the decision to "tell or not tell" the prospective employer about his or her substance abuse history. Although lying on a job application is grounds for dismissal, the decision to reveal or not reveal a history of disability and substance abuse or addiction is ultimately up to the client. Clients are afforded some protection under Title I of the Americans with Disabilities Act (1990) if certain conditions are met:

> Under the provisions of the ADA, an employer may not discriminate against a substance abuser who is not currently using drugs, who has been rehabilitated, or who is participating in a supervised program of rehabilitation. . . . Generally, employers may not ask about past disabilities, such as alcohol or drug addiction. However, employers may ask about past abuse and treatment for a position in which such information is job-related and consistent with business necessity (e.g., nursing, pharmacy). (p. 7.9, RRTCDD, 1996)

The client who chooses to disclose his or her history of substance abuse should do so in the least damaging way. If the application form asks about disabilities, it is a good idea to write "Will explain in interview." (There is never enough room on an application form to adequately answer this question anyway.) Then be prepared to address the issue in the least damaging way possible in the subsequent interview by emphasizing the learning and positive change that has taken place with rehabilitation and an eagerness to get on with a new life. Answer all questions as simply and completely as possible, then quickly move on to a discussion of skills, abilities, and potential as a new employee.

A well-written application form should be supplemented by a one-page resume that summarizes the client's work history. A chronological resume lists past employment in historical order. This type of resume emphasizes education, former employers, and former job titles. A functional resume emphasizes the skills and abilities gained through employment and education and consists primarily of broad skill descriptions such as organizational and management skills, clerical abilities, and custodial skills. Each area consists of descriptions of the client's skill in each area. The chronology of education and employment then follows, using only a line for each job held or degree earned. Typically, the chronological resume is most appropriate for people who have had a solid work history, been employed by prestigious companies, or held jobs with titles similar to the work being applied for. Functional resumes, for the most part, will be most appropriate for substance abuse clients because they deemphasize work history and stress the capabilities or skills that the applicant will bring to the job. Resumes should be prepared in a simple and clear style that draws attention to the most saleable characteristics of the applicant. Popular wisdom holds that employers spend less than 60 seconds reading a resume, so it is important for it to be short, uncluttered, and to the point.

Like the application form and resume, letters of application should clearly identify the job being applied for and highlight the client's qualifications for the job. Poor spelling, grammar, or crumpled or messy letters will quickly move the client's application to the bottom of the pile, regardless of the applicant's qualifications. Employers believe that motivation for the job and attention to simple detail, as reflected in the letter of application, are minimal criteria for considering the applicant further.

All of the client's job-seeking skills and job search efforts are aimed at obtaining a job interview because decisions for hiring are made only after one has met with the employer face to face. There are several guidelines for interviewing, but in general, the applicant should (1) emphasize assets or why the employer should hire the applicant; (2) minimize or explain away deficits or reasons why one shouldn't be hired; (3) handle difficult questions, such as those about disability, in a positive but brief manner; and (4) end the interview with a "call-back" response that allows the applicant to telephone the employer sometime in the near future to follow up on the hiring decision. Even with a negative interview outcome, the follow-up telephone call will provide useful information because the client can use this opportunity to solicit feedback and hone interviewing skills. A final follow-up thank you letter should also be sent to all employers who took the time and effort to interview the applicant. This letter will leave the employer with a positive impression and may be helpful if future openings develop.

SUMMARY

Work is a major life area for most people and has a number of benefits beyond its financial rewards. Work contributes to the development of one's self-concept, builds and maintains self-esteem, provides a sense of belongingness to society, and gives an objective structure to one's waking hours. Although many people may be unemployed because of substance abuse or dependence problems, there are probably many more who bring their substance abuse problems to work with them. Research indicates that 10 percent to 12 percent of the workforce may be classified as substance abusers and that these workers have a significant negative impact on their employers, including increased numbers of absences and use of sick leave, higher probability of filing workers' compensation claims and being involved in on-the-job accidents, and using and dealing drugs while at work.

The ability to hold a job requires more than the ability to perform essential job functions. In addition, the successful worker must demonstrate critical vocational behaviors such as adhering to attendance and punctuality standards, meeting dress and grooming expectations, and demonstrating appropriate interactions with coworkers and supervisors. These behaviors are often negatively impacted by substance abuse problems and are more likely the reason for job termination than the inability to do the work.

Vocational counseling became necessary when work became more complex and diversified after the industrial revolution. A number of vocational counseling theories exist with techniques based on sociological, developmental, personality traits, and behavioral principles. The basic areas of agreement between the various theories are that people and jobs vary in terms of their abilities and requirements, occupational choice is important to success in life, a number of factors influence the decision-making process, and although most people will gravitate toward work that is appropriate for them, they would benefit from vocational counseling because it increases efficiency and effectiveness, resulting in better vocational choices.

People with substance abuse problems often have underdeveloped vocational identities because alcohol or drug use prevented them from gaining work-related experiences, behaviors, skills, and a solid work history. Those who were able to get and keep a job while struggling with alcohol or drug problems face the threatened loss of social status, home, income, and even their family because of substance abuse. The recommended sequence for engaging substance abuse clients in vocational counseling is exploration of the self and the world of work, identification of a vocational goal, development of a job placement plan, and implementation and follow-up of the job placement plan. The development of a job placement plan, separate from any other treatment of rehabilitation, was viewed as important to successful vocational outcomes. Critical to placement success for most clients is job-seeking skills instruction and implementation. These skills assist the substance abuser in recovery with job applications, developing a resume, presenting a positive image in the interview, and handling difficult questions regarding their substance abuse histories.

References

Abadinsky, H. (1997). *Drug abuse: An introduction* (3d ed.). Chicago: Nelson-Hall.

Abbott, A. (1992). Neurobiological perspectives on drugs of abuse. *Trends in Pharmacological Science, 13,* 169.

Ackerman, D. L. (1995). Drug testing. In R. H. Coombs & D. C. Ziedonis (Eds.), *Handbook on drug abuse prevention* (pp. 473–490). Needham Heights, MA: Allyn & Bacon.

Agranoff, R. (1977). Services integration. In W. F. Anderson, B. F. Frieden, & M. J. Murphy (Eds.), *Managing human services.* Washington, DC: International City Management Association.

Aiken, L. R. (1976). *Psychological testing and assessment.* Boston: Allyn & Bacon.

Akil, H., Madden, J., Patrick, R. L., & Barchas, J. D. (1976). Stress induced increase in endogenous opiate peptides: Concurrent analgesia and its partial reversal by Naloxone. In H. W. Kosterlitz (Ed.), *Opiates and endogenous opioid peptides.* Amsterdam: North-Holland Publishing Co.

Alcohol Alert. (1994, Jan.) *Alcohol and Minorities, 23* (PH347), Washington, DC: National Institute on Alcohol Abuse and Alcoholism.

Alcohol and Health (1990). *Seventh special report to the U.S. Congress from the Secretary of Health and Human Services.* Alexandria, VA: National Institute on Alcohol Abuse and Alcoholism (publication prepared by Editorial Experts Inc.).

Alcoholics Anonymous World Services, Inc. (1957). *Alcoholics Anonymous comes of age: A brief history of AA.* New York: Author.

Alcoholics Anonymous World Services, Inc. (1976). *Alcoholics Anonymous* (3d ed.). New York, NY: Author.

Alcoholics Anonymous World Services, Inc. (1990). *Alcoholics Anonymous 1989 membership survey* [Brochure]. New York, NY: Author.

Alcoholics Anonymous World Services, Inc. (1993). *Alcoholics Anonymous 1992 membership survey* [Brochure]. New York, NY: Author.

Alcoholics Anonymous World Services, Inc. (1997, Winter /Spring). *A.A. around the world. About A.A.*

Alcoholics Anonymous World Services, Inc. (1997). A.A. fact file. *In Alcoholics Anonymous* [Online]. Available: http://www.alcoholics-anonymous.org.

Aliesan, K., & Firth, R. C. (1990). A MICA program: Outpatient rehabilitation services for individuals with concurrent mental illness and chemical abuse disorders. *Journal of Applied Rehabilitation Counseling, 21*(3), 25–29.

Allen, J. P., Eckardt, M. J., & Wallen, J. (1988). Screening for alcoholism: Techniques and issues. *Public Health Reports, 103,* 586–592.

Alston, R. J., & Turner, W. L. (1994). A family strengths model of adjustment to disability for African American clients. *Journal of Counseling and Development, 72,* 378–383.

American Medical Association, Council on Scientific Affairs (1996). Alcoholism in the elderly. *Journal of the American Medical Association, 275,* 797–801.

American Medical Association (1992). The definition of alcoholism, *Journal of the Medical Association, 268(8),* 1012–1014.

American Society of Addiction Medicine (1996). *Patient placement criteria for the treatment of psychoactive substance use disorders* (2d ed.).

American Society of Addiction Medicine (1997). Information about ASAM [Online]. Available at http://207.201.181.5/info/info.htm#History.

American Psychiatric Association (1994). *Diagnostic and statistical manual of mental disorders* (4th ed). Washington DC: American Psychiatric Association.

Americans with Disabilities Handbook (1991). *Americans with Disabilities Handbook,* Equal Employment Opportunities Commission and the U.S. Department of Justice. Washington, DC: Author.

Anastasi, A. (1988). *Psychological testing* (6th ed.). New York: Macmillan.

Anderson, D., & Berlant, J. (1995). Managed mental health and substance abuse services. In P. Kongstvedt (Ed.), *Essentials of managed health care.* Gaithersburg, MD: Aspen Publications, Inc.

Angarola, R. T., & Rodriguez, S. N. (1989). State legislation: Effects on drug programs. In S. W. Gust, & J. M Walsh (Eds.), *Drugs in the workplace: Research and evaluation data [National Institute on Drug Abuse Research Monograph Series—No. 91] (pp.305–318).* Rockville, MD: National Institute on Drug Abuse.

Apfeldorf, M., & Hunley, P. J. (1981). The MacAndrew Scale: A measure of the diagnosis of alcoholism. *Journal of Studies on Alcohol, 42(1),* 80–86.

Armstrong, M. J., & Fitzgerald, M. H. (1996). Culture and disability studies: Anthropological perspective. *Rehabilitation Education, 10,* 274–304.

Arokiasamy, C.V. (1993). A theory for rehabilitation? *Rehabilitation Education, 7*(2), 77–98.

Atchley, R. C. (1994). *Social forces and aging: An introduction to social gerontology.* Belmont, CA: Wadsworth.

Austin, C. (1983). Case management in long-term care: Options and opportunities. *Health and Social Work, 8 (1),* 16–30.

Azrin, N. H., Philip, R. A., Thienes-Hontos, P., & Besalel, V. A. (1980). Comparative evaluation of the Job Club Program with welfare recipients. *Journal of Vocational Behavior, 16,* 133–145.

Babor, T. F. (1992). Avoiding the horrible and beastly sin of drunkenness: Does dissuasion make a difference? Unpublished manuscript, University of Connecticut School of Medicine.

Backer, T. E. (1988). The future of rehabilitation in the workplace: Drug abuse, AIDS & disability management. *Journal of Rehabilitation, 19*(2), 38–40.

Backer, T. E. (1995). Mass media. In R. H. Coombs & D. C. Ziedonis (Eds.), *Handbook on drug abuse prevention* (pp. 249–264). Needham Heights, MA: Allyn & Bacon.

Backer, T. E., & Newman, S. S. (1994). Organizational linkage and information dissemination: Strategies to integrate the substance abuse and disabilities field. *Rehabilitation Counseling Bulletin, 38,* 93–107.

Bagarozzi, D., & Kurtz, L. (1983). Administrators' perspectives on case management. *Arete, 8,* 13–21.

Ballew, J. R., & Mink, G. (1986). *Case management in the human services.* Springfield, IL: Thomas.

Bandler, R., Grinder, J., & Satir, V. (1976). *Changing with families.* Palo Alto: Science and Behavior Books.

Banta, W. F., & Tennant, F., Jr. (1989). *Complete handbook for combating substance abuse in the workplace.* Lexington, MA: Lexington.

Bartecchi, C. E., MacKenzie, T. D., & Schrier, R. W. (1994). The human costs of tobacco use. *New England Journal of Medicine, 330,* 907–919.

Bayh, B. (1979). Employment rights of the handicapped. *Journal of Rehabilitation, 3,* 57–61.

Beale, A. V. (1984). The continuing education and renewal of employee assistance program counselors. *Journal of Employment Counseling, 21,* 83–88.

Beaman, D. (1994). Black English and the therapeutic relationship. *Journal of Mental Health Counseling, 6*(3), 379.

Beattie, M. (1987). *Codependent no more.* New York: HarperCollins.

Beaumont, J. G. (1983). *Introduction to neuropsychology.* The Guilford Press, NY.

Beck, A. T., Wright, F. D., Newman, C. F., & Liese, B. S. (1993). *Cognitive therapy of substance abuse.* New York: Guilford Press.

Becker, R. L. (1981). *Revised Reading Free Vocational Interest Inventory.* Columbus, OH: Elbern.

Bellah, R. N., Madsen, R., Sullivan, W. M., Swidler, A., & Tipton, S. M. (1985). Habits of the heart. New York: Harper & Row

Benshoff, J. J. (1996). Peer self-help groups. In W. Crimando & T. F. Riggar (Eds.), *Utilizing community resources: An overview of human services.* (pp. 57–66) Delray Beach, FL: St. Lucie Press.

Benshoff, J. J., Grissom, J., & Nelson, R. (1990). Job placement practices with clients who are substance abusers: National trends. *Journal of Job Placement, 6*(2), 16–21.

Benshoff, J. J., & Riggar, T. F. (1990). Cocaine: A primer for rehabilitation counselors. *Journal of Applied Rehabilitation Counseling, 21*(3), 21–24.

Benshoff, J. J., & Roberto, K. A. (1987). Alcoholism in the elderly: Clinical issues. *Clinical Gerontologist, 7*(2), 3–13.

Bernstein, M., & Mahoney, J. J. (1989). Management perspectives on alcoholism: The employers stake in alcoholism treatment. *Occupational Medicine, 4,* 223–232.

Black, C. (1982). *It will never happen to me.* Denver: M.A.C. Printing.

Blum, T. C. (1989). The presence and integration of drug abuse intervention in human resource management. In S. W. Gust, & J. M Walsh (Eds.), *Drugs in the workplace: Research and evaluation data [National Institute on Drug Abuse Research Monograph Series—No. 91] pp. 245–270).* Rockville, MD: National Institute on Drug Abuse.

Blum, T. C., & Roman, P. M. (1987). Social constructions and ideologies of substance abuse, 2. *Journal-of-Drug-Issues, 17*(4), 1–5.

Blume, S. B. (1988). Alcohol/drug dependent women: *New insights into their special problems, treatment, recovery,* Minneapolis: Johnson Institute.

Bowe, F. (1980). *Rehabilitating America: Toward independence for disabled and elderly people.* New York: Harper & Row.

Bradshaw, J. (1988). *Bradshaw on the family: A revolutionary way of self-discovery.* Deerfield Beach, FL: Health Communications, Inc.

Bratter, T. E., Collabolletta, E. A., Fossbender, A. J., Pennachia, M. C., & Rubel, J. R. (1985). The American self-help residential therapeutic community: A pragmatic treatment approach for addicted character-disordered individuals. In T. E. Bratter & G. G. Forrest (Eds.), *Alcoholism and substance abuse: Strategies for clinical intervention .* New York: The Free Press.

Bratter, T. E., Pennacchia, M. C., & Gauya, D. C. (1985). From methadone maintenance to abstinence: The myth of the metabolic disorder theory. In T. E. Bratter & G. G. Forrest (Eds.), *Alcoholism and substance abuse: Strategies for clinical intervention.* New York: The Free Press.

Brecher, E. M. (1972). Licit and illicit drugs. Boston: Little, Brown and Company.

Brown, S. (1985). *Treating the alcoholic: A developmental model of recovery.* New York: John Wiley & Sons.

Brown, B. B. (1982). Professional's perceptions of drug and alcohol abuse among the elderly. *The Gerontologist, 22,* 519–524

Brown, S. (1985). *Treating the alcoholic: A developmental model of recovery.* New York: John Wiley & Sons.

Brown, S. (1988). *Treating adult children of alcoholics: A developmental perspective.* New York: Wiley.

Buehler, C. (1933). *Der menschliche lebenslauf als psychologisches problem.* Leipzig: Hirzel.

Buelow, G. (1995). Comparing students from substance abusing and dysfunctional families: Implications for counseling. *Journal of Counseling and Development, 73,* 327–330.

Buelow, G., & Herbert, S. (1995). Counselor's resource on psychiatric medications. Pacific Grove, CA: Brooks/Cole Publishing Co.

Burgess, K. M., Benshoff, J. J., Early, J. K., & Taricone, P. F. (1990). Field experiences for rehabilitation students in EAP settings. *Rehabilitation Education, 4,* 109–119.

Burgess, K. M., Fried, J. H., & Benshoff, J. J. (1989). Employee assistance programs: Challenges to education and business. *Journal of Job Placement, 5*(2), 16–20.

Burke, T. R. (1988). The economic impact of alcohol abuse and alcoholism. *Public Health Reports, 103,* 567.

Butler, J. P. (1992). Of kindred minds: The ties that bind. In M. A. Orlandi, R. Weston, & L. G. Epstein (Eds.), *Cultural competence for evaluators: A guide for alcohol and other drug prevention practitioners working with ethnic/racial communities* (pp. 23–54). Rockville, MD: U.S. Department of Health and Human Services, Office for Substance Abuse Prevention.

Campbell, J., Gabrielli, W., Laster, L. J, & Liskow, B. I. (1997). Efficacy of outpatient intensive treatment for drug abuse. *Journal of Addictive Diseases, 16*(2).

Carey, K. B. (1996). Treatment of co-occurring substance abuse and major mental illness. In R. E. Drake & K. T. Myeser (Eds.), *Dual diagnosis of major mental illness and substance abuse: Volume 2, Recent research and clinical implications* (pp. 19–31).

Casas, J. M. (1992). A culturally sensitive model for evaluating alcohol and other drug abuse prevention programs: A Hispanic perspective. In M. A. Orlandi, R. Weston, & L. G. Epstein (Eds.), *Cultural competence for evaluators: A guide for alcohol and other drug prevention practitioners working with ethnic/racial communities* (pp. 75–116). Rockville, MD: U.S. Department

of Health and Human Services, Office for Substance Abuse Prevention.

Cermack, T. L. (1986) Diagnostic criteria for codependency. *Journal of Psychoactive drugs, 18,* 15–20.

Clopton, J. R., & Klein, G. L. (1978). An initial look at the redundancy of specialized MMPI scales. *Journal of Consulting & Clinical Psychology, 46,* 1436–1438.

Cocaine Anonymous (1997). *Cocaine Anonymous World Services.* Available online: http://www.ca.org.

Cole, M. (1993). *Group dynamics in occupational therapy: The theoretical basis and practice application of group treatment.* Thorofare, NJ: Slack, Incorporated.

Collum, C. M., Kuck, J., & Ruff, R. M. (1990). Neuropsychological assessment of traumatic brain injury in adults. In E. D. Bigler (Ed.), *Traumatic brain injury: Mechanisms of damage, assessment, intervention and outcome* (pp. 129–164). Austin, TX: PRO-ED.

Commission on Rehabilitation Counselor Certification (1987). *Code of professional ethics for rehabilitation counselors.* Rolling Meadows, IL.

Connor, R. I., & Burns, P. (1995). Law enforcement and regulatory agencies. In R. H. Coombs & D. C. Ziedonis (Eds.), *Handbook on drug abuse prevention* (pp. 47–68). Needham Heights, MA: Allyn & Bacon.

Constantine, L. (1978). *Family Paradigms: The practice of theory in family therapy.* New York: Guilford.

Constantine, L. (1986). *Family paradigms: The practice of theory in family therapy.* New York: Guilford.

Cook, R. F. (1989). Drug abuse among working adults: Prevalence rates and estimation methods. In S. W. Gust & J. M. Walsh (Eds.), *Drugs in the workplace: Research and evaluation data* (Research Monograph No. 91, pp. 17–32). Rockville, MD: National Institute on Drug Abuse.

Cooper, P. G., & Davis, S. (1979). Case flow modeling: A program management innovation for planning services to the severely disabled. In B. Bolton & P. G. Cooper *Readings in rehabilitation counseling research.* Baltimore: University Park Press.

Cooper, S. E., & Robinson, D. A.G. (1987). Use of the Substance Abuse Subtle Screening Inventory with a college population. *Journal of American College Health, 36,* 180–184.

Corey, G. (1995). *Theory and practice of group counseling* (4th ed.). Pacific Grove, CA: Brooks/Cole.

Craddock, S., Hubbard, R., Bray, R., Cavanaugh, E., & Rachal, J. (1982). *Client characteristics, behaviors and in-treatment outcomes: 1980 TOPS admission cohort.* Rockville, MD: National Institute on Drug Abuse.

Craig, R. J. (1980). Effectiveness of low dose methadone maintenance for the treatment of inner-city heroin addicts. *International Journal of the Addictions, 15,* 701–710.

Crandall, R. C. (1991). *Gerontology: A behavioral science approach.* New York: McGraw-Hill.

Crew, N., & Athelstan, G. (1984). *Functional assessment inventory manual.* Materials Development Center, Stout Vocational Rehabilitational Institute, University of Wisconsin-Stout.

Crimando, W. (1996). Case management implications. In W. Crimando & T. F. Riggar (Eds.), *Utilizing community resources: An overview of human resources.* Delray Beach, FL: St. Lucie Press, Inc.

Crimando, W., & Riggar, T. F. (Eds.). (1996). *Utilizing community resources: An overview of human resources,* Delray Beach, FL: St. Lucie Press, Inc.

Crump, M. T., & Milling, R. N. (1996). The efficacy of substance abuse educatiom among dual diagnosis patients. *Journal of Substance Abuse Treatment, 13,* 141–144.

CTB/McGraw-Hill. (1976). *Tests of Adult Basic Education technical report.* Monterey, CA: Author.

Darke, S., Hall, W., Wodak, A., Heather, N., & Ward, J. (1992). Development and validation of a multi-dimensional instrument for assessing outcome of treatment among opiate users: The Opiate Treatment Index. *British Journal of Addiction, 87,* 733–742.

Davidson, G. C., & Neale, J. M. (1986). *Abnormal psychology: An experimental clinical approach (4th ed.).* New York: John Wiley & Sons.

DeLeon, G. (1984). Program-based evaluation research in therapeutic communities. In F. M. Timms & J. P. Ludford (Eds.), *Drug abuse treatment evaluation: Strategies progress, and prospects* (NIDA Research Monograph No. 51, pp. 69–87). Rockville, MD: National Institute on Drug Abuse.

Deren, S., & Randell, J. (1990). The vocational rehabilitation of substance abuser. *Journal of Applied Rehabilitation Counseling, 21(2),* 4–6.

Desmond, R. E. (1985). Careers in employee assistance programs. *Journal of Applied Rehabilitation Counseling, 16(2),* 26–30.

DeSouza, E. B., Battaglia, G., & Insel, T. R. (1990). Neurotoxic effects of MDMA on brain serotonin neurons: Evidence from neurochemcial and radiologic and binding studies. *Annals of the New York Academy of Science, 600,* 682–689.

DeWit, H., Pierri, J., & Johanson, C. E. (1989). Assessing individual differences in ethanol preferences using a cumulative dosing procedure. *Psychopharmacology, 98(1),* 113–119.

Diagnostic and statistical manual of mental disorders (4th ed.). (1994). Washington, D. C.: American Psychiatric Association.

Dial, J., Mezger, C., Gray, S., Massey, T., Chan, F., & Hull, J. (1992). *The Comprehensive Vocational Evaluation System.* Dallas, TX: McCarron-Dial Systems.

DiChiara, G., & North, R. A. (1992). Neurobiology of opiate abuse. *Trends in Pharmacological Science, 13,* 185–193.

Dickerson, L. R., Smith, P B., & Moore, J. E. (1997). An overview of blindness and visual impairment. In J. E. Moore, W. H. Graves, & J. B. Patterson (Eds.). *Foundations of rehabilitation counseling with persons who are blind or visually impaired* (pp. 3–23). New York: AFB Press.

Dickman, F. (1985). Employee assistance programs: History and philosophy. In J. F. Dickman, W. G. Emener, & W. S. Hutchinson, Jr. (Eds.), *Counseling the troubled person in industry: A guide to the organization, implementation and evaluation of employee assistance programs* (pp. 7–12). Springfield, IL: Charles C. Thomas.

Dickman, F. (1985). Ingredients of an effective EAP. In F. Dickman, W. G. Emener, & W. S. Hutchinson (Eds.), *Counseling the* troubled person in industry. Springfield, IL: Charles C. Thomas.

Dickman, F., & Challenger, B. R. (1988). Employee assistance prgrams: A historical sketch. In F. Dickman, B. R. Challenger, W. G. Emener, & W. S. Hutchinson (Eds.), *Employee Assistance Programs: A basic text* (pp. 48–53). Springfield, IL: Charles C. Thomas.

DiNitto, D. M., & Swabb, A. J. (1993). Screening for undetected substance abuse among vocational rehabilitation clients. *American Rehabilitation, 19,* 12–20.

Dinkmeyer, D. C., Pew, W. L., & Dinkmeyer, D. C., Jr. (1979). *Adlerian counseling and psychotherapy.* Monterey, CA: Brooks/Cole.

Dittrich, J. R. (1993). A group program for wives of treatment-resistant alcoholics. In T. J. O'Farrell (Ed.), *Treating alcohol problems: Marital and family interventions* (pp. 78–116). New York: The Guilford Press.

DiVito, J. A. (1995). *The interpersonal communication book* (7th ed.). New York: Harper Collins.

Dole, V. P., & Nyswander, M. (1967). Rehabilitation of the street addict. *Archives of Environmental Health, 14,* 477–480.

Doweiko, H. E. (1996). Concepts of chemical dependency. (3rd ed.). Pacific Grove, CA: Brooks/Cole.

Dreikurs, R. (1981). The three life tasks. In L. Baruth & D. Eckstein (Eds.), Lifestyle: *Theory, practice and research* (2d ed.). Dubuque, IA: Kendall/Hunt.

Drugs At Work, (1985). National Institute of Drug Abuse (NIDA), Washington, DC: SAMHSA Media Services.

Duvall, E. M. (1977). *Marriage and family development* (5th ed.). New York: Lippincott.

Duvall, E. M., & Miller, B. C. (1985). *Marriage and family development* (6th ed.). New York: Harper & Row.

Egan, G. (1990). *The skilled helper.* Pacific Grove, CA: Brooks/Cole Publishing Company.

Ellickson, P. L. (1995). Schools. In R. H. Coombs & D. Ziedonis (Ed.) *Handbook on drug abuse prevention* (pp. 93–120). Needham Heights, MA: Allyn & Bacon.

Emrick, C. D. (1987). Alcoholics Anonymous: Affiliation processes and effectiveness as

treatment. *Alcoholism Clinical and Experimental Research, 11,* 416–423.

England, G. W. (1991). The meaning of work in the USA: Recent changes. *European Work and Organizational Psychologist, 1,* 111–124.

Enns, C. Z. (1992). Self-esteem groups: A synthesis of consciousness-raising and assertiveness training. *Journal of Counseling and Development, 71,* 7–13.

Erikson, E. (1963). *Childhood and society.* New York: W. W. Norton & Co.

Erikson, E. H. (1968). *Identity: Youth and crisis.* New York: W. W. Norton.

Estroff, T. W. (1987). Medical and boilogical consequences of cocaine abuse. In A. M. Washton & M. S. Gold (Eds.), *Cocaine: A clinician's handbook* (pp. 23–32). New York: The Guilford Press.

Extein, I., & Dackis, C. A. (1987). Brain mechanism in cocaine dependency. In A. M. Washton & M. S. Gold (Eds.), *Cocaine: A clinician's handbook* (pp. 73–84). New York: The Guilford Press.

Fagan, J. (1993). Set and setting revisited: influences of alcohol and illicit drugs on the social context of violent events. In S. F. Martin (Ed.), *Alcohol and interpersonal violence: Fostering multidisciplinary perspectives* (Research monograph 24, pp. 161–192). Rockville, MD: National Institute on Alcohol Abuse and Alcoholism, U.S. Department of Health and Human Services.

Falvo, D. R., Hollard, B., Brenner, J., & Benshoff, J. J. (1990). Medication use practices in the ambulatory elderly. *Health Values, 14*(3), 10–16.

Farr, C. L., Bordieri, J. E., Benshoff, J. J., & Taricone, P. F. (1996). Rehabilitation needs of individuals in treatment for alcohol dependency. *Journal of Applied Rehabilitation Counseling, 27*(1), 17–22.

Feldblum, C. R. (1991). Employment protections. In J. West (Ed.), *The Americans with Disabilities Act: From policy to practice.* (pp. 81–110). New York: Milbank Memorial Fund.

Fenell, D. L., & Weinhold, B. K. (1989). *Counseling families: An introduction to marriage and family therapy.* Denver: Love Publishing.

Fingarette, H. (1988). *Heavy drinking: The myth of alcoholism as a disease.* Berkeley: University of California Press.

Finnegan, D. G., & McNally, F. B. (1989). The lonely journey: Lesbians and gay men who are co-dependent. In B. Carruth and W. Mendenhall (Eds.), *Co-dependency: Issues in Treatment and Recovery* (pp. 121–134). Binghamton, NY: Haworth Press, Inc.

Finney, J. C., Smith, D. F., Skeeters, D. E., & Auvenshine, C. D. (1971). MMPI alcoholism scales: Factor structure and content analysis. *Quarterly Journal of Studies on Alcohol, 32,* 1055–1060.

Fishbein, D. H., & Pease, S. E. (1996). *The dynamics of drug abuse.* Boston: Allyn & Bacon.

Fisher, G. L., & Harrison, T. C. (1997). *Substance abuse: Information for school counselors, social workers and therapists.* Needham Heights, MA: Allyn & Bacon.

Forrest, G. G. (1985). *Antabuse* treatment. In T. E. Bratter & G. G. Forrest (Eds.), *Alcoholism and substance abuse: Strategies for clinical intervention* (pp. 307–336). New York: The Free Press.

Foulks, E. F., & Pena, J. M. (1995). Ethnicity and psychotherapy: A component in the treatment of cocaine addiction in African Americans. *Psychiatric Clinics of North America, 18,* 607–620.

Freddolino, P. P. (1983). Findings from the national mental health advocacy survey. *Mental Disability Law Reporter, 7(5),* 416–421, 435.

French, J. R. P., & Raven, B. (1968). The bases of social power. In D. Cartwright & A. Zander (Eds.), *Group dynamics: Research and theory.* New York: Harper & Row.

Frezza, C., DiPadova, C. Pozzeto, G., Terpin, M., Baraono, E., & Lieber, C. S. (1990). Higher blood alcohol levels in women: The role of decreased gastric alcohol dehydrogenase activity and first-pass metabolism. *The New England Journal of Medicine, 322*(2), 95–99.

Friedrich, W. N., & Loftsgard, S. O. (1978). A comparison of the MacAndrew Alcoholism Scale and the Michigan Alcoholism Screening Test in a sample of problem drinkers. *Journal of Studies on Alcohol, 39,* 1940–1944.

Fulgham, R. (1990) *All I really need to know I learned in kindergarten: Uncommon thoughts on common things.* New York: Random House.

Fuller, R. K. (1995). Antidipsotropic medications. In R. K. Hester & W. R. Miller (Eds.), *Handbook of alcoholism treatment approaches: Effective Alternatives* (2d ed.). Needham Heights, MA: Allyn & Bacon.

Fureman, B., Parikh, G., Bragg, A., & McLellan, A. I. (1990). *Addiction severity index: 5th ed. with preface. A guide to training and supervising ASI interviews based on the past ten years.* Philadelphia: The University of Pennsylvania/Veterans Administration Center for Studies of Addiction.

Garvin, R. E. (1985). The role of the rehabilitation counselor in industry. Journal of *Applied Rehabilitation Counseling, 16(4),* 44–47, 50.

Gerstein & Bayer (1988).

Gerstein, L. H., & Bayer, G. A. (1988). Employee assistance programs: A systematic investigation of their use. *Journal of Counseling and Development, 66,* 294–297.

Gerstein, L. H., & Bayer, G. A. (1991). Counseling and the bystander–equity model of supervisory helping behavior: Directions for EAP research. *Journal of Counseling and Development, 69,* 241–247.

Gierymski, T., & William, T. (1986). Co-dependency. *Journal of Psychoactive Drugs, 18,* 7–13.

Ginzberg, E. (1952). Toward a theory of occupational choice. *Occupations, 30,* 491–494.

Glasser, W. (1967). *Reality Therapy.* New York: Julian Press.

Glasser, W. (1998). *Choice Theory: A new psychology of personal freedom.* New York: HarperCollins.

Gleick, E. (1996, February 5). Rehab centers run dry. *Time Magazine, 147(6),* 44–45.

Glover, N., Janikowski, T. P., & Benshoff, J. J. (1995). The incidence of incest histories among clients receiving substance abuse treatment. *Journal of Counseling and Development, 73,* 475–480.

Glover, N. M., Janikowski, T. P., & Benshoff, J. J. (1996). Substance abuse and past incest contact: A national perspective. *Journal of Substance Abuse Treatment, 3,* 185–193.

Godley, M. D., Cronk, B. C., & Landrum, E. (1996). In W. Crimando & T. F. Riggar

(Eds.), *Utilizing community resources: An overview of human service.* Delray Beach, FL: St. Lucie Press.

Goldberg, R. (1997). *Drugs across the spectrum.* Englewood, CO: Morton Publishing Co.

Goldenberg, I., & Goldenberg, H. (1996). *Family therapy: An overview* (4th ed.). Pacific Grove, CA: Brooks/Cole.

Goldstein, A. (1989). *Molecular and cellular aspects of the drug addictions.* New York: Springer-Verlag.

Gomberg, E. S. L. (1988). Alcoholic women in treatment: The question of stigma and age. *Alcohol & Alcoholism, 23*(6), 507–514.

Gordon, E. T., Gordon, E. W., & Nembhard, J. G. G. (1994). Social science literature concerning African American men. *Journal of Negro Education, 1994, 63*(4), 508–531.

Gorman, M. (1996). *Speed use and HIV transmission.* Available online: *http//www.tweaker.org/science.html.*

Grace, C. A. (1992). Practical considerations for program professionals and evaluators working with African American communities. In M. A. Orlandi, R. Weston, & L. G. Epstein (Eds.), *Cultural competence for evaluators* (pp. 55–74). Rockville, MD: U.S. Department of Health and Human Services.

Grosser, G. H., & Paul, N. L. (1971). Ethical issues in family group therapy. In J. Haley (Ed.), *Changing families: A family therapy reader.* New York: Grune & Stratton.

Guthman, D., Lybarger, R., & Sandberg, K. A. (1993). Providing chemical dependency treatment to the deaf or hard of hearing mentally ill client. *Journal of the American Deafness and Rehabilitation Association, 27*(1), 1–15.

Guthman, D., & Sandberg, K. A. (1997). Deaf cultures and substance abuse. *The Counselor, 15*(1), 29–32.

Haaga, J. G., & Reuter, P. H. (1995). Prevention: The (lauded) orphan of drug policy. In R. H. Coombs & D. C. Ziedonis (Eds.), *Handbook on drug abuse prevention.* Needham Heights, MA: Allyn & Bacon.

Hale, J., & Hunter, M. (1988). *From HMO movement to managed care industry: The future of HMO's in a volatile healthcare market.* Monograph published by the InterStudy Center for Managed Care Research.

Hale-Benson, J. E. (1986). *Black children: Their roots, cultures and learning styles.* Baltimore, MD: John Hopkins University Press.

Haley, J. (1963). *Strategies of psychotherapy.* New York: Grune & Stratton.

Haley, J. (1976). *Problem-solving therapy.* San Francisco: Jossey-Bass.

Hanna, S. M., & Brown, J. H. (1995). *The practice of family therapy: Key elements across models.* Pacific Grove, CA: Brooks/Cole.

Hanson, G., & Venturelli, P. J. (1995). *Drugs and society* (4th ed.). Boston: Jones and Bartlett.

Hanson, J. C., & Campbell, D. P. (1992). *Manual for the Strong Interest Inventory* (4th ed.). Stanford, CA: Stanford University Press.

Hanson, M. (1983). Use of the job placement plan in vocational rehabilitation. *Dissertation Abstracts International, 44,* 23–61. (University Microfilms No. ADG83–28, 495).

Harford, T. C., & Brooks, S. D. (1992). Cirrhosis mortality and occupation. *Journal of Studies on Alcohol,* September, 463–468.

Harney, R. B., & Harger, R. N. (1965). The alcohols. In J. R. DiPalma (Ed.), *Drill's pharmacology in medicine* (3d ed.). New York: McGraw-Hill.

Harris, T. A. (1969). *I'm OK—You're OK.* New York: Harper & Row, Pub.

Hartog, S. B., Hickey, D., Reichman, W., & Gracin, L. (1993). EAP referral and the supervisor: An examination of perceptions of situational constraints and organizational barriers. *Journal of Employee Assistance Research, 2, (1),* 47–63.

Haskell, R. E. (1993). Realpolitik in the addictions field: treatment-professional, popular-culture ideology, and scientific research. *Journal-of-Mind-and-Behavior, 14*(3), 275–276.

Havighurst, R. (1948). *Developmental tasks and education.* Michigan: Edwards Brothers.

Hawkins, J. D., Catalano, R. F., & Miller, J. Y. (1992). Risk and protective factors for alcohol and other drug problems in adolesence and early adulthood. Implications for sustance abuse prevention. *Psychological Bulletin, 112.* 64–105.

Heather, N., & Robertson, I. (1981). *Controlled drinking.* London: Methuen.

Heinrich, R. K., Corbine, J. L., & Thomas, K. R. (1990). Counseling Native Americans. *Journal of Counseling and Development, 69,* 128–133.

Heller, K. W., Alberto. P. A. , Forney, P. E., & Schwartzman, M. N. (1996). *Understanding physical, sensory and health impairments: Characteristics and educational implications.* Pacific Grove, CA: Brooks/Cole ITP.

Helwig, A. A., & Holicky, R. (1994). Substance abuse in persons with disabilities: Treatment considerations. *Journal of Counseling and Development, 72,* 227–233.

Herbert, J. T. (1989). Assessing the need for family therapy: A primer for rehabilitation counselors. *Journal of Rehabilitation, 55(1),* 45–51.

Herkenham, M., Lynn, A. B., Little, M. D., Johnson, M. R., Melvin, L. S., de Costa, B. R., & Rice, K. C. (1990). Cannabinoid receptor localization in the brain. *Proceedings of the National Academy of Sciences, 87,* 1932–1936.

Hester, R. K., & Miller, W. R. (Eds.). (1995). *Handbook of alcoholism treatment approaches:* Effective alternatives (2nd ed.). Boston: Allyn & Bacon.

Hoffman, J. A., Caudill, B. D., Koman, J. J., Luckey, J. W., Flynn, P. M., & Mayo, D. W. (1996). Psychosocial treatment for cocaine abuse: 12-month treatment outcomes. *Journal of Substance Abuse Treatment, 13,* 3–11.

Hoffmann, H., Loper, R. G., & Kammeier, M. L. (1974). Identifying future alcoholics with MMPI alcoholism scales. *Quarterly Journal of Studies on Alcohol, 35,* 490–498.

Hoffmann, N. G., Harrison, P. A., & Bellile, C. A. (1983). Alcoholics Anonymous after treatment: Attendance and abstinence. *The International Journal of Addictions, 18,* 311–318.

Hoffmann, N. G., Halikas, J. A., & Mee-Lee, D. (1987). *The Cleveland Admission, Discharge, and Transfer Criteria: Model for Chemical Dependency Treatment Programs.* The Northern Ohio Chemical Dependency Treatment Directors Association, Cleveland, Ohio.

Holland, J. L. (1959). A theory of vocational choice. *Journal of Counseling Psychology, 6,* 35–45.

Holland, J. L. (1987). Current status of Hollands' theory of careers: Another perspective. *Career Development Quarterly, 36,* 31–44.

Hollingshead, A. B. (1949). *Elmtown's youth.* New York: Wiley.

Homer, A. L., & Dillon, D. (1997). *Web of Addictions.* Available online: http://www.well.com/user/woa/aodsites.htm# Self Help News Group.

Hoppock, R. (1976). *Occupational information* (4th ed.). New York: McGraw-Hill.

Hosie, T. W., West, J. D., & Mackey, J. A. (1993). Employment and roles of counselors in employee assistance programs. *Journal of Counseling and development, 71,* 355–359.

Hull, C. L. (1928). *Aptitude testing.* Yonkers-on-Hudson, NY: World.

Hutchins, D. E., & Cole, C. G. (1992). *Helping relationships and strategies* (2nd ed.). Pacific Grove, CA: Brooks/Cole.

Illinois Women's Substance Abuse Coalition (1985). *Report of the Prevention/Treatment Committee.* Unpublished manuscript.

Inaba, D. S., & Cohen, W. E. (1989). *Uppers, downers and all arounders.* (1st ed.). Ashland, OR: Cineme.

Inaba, D. S., & Cohen, W. E. (1997). *Uppers, downers, all arounders: Physical and Mental effects of drugs of abuse.* (3rd ed.). Ashlanuma, 24, 40–44.

Inciardi, J. A., Isenberg, H., Lockwood, D., Martin, S. S., & Scarpitti, F. R. (1992). Assertive community treatment with a parolee population: An extension of case management. In R. Ashery (Ed.), *Progress and issues in case management* (Research monograph No. 127, pp. 350–367). Rockville, MD: National Institute on Drug Abuse.

Independent Living Center Resource Handbook (1993, January 21). *Change* [Brochure]. Washington, DC: Author.

International Labor Office (1973). *Basic principles of vocational rehabilitation of the disabled* (2nd ed.). Geneva: Author.

Isaacson, L.E. (1986). *Career information in counseling and career development,* (4th ed.). Boston: Allyn & Bacon.

Issacson, L. E., Brown, D. (1993). Career information, career counseling, & career development (5th ed.). Boston: Allyn & Bacon.

Jagger, J., Levine, J. I., Jane, J., & Rimel, R. W. (1984). Epidemiologic features of head injury in a predominately rural population. *Journal of Trauma, 24,* 40–44.

Jaques, M. E. (1970). *Rehabilitation counseling: Scope and services.* Boston: Houghton-Mifflin.

Jarvis, T. J., Tebbutt, J., & Mattick, R. P. (1995). *Treatment approaches for alcohol and drug dependence: An introductory guide.* West Sussex, UK: John Wiley & Sons Ltd.

Jellinek, E. M. (1952). Phases of alcohol addiction. *Quarterly Journal of Studies on Alcohol, 13,* 673–674.

Jellinek, E. M. (1960). *The disease concept of alcoholism.* New Haven, CT: Hillhouse Press.

Jenkins, W. M., Patterson, J. B., & Szymanski, E. M. (1992). Philosophical, historical, and legislative aspects of the rehabilitation counseling profession. In R. M. Parker & E. M. Szymanski (Eds.), *Rehabilitation counseling: Basics and beyond* (2d ed.). Austin, TX: PRO-ED.

Jerrell, J. M. (1996). Toward cost effective care for persons with dual diagnoses. *Journal of Mental Health Administration, 23,* 329–337.

Johnson, D. W., & Johnson, F. P. (1975). *Joining together: Group theory and group skills.* Englewood Cliffs, NJ: Prentice-Hall.

Johnson, L., & Associates, Inc. (1984). *Final report: Evaluation of the delivery of services to select disabled people by the vocational rehabilitation service system* (RSA Contract #300-81-0267). Washington, DC: Department of Education, Office of Special Education and Rehabilitative Services.

Johnson, P., & Rubin, A. (1983). Case management in mental health: A social work domain? *Social Work, 1,* 49–55.

Johnson, Jr., S. D. (1990). Toward clarifying culture, race, and ethnicity in the context of multi-cultural counseling. *Journal of Multi-cultural Counseling and Development, 18,* 41–50.

Johnson, V., & White H. (1995). The relationship between work-specific and generalized stress and alcohol and marijuana use among recent entrants to the labor force. *Journal of Drug Issues, 25(2),* 237–251.

Jones, R. T. (1987). Psychopharmacology of cocaine. In A. M. Washington & M. S. Gold (Eds.), *Cocaine: A clinicians handbook.* New York: The Guilford Press.

Jung, J. (1994). *Under the influence: Alcohol and human behavior.* Pacific Grove, CA: Brooks/Cole.

Kalat, J. W. (1998). *Biological psychology* (6th ed.). Pacific Grove, CA: Brooks/Cole.

Kantor, D., & Lehr, W. (1975). *Inside the family.* San Francisco: Jossey-Bass.

Kantor, G. K. (1993). Refining the brushstrokes in portraits of alcohol and wife assaults. In S. E. Martin (Ed.), *Alcohol and interpersonal violence: Fostering multidisciplinary perspectives* (Research monograph no. 24, pp. 281–291). Rockville, MD: National Institutes of Alcoholism and Alcohol Abuse.

Kelley, S. D. M., & Benshoff, J. J. (1997). Dual diagnosis of mental illness and substance abuse: Contemporary challenges for rehabilitation. *Journal of Applied Rehabilitation Counseling, 28(3),* 43–49.

Kemp, D. R. (1985). State employee assistance programs: Organization and services. *Public Administration review, 45,* 378–382.

Kerr, B. (1994). Substance Abuse Subtle Screening Inventory. In J. C. Conoley & J. C. Impara (Eds.), *The supplement to the eleventh mental measurements yearbook.* Lincoln, NE: The University of Nebraska Press.

Kinney, J. & Leaton, G. (1995). *Loosening the grip: A handbook of alcohol information* (5th ed.). St. Louis: Mosby.

Kirstein, L. S. (1987). Inpatient cocaine abuse treatment. In A. M. Washton & M. S. Gold (Eds.), *Cocaine: A clinicians's handbook.* New York: The Guilford Press.

Kitson, H. D. (1925). *The psychology of vocational adjustment.* Philadelphia: Lippincott.

Knowlton, L. (1995). *Public and research views of dual diagnosis explored.* MHI. (OnLine). Available: http//www.mhsource.co/edu/psytimes/p950536.html.

Kolata, G. (1986). New drug counters alcohol intoxication. *Science, 234,* 1198–1199.

Koob, G. F. (1992). Drugs of abuse: Anatomy, pharmacology and function of reward pathways. *Trends in Pharmacological Science, 13,* 177–184.

Kostyk, D., Lindblom, L., Fuchs, D., Tabiz, E., & Jacyk, W. R. (1994). Chemical dependency in the elderly: Treatment phase. *Journal of Gerontological Social Work, 22,* 175–191.

Kottler, J. A. (1992). Confronting our own hypocrisy: Being a model for our students and clients. *Journal of Counseling and Development, 70,* 475–476.

Kramer Communications. (1990). *Co-dependency: How far does the shadow of chemical dependency reach?* [Booklet]. San Bruno, CA: Author.

Krantz, G. (1971). Critical vocational behaviors. *Journal of Rehabilitation, 37,* 14–16.

Kurtz, N. R., Googins, B., & Howard, W. C. (1984). Measuring the success of occupational alcoholism programs. *Journal of Studies on Alcohol, 45,* 33–45.

Lam, C. S. (1986). Comparison of sheltered and supported work programs: A pilot study. *Rehabilitation Counseling Bulletin, 30(2),* 66–82.

Lawson, G., Peterson, J. S., & Lawson, A. (1983). *Alcoholism and the family.* Rockville, MD: Aspen Publications, Inc.

Lazarus, A. A. (1983). *The practice of multimodal therapy.* New York: McGraw-Hill.

Lemons, S. L., & Sweeny, P. (1981). Vocational rehabilitation professionals in the veterans administration. *Journal of Applied Rehabilitation Counseling, 12(3),* 151–155.

Levine, I. S., & Fleming, M. (1985). *Issues in case management.* Rockville, MD: National Institute of Mental Health.

Lewis, J. A., Dana, R. Q., & Blevins, G. A. (1994). *Substance abuse counseling: An individualized approach* (2d ed.), Pacific Grove, CA: Brooks/Cole Publishing.

Linkowski, D. C., & Szymanski, E. M. (1993). Accreditation in rehabilitation counseling: Historical and current context and process. *Rehabilitation Counseling Bulletin, 37(2),* 81–91.

Livneh, H., & Male, R. (1993). Functional limitations: A review of their characteristics and vocational impact. *Journal of Rehabilitation, October/November/December,* 44–50.

Locke, E. A., & Latham, G. P. (1984). *Goal setting: A motivational technique that works.* Englewood Cliffs, NJ: Prentice-Hall.

Loftquist, L. H., & Dawis, R. V. (1978). Values as second-order needs in the Theory of Work Adjustment. *Journal of Vocational Behavior, 12,* 12–18.

Longabaugh, R. (1988). Longitudinal outcome studies. In R. M. Rose & J. Barrett (Eds.), *Alcoholism: Origins and outcome.* New York: Raven Press, Ltd.

Luxton, L., Bradfield, A., Maxson, B. J., & Starkson, B. C. (1997). The rehabilitation team. In J. E. Moore, W. H. Graves, & J. B. Patterson (Eds.). *Foundations of rehabilitation counseling with persons who are blind or visually impaired.* New York: AFB Press.

Lynch, R. K., & Herbert, J. T. (1984). Employment trends for rehabilitation counselors. *Journal of Applied Rehabilitation Counseling, 15(3),* 43–46.

MacAndrew, C. (1965). The differentiation of male alcoholic outpatients from non-alcoholic outpatients by means of the MMPI. *Quarterly Journal of Studies on Alcohol, 26(2),* 238–246.

MacAndrew, C. (1981). What the MAC scale tells us about men alcoholics: An interpretive review. *Journal of Studies on Alcohol, 42,* 604–625.

MacLeod, G. K. (1995). An overview of managed health care. In P. Kongstvedt (Ed.), *Essentials of managed health care.* Gaithersburg, MD: Aspen Publications, Inc.

Margolin, G. (1982). Ethical and legal considerations in family therapy. *American Psychologist, 37,* 788–801.

Marquardt, T. P., Stoll, J., & Sussman, H. (1990). Disorders of communication in traumatic brain injury. In E. D. Bigler (Ed.), *Traumatic brain injury: Mechanisms of damage, assessment, intervention and outcome.* Austin, TX: PRO-ED.

Marshall, C. A., Johnson, M. J., Martin, Jr., W. E., Saravanabhavan, R. C., & Bradford, B. (1992). The rehabilitation needs of American Indians with disabilities in an urban setting. *Journal of Rehabilitation, X(xx),* 13–21.

Marshall, C. A., Martin, Jr., W. E., & Johnson, M. J. (1990). Issues to consider in the provision of vocational rehabilitation services to American Indians with alcohol problems. *Journal of Applied Rehabilitation Counseling, 21(3),* 45–48.

Marshall, C. A., Martin, Jr., W. E., Thomason, T. C., & Johnson, M. J. (1991). Multiculturalism and rehabilitation counselor training: Recommendations for providing culturally appropriate counseling services to American Indians with disabilities. *Journal of Counseling and Development, 70,* 225–234.

Martin, S. (1993). *Alcohol and interpersonal violence: Fostering multidisciplinary perspectives* (Research monograph No. 24, NIH Publication No. 93-3496) Rockville, MD: National Institute on Alcohol Abuse and Alcoholism.

Matkin, R. E. (1983). The roles and functions of rehabilitation specialists in the private sector. *Journal of Applied Rehabilitation Counseling, 14(1),* 14–27.

Matkin, R. E., Riggar, T. F. (1986). The rise of private sector rehabilitation and its effects on training programs. *Journal of Rehabilitation, 52(2),* 50–52.

Matuschka, E. (1985). Treatment, outcomes and clinical evaluation. In T. E. Bratter & G. G. Forrest (Eds.), *Alcoholism and substance abuse: Strategies for clinical intervention.* New York: The Free Press.

McBride, M. C. (1990). Autonomy and the struggle for female identity: Implications for counseling women. *Journal of Counseling and Development, 69,* 22–26.

McCrady, B. S., & Delaney, S. I. (1995). Self-help groups. In R. K. Hester & W. R. Miller (Eds.), *Handbook of alcoholism treatment approaches: Effective Alternatives* (2nd ed.). Needham Heights, MA: Allyn & Bacon.

McDonough, R. L., & Russell, L. (1994). Alcoholism in women: A holistic comprehensive care model. *Journal of Mental Health Counseling, 16,* 459–474.

McGuire, T. L., & Sylvester, C. E. (1990). Neuropsychiatric evaluation and treatment of traumatic brain injury. In E. D. Bigler (Ed.), *Traumatic brain injury: Mechanisms of damage, assessment, intervention and outcome.* Austin, TX: PRO-ED.

McKay, J. R., & Maisto, S. A. (1993). An overview and critique of advances in the treatment of alcohol use disorders. In G. J. Connors (Ed.), *Innovations in alcoholism treatment: State of the art reviews and their implications for clinical practice.* New York: The Haworth Press, Inc.

McKay, J. R., McLellan, A. T., & Alterman, A. I. (1992). An evaluation of the Cleveland Criteria for inpatient substance abuse treatment. *American Journal of Psychiatry, 149,* 1212–1218.

McKirnan, D. J., & Peterson, P. L. (1989). Alcohol and drug use among homosexual men and women: Epidemiology and population characteristics. *Addictive Behaviors, 14,* 545.

McLellan, A. T., Hagan, T. A., Meyers, K, Randall, M., & Durell, J. (1997). Intensive outpatient substance abuse treatment: Comparisons with traditional outpatient treatment. *Journal of Addictive Diseases, 16, (3).*

McLellan, A. T., Woody, G. E., Luborsky, L., O'Brien, C. P., & Druley, K. A. (1983). Increased effectiveness of substance abuse treatment: A prospective study of patient-treatment matching. *Journal of Nervous and Mental Disease, 171,* 597–605.

McNair, L. D., & Roberts, G. W. (1997). Pervasive and persistent risk: factors influencing African American women's HIV/AIDS vulnerability. *Journal of Black Psychology, 27,* 180–192.

Mejta, C. L., & Bokos, P. J. (1992, February). *The effectiveness of a case management approach with intravenous drug users: Preliminary results.* Paper presented at the National Institute on Drug Abuse Technical Review Meeting, Progress in Case Management. Bethesda, MD.

Mejta, C. L., Bokos, P. J., Mickenberg, J. H., Maslar, E. M., Hasson, A. L., Gil, V., O'Keefe, Z., Martin, S. S., Isenberg, H., Inciardi, J. A., Lockwood, D., Rapp, R. C., Siegal, H. A., Fisher, J. H., & Wagner, J. H. (1994). Approaches to case management with substance-abusing populations. In J. Lewis (Ed.), *Addictions: Concepts and strategies for treatment.* Gaithersburg, MD: Aspen.

Mendelson, J. H., & Mello, N. K. (1966). Experimental analysis of drinking behavior of chronic alcoholics. *Annals of the New York Academy of Science, 133,* 828–831.

Miller, D. C., & Form, W. H. (1951). *Industrial sociology.* New York: Harper & Row.

Miller, G. A. (1985). *The Substance Abuse Subtle Screening Inventory manual.* Bloomington, IN: Addiction Research & Consultation.

Miller, L. M. (1992). *Codependency: An analysis of Cermak's diagnostic criteria.* Unpublished Master of Science Research Paper: Southern Illinois University at Carbondale.

Miller, N. S., & Gold, M. S. (1993). A neurochemical basis for alcohol and other drug addiction. *Journal of Psychoactive Drugs, 25(2),* 121–128.

Miller, W. R. (1976). Alcoholism scales and objective measures. *Psychological Bulletin, 83,* 649–674.

Miller, W. R. (1989). Matching individual with interventions. In R. K. Hester & W. R. Miller (Eds.), *Handbook of alcoholism treatment approaches.* New York: Pergamon Press.

Miller, W. R. (1992). The evolution of treatment for alcohol problems since 1945. In P. G. Erickson & H. Kalan (Eds.), *Windows on science.* Toronto: Addiction Research Foundation.

Miller, W. R., Brown, J. M., Simpson, T. L., Handmaker, N. S., Bien, T. H., Luckie, L. F., Montgomery, H. A., Hester, R. K., & Tonigan, J. S. (1995). What works? A methodological analysis of the alcohol treatment outcome literature. In R. K. Hester & W. R. Miller (Eds.), *Handbook of alcoholism treatment approaches: Effective Alternatives* (2d ed.). Needham Heights, MA: Allyn & Bacon.

Miller, W.R., & Hester, R. K. (1986). Inpatient alcoholism treatment: Who benefits? *American Psychologist, 41,* 794–806.

Miller, W. R., & Hester, R. K. (1989). Treating alcohol problems: Toward an informed eclecticism. In R. K. Hester & W. R. Miller (Eds.), *Handbook of alcoholism treatment approaches.* Needham Heights, MA: Allyn & Bacon.

Miller, W. R., & Marlatt, G. A. (1984). *Comprehensive Drinker Profile.* Odessa Florida: Psychological Assessment Resources.

Minuchin, S., & Fishman, H. C. (1981) *Family therapy techniques.* Cambridge, MA: Harvard University Press.

Mitchell, A. M., Jones, G. B., & Krumboltz, J. D. (1979). *Social learning and career decision making.* Cranston, RI: Carroll Press.

Monti, P. M., Rohsenow, D. J., Colby, S. M., & Abrams, D. B. (1995). Coping and social skills training. In R. K. Hester & W. R. Miller (Eds.), *Handbook of alcoholism treatment approaches: Effective Alternatives* (2d ed.). Needham Heights, MA: Allyn & Bacon.

Moore, D., & Li, L. (1994). Substance use among rehabilitation consumers of vocational rehabilitation services. *Journal of Rehabilitation, 60 (4),* 48–53.

Moore, J. E. (1997). Blindness and vision disorders. In A. E. Dell Orto & R. P. Marinelli (Eds.), *Encyclopedia of disability and rehabilitation.* New York: Simon & Schuster Macmillan.

Moos, R. H., & Moss, B. (1986). *Family Environmental Scale manual: Second edition.* Palo Alto: Consulting Psychologists Press.

Morey, L.C. (1996). Patient Placement Criteria—Linking typologies to managed care. *Alcohol Health & Research World, 20(1),* 36–44.

Morgan, T. J. (1996). Behavioral treatment techniques for psychoactive substance use disorders. In F. Rotgers, D.S. Keller, & J. Morgenstern (Eds.), *Treating substance abuse: Theory and technique.* New York: The Guilford Press.

Morrison, J. K., Layton, D., & Newman, J. (1982). Ethical conflict in decision making. In J. C. Hanson & L. L'Abate (eds.), *Values, ethics, legalities and the family therapist.* Rockville, MD: Aspen.

Morse, R. M., & Flavin, D. K. (1992). The definition of alcoholism. *Journal of the American Medical Association, 268(8),* 1012–1014.

Myers, P. S., & Myers, D. W. (1985, May). EAPs: The benefit that creates new risks. *Risk Management,* 46–52.

Nace, E. P. (1990). Inpatient treatment of alcoholism: A necessary part of the therapeutic armamentarium. *The Psychiatric Hospital, 21,* 9–31.

Nagler, M., & Wilson, W. (1995). Disability. In A. E. Dell Orto, & R. P. Marinelli (Eds.), *Encyclopedia of disability and rehabilitation* (pp. 257–260). New York: Simon & Schuster Macmillan.

Narcotics Anonymous (1997). *Facts about Narcotics Anonymous.* Available online: *http://www.wsoinc.com/berlbull.htm.*

National Alliance for the Mentally Ill. (1997). *A legacy of failure: The inability of the state-federal rehabilitation system to serve people with severe mental illnesses* (Report summary) Arlington, VA: Author.

National Clearinghouse for Alcohol and Drug Information. (1997). Drug use among American teens shows some signs of leveling after a long rise. *Monitoring the Future Study.* Available online: http://www.healthorg/pressrel/dec97/10.html.

National Council on Alcohol and Drug Dependence. (1997a) *Significant events in the field of alcoholism and other drug addictions* [Online]. Available at http://www.ncadd.org/events.html.

National Council on Alcohol and Drug Dependence. (1997b). *Definition of alcoholism* [Online]. Available at http://ncadd.org/defalc.html.

National Council on Alcohol and Drug Dependence. (1997c) *Alcohol and other drugs in the workplace* [Online]. Available at http://ncadd.org/workplac.html.

National Head Injury Foundation (1988). *Substance abuse task force white paper.* Southborough, MA: Author.

National Information Center for Children and Youth with Disabilities. (1994). *General information about spina bifida.* Fact sheet no. 12.

National Institute on Alcohol Abuse and Alcoholism. (1987). *Screening for alcoholism in primary care settings.* Public Health Service, Rockford, MD.

National Institute on Alcohol Abuse and Alcoholism. (1990, Oct.), Alcohol and women, *Alcohol Alert,* No. 10 PH 290.

National Institute on Alcohol and Alcoholism. (1997, January). Alcohol metabolism. *Alcohol Alert, 35,* 1–4.

National Institute on Alcoholism and Alcohol Abuse. (1995). *NIAAA Press Release: Naltrexone approved for alcoholism treatment.* Available: http://www.niaaa.nih.gov/events/naltre.htm.

National Institute on Disability and Rehabilitation Research. (1994). Community integration of individuals with traumatic brain injury. *Rehab: Bringing research into effective focus, XVI(8),* 1–4.

National Institute on Drug Abuse (1990). *Research on drugs in the workplace.* U.S. Department of Health and Human Services, Rockville, MD.

National Occupational Information Coordinating Committee. (1986). *Using labor market information in career exploration and decision making: A resource guide.* Garrett Park, MD: Garrett Park Press.

Naugle, R. I. (1990). Epidemiology of traumatic brain injury in adults. In E. D. Bigler (Ed.), *Traumatic brain injury: Mechanisms of damage, assessment, intervention*

and outcome (pp. 69–106). Austin, TX: PRO-ED.

Neff, W.S. (1977). *Work and human behavior* (2d ed.). Chicago: Aldine.

Nelson, N. (1971). *The services of workshops for the handicapped in the United States: An historical and developmental perspective.* Springfield, IL: Charles C. Thomas.

Nisbet, R. A. (1966). *The sociological tradition.* New York: Basic Books.

Nixon, S. J. (1994). Cognitive deficits in alcoholic women. *Alcohol Health & Research World, 18,* 228–232.

Noelle, D. (1997). *Secular Organizations for Sobriety home page.* Available online: *http://www.SecularHumanism.org/sos/.*

Normand, J., Lempert, R. O, & O'Brien, C. P. (1994). *Under the influence? Drugs and the American work force. Committee on Drug Use in the Workplace,* Washington, DC: National Academy Press.

Nosek, M. A. (1992) Independent living. In R. M. Parker & E. M. Szymanski (Eds.), Rehabilitation counseling: *Basics and beyond* (2nd ed.). Austin, TX: PRO-ED.

Obermann, C. E. (1965). *A history of vocation rehabilitation in America.* Minneapolis: The Dennison Company.

O'Brien, C. P., Woody, G. E., & McLellan, A. T. (1995). Enhancing the effectiveness of methadone using psychotherapeutic interventions. In L. S. Onken, J. D. Blaine, & J. J. Boren (Eds.). *Integrating behavioral therapies with medications in the treatment of drug dependence* (NIDA Research Monograph 150). Rockville, MD: National Institute on Drug Abuse, U.S. Department of Health and Human Services.

O'Farrell (Ed.), (1995) *Treating alcohol problems: Marital and family interventions.* New York: The Guilford Press.

Office of National Drug Control policy cited in Abadinsky, 1977.

Ogborne, A. C., & Glaser, F. B. (1981). Characteristics of affiliates of Alcoholics Anonymous: A review of the literature. *Journal of Studies on Alcohol, 42,* 661–675.

Olson, D. H. (1986). Circumplex model VII: Validation studies and FACES II. *Family Process, 26,* 337–351.

Ontario Ministry of Health. (1985). *Addictions services policy.* Toronto, Ontario: Author.

Orford, J., Oppenheimer, E., & Edwards, G. (1976). Abstinence or control: The outcome for excessive drinkers two years after consultation. *Behavior Research and Therapy, 14,* 409–419.

Orlandi, M. A. (1992a). The challenge of evaluating community based prevention programs: A cross-cultural perspective. In M. A. Orlandi, R. Weston, & L. G. Epstein (Eds.), *Cultural Competence for evaluators: A guide for alcohol and other drug prevention practitioners working with ethnic/racial communities.* Rockville, MD: U.S. Department of Health and Human Services, Office for Substance Abuse Prevention.

Orlandi, M. A. (1992b). Defining cultural competence: An organizing framework. In M. A. Orlandi, R. Weston, & L. G. Epstein (Eds.), *Cultural Competence for evaluators: A guide for alcohol and other drug prevention practitioners working with ethnic/racial communities.* Rockville, MD: U.S. Department of Health and Human Services, Office for Substance Abuse Prevention.

Osipow, S. H. (1983). *Theories of career development* (3d ed.). Englewood Cliffs, NJ: Prentice-Hall.

Pabis-Mock, A. (1997). *Profile of Jean Kirkpatrick* [Online]. Available: http//www.mediapulse.co/wfw/wfs-jean.html.

Padilla, A. M., Duran, D., & Nobles, W. W. (1995). Inner-city youth. In R. H. Coombs & D. C. Ziedonis (Eds.), *Handbook on drug abuse prevention.* Needham Heights, MA: Allyn & Bacon.

Padilla, A. M., & Salgado de Snyder, V. N. (1992). Hispanics: What the culturally informed evaluator needs to know. In M. A. Orlandi, R. Weston, & L. G. Epstein (Eds.), *Cultural Competence for evaluators: A guide for alcohol and other drug prevention practitioners working with ethnic/racial communities.* Rockville, MD: U.S. Department of Health and Human Services, Office for Substance Abuse Prevention.

Palfai, T., & Jankiewicz, T. I. (1997). *Drugs and Human Behavior* (2nd Ed.). Dubuque, IA: Brown and Benchmark Publishers.

Parker, D. A., & Broady, J. A. (1982). Risk factors for alcoholism and alcohol problems among employed women and men. In National Institute on Alcohol Abuse and Alcoholism. *Occupational alcoholism: A review of Research Issues* (Research Monograph No. 8, DHHS Publication No. ADM 82-1184, pp. 99–133). Washington: Government Printing Office.

Parsons, F. (1909). *Choosing a vocation.* Boston: Houghton Mifflin.

Patient Placement Criteria 2 (1996). *American Society of Addiction Medicine patient placement for the treatment of substance-related disorders* (2nd ed.). Annapolis, MD: EJP Inc.

Patterson, C. H. (1957). Counselor or coordinator? *Journal of Rehabilitation, 23(5),* 9–10, 27–28.

Patterson, J. B. (1996). Occupational and labor market information and analysis. In E. M. Szymanski & R. M. Parker (Eds.), *Work and disability: Issues and strategies in career development and job placement.* Austin, TX: PRO-ED.

Paul, J. P., Stall, R., and Bloomfield, K. A. (1991). Gay and Alcoholic Epidemiologic and Clinical Issues. *Alcohol Health & Research World, 15(2).*

Peele, S. (1990). *Diseasing of America: Addiction treatment out of control.* Lexington, MA: Lexington Books.

Peluso, E., & Peluso, L. S. (1989). Alcohol and the elderly. *Professional Counselor, 4(2),* 44–46.

Phillips, B., Kemper, P., & Applebaum, R. (1988). The evaluation of the national long term care demonstration. 4: Case management under channeling. *Health Services Research, 23(1),* 67–81.

Piaget, J. (1952). *The origins of intelligence in children.* New York: International Universities Press.

Pinson-Millburn, N. M., Fabian, E. S., Schlossberg, N. K., & Pyle, M. (1996). Grandparents raising grandchildren. *Journal of Counseling and Development, 74,* 548–554.

Pisani, R. G. (1995). Advertising industry. In R. H. Coombs & D. C. Ziedonis (Eds.), *Handbook on drug abuse prevention.* Needham Heights, MA: Allyn & Bacon.

Platt, J. J. (1995). Vocational rehabilitation of drug abusers. *Psychological Bulletin, 117,* 416–433.

Platt, J. J., & Metzger, D.S. (1987). *Final report, role of work in the rehabilitation of methadone clients.* Rockville, MD: National Institute on Drug Abuse.

Pohl, M. I. (1991, Nov.–Dec.). Gay men, lesbians and sexuality: Not just another special issue. *The Counselor,* 6–7.

Pokorny, M. D., Miller, B. A. & Kaplan, H. B. (1972). The brief MAST: A shortened version of the Michigan Alcoholism Screening Test. *American Journal of Psychiatry, 129,* 343–345.

Power, P. W. (1991). *A guide to vocational assessment.* Austin, TX: PRO-ED.

Prochaska, J. O., DiClemente, C. O., & Norcross, J. C. (1992). In search of how people change: Applications to addictive behaviors. *American Psychologist, 47,* 1102–1114.

Project MATCH Research Group (1997). Matching alcoholism treatments to client heterogeneity: Project MATCH post-treatment drinking outcomes. *Journal of Studies on Alcohol, 58,* 7–29.

Randall, T. (1992). Cocaine, alcohol mix in body to form even longer lasting, more lethal drug. *Journal of the American Medical Association, 267,* 1043–1044.

Rapp, C. A. (1996). The active ingredients of effective case management: A research synthesis. In L. J. Giesler (Ed.), *Case management for behavioral managed care.* Available from NACM, Suiete 306, 10050 Montgomery Road, Cincinnati, OH 45242.

Rapp, C. A., & Chamberlain, R. (1985). Case management services for the chronically mentally ill. *Social Work, 30,* 417–422.

Rational Recovery Systems (1997). *The Worldwide Web Rational Recovery Center.* Available online: http://www.rational.org/ recovery/index.html.

Ray, O., & Ksir, C. (1996). *Drugs, society, and human behavior* (7th ed.). St. Louis: Mosby-Year Book, Inc.

Regier, D., Farmer, M., & Rae, D. (1990). Co-morbidity of mental disorders with alcohol and other drug abuse: Results form an Epidemiologic Catchment Area (ECA) Study. *Journal of the American Medical Association, 264,* 2511–2518.

Rehabilitation Institute of Chicago (1991). *Alcohol and Other Drug Abuse Prevention for People with Traumatic Brain and Spinal Cord Injuries.* Chicago: Author.

Rehabilitation Research and Training Center on Drugs and Disability (1996). *Substance abuse, disability and vocational rehabilitation.* SARDI/Wright State University/New York University: Author.

Rendon, M. E. (1992). Deaf culture and alcohol and substance. *Journal of Substance Abuse Treatment, 9,* 103–110.

Reuler, J. B., Girard, D. E., & Cooney, T. G. (1985). Wernicke's encephalopathy. *New England Journal of Medicine, 312,* 1035–1039.

Rhodes, S. S., & Jasinski, D. R. (1990). Learning disabilities in alcohol dependent adults: A preliminary study. *Journal of Learning Disabilities, 23,* 551–556.

Rice, D., Kelman, S., Miller, L., & Dunmeyer, S. (1990). *The economic costs of alcohol and drug abuse and mental illness: 1985.* San Francisco: Institute for Health and Aging, University of California.

Richmond, C. (1972). Therapeutic housing. *Rehabilitation Record, November–December,* 8–13.

Rieske, R. J., & Holstege, H. (1996). *Growing older in America.* New York: McGraw-Hill.

Rimmele, C. T., Howard, M. O., & Hilfrink, M. L. (1995). Aversion therapies. In R. K. Hester & W. R. Miller (Eds.), *Handbook of alcoholism treatment approaches: Effective Alternatives* (2d ed.). Needham Heights, MA: Allyn & Bacon.

Riordan, R. J. (1992). The use of mirror image therapy in substance abuse treatment. *Journal of Counseling and Development, 71,* 101–102.

Robe, M. P., Russell-Einhorn, M., & Baker, M. A. (1986). The fear of AIDS. *Harvard Business Review, 64 (4),* 28–36.

Robertson, J. C. (1989). Cocaine addiction and cocaine anhedonia. *Professional Counselor, 4 (3),* 31–34.

Robinson, G., & Bergman, G. (1989). *Choices in case management: A review of current knowledge and practice for mental health programs.* Washington, DC: Policy Resources Incorporated.

Robinson, T. E., & Berridge, K.C. (1993). The neural basis of drug craving: an incentive-sensitization theory of addiction. *Brain Research Reviews, 18,* 247–291.

Roe, A. (1957). Early determinants of vocational choice. *Journal of Counseling Psychology, 4,* 212–217.

Roessler, R. T. (1983). The role of the rehabilitation counselor in independent living. *Rehabilitation Counseling Bulletin, 26(3),* 174–180.

Roessler, R. T., & Rubin, S. E. (1992). *Case management and rehabilitation counseling.* Austin, TX: PRO–ED.

Rogers Memorial Hospital (1988). *The progression of chemical dependency: The family illness.* Oconomowac, WI: Author.

Roman, P. (1981). From employee alcoholism to employee assistance. *Journal of Studies on Alcohol, 42,* 244–272.

Rone, L. A., Miller, S. I., & Frances, R. J. (1995). Psychotropic medications. In R. K. Hester, & W. R. Miller (Eds.), *Handbook of alcoholism treatment approaches: Effective alternatives* (2nd ed.) (pp. 267–277). Boston: Allyn & Bacon.

Rose, S. D. (1977). *Group therapy: A behavioral approach.* Englewood Cliffs, NJ: Prentice-Hall.

Rosenhan, D. L., & Seligman, M. E. P. (1995). *Abnormal psychology.* New York: W. W. Norton & Co.

Rotgers, F., Keller, D. S., & Morgenstern, J. (1996). *Treating substance abuse: Theory and technique.* New York: The Guilford Press.

Rothman, R. A. (1987). *Working: Sociological perspectives.* Englewood Cliffs, NJ: Prentice-Hall.

Rubin, S. E., Matkin, R. E., Ashley, J., Beardsley, M. M., May, V. R., Onstott, K., & Puckett, F. D. (1984). Roles and functions of certified rehabilitation counselors. *Rehabilitation Counseling Bulletin, 27(4),* 199–224.

Rubin, S. E., Pusch, B. D., Fogarty, C., & McGinn, F. (1995). Enhancing the cultural sensitivity of rehabilitation counselors. *Rehabilitation Education, 9,* 253–264.

Rubin, S. E., & Roessler, R. T. (1995). *Foundations of the vocational rehabilitation process* (4th ed.). Austin, TX: PRO-ED.

Rutan, J. S., & Stone, W. N. (1993). *Psychodynamic Group Psychotherapy* (2d ed.). New York: The Guilford Press.

Sacks, S. Z., Barrett, S. S., & Orlansky, M. D. (1997). People with multiple disabilities. In J. E. Moore, W. H. Graves, & J. B. Patterson (Eds.). *Foundations of rehabilitation counseling with persons who are blind or visually impaired.* New York: AFB Press.

Salamone, P. R. (1996). Career counseling and job placement: Theory and practice. In E. M. Szymanski and R. M. Parker (Eds.), *Work and disability: Issues and strategies in career development and job placement.* Austin, TX: PRO-ED.

Santrock, J. W. (1990). *Adolescence* (4th ed.). Dubuque, IA: William C. Brown Publishers.

Scanlon, W. (1991). *Alcoholism and drug abuse in the workplace* (2d ed.). New York: Praeger.

Schaef, A. W. (1986). Co-dependence: Misunderstood–mistreated. San Francisco: Harper & Row.

Schene, A., & Gersens, V. (1986). Effectiveness and application of partial hospitalization. *Acta Psychiatrica Scandanavia, 74,* 335–340.

Scofield, M. E., & Andrews, J. A. (1981). Finding a job in human services: The value of rehabilitation counselor competencies. *Journal of Applied Rehabilitation Counseling, 12(3),* 146–151.

Sears, S. (1982). A definition of career guidance terms: A National Vocational Guidance Association perspective. *Vocational Guidance Quarterly, 31,* 137–143.

Secretary of Health and Human Services. (1990). *Seventh Special Report to the U.S. Congress on Alcohol and Health* (DHHS Publication No. ADM 281-88-0002). Washington, DC: U.S. Government Printing Office.

Segal, R., & Sisson, B. V. (1985) Medical complications associated with alcohol use and the assessment of risk of physical damage. In T. E. Bratter, & G. G. Forrest (Eds.), *Alcoholism and substance abuse: Strategies for clinical intervention.* New York: The Free Press.

Selzer, M. L. (1971). The Michigan Alcoholism Screening Test: The quest for a new diagnostic instrument. *American Journal of Psychiatry, 127,* 1653–1658.

Selzer, M. L., Vinokur, A., & Van Rooijen, L. A. (1974). Self-administered Short Michigan Alcoholism Screening Test (SMAST). *Journal of Studies on Alcohol, 15,* 276–280.

Sewell, W. H., & Hauser, R. M. (1975). *Education, occupation, and earnings.* New York: Academic Press.

Shartle, C. L. (1959). *Occupational information—its development and applications* (3d ed.). Englewood Cliffs, NJ: Prentice-Hall.

Shaw, L. R., MacGillis, P. W., & Dvorchik, K. M. (1994). Alcoholism and the Americans with Disabilities Act: Obligations and accommodations. *Rehabilitation Counseling Bulletin, 38(2),* 108–123.

Shipley, R. W., Taylor, S. M., & Falvo, D. R. (1990). Concurrent evaluation and rehabilitation of alcohol abuse and trauma. *Journal of Applied Rehabilitation Counseling, 21(3),* 37–39.

Shoenfeld, E. (1975). Deinstituionalization/Community alternatives. In K. Mallik, S. Yuspeh, & J. Mueller (Eds.), *Comprehensive vocational rehabilitation for severely disabled persons.* Washington, DC: George Washington University Medical Center, Job Development Laboratory.

Shrey, D. E. (1979). The rehabilitation counselor in industry: A new frontier. *Journal of Applied Rehabilitation Counseling, 9(4),* 168–172.

Siegal, H. A., Rapp, R. C., Kelliher, C. W., Fisher, J. H., Wagner, J. H., & Cole, P. A. (1995). The strengths perspective of case management: A promising inpatient substance abuse treatment enhancement. *Journal of Psychoactive Drugs, 27(1),* 67–72.

Siegel, R. K. (1987). Cocaine smoking: Nature and extent of coca paste and cocaine free-base abuse. In A. M. Washton & M. S. Gold (Eds.), *Cocaine: A clinician's handbook* (pp. 175–191). New York: The Guilford Press.

Simon, S. B., Howe, L. W., & Kirschenbaum, H. (1995). *Values clarification.* New York: Warner Books.

Skinner, H. A. (1994). *The Computerized Lifestyle Assessment.* Toronto, Canada: Multi-Health Systems.

Smith, G. (1991, Feb. 18). Shadow of a nation. *Sports Illustrated,* 60–74.

Smith, J. W. (1982). Neurological disorders in alcoholism. In N. J. Estes, & M. E. Heineman (Eds.), *Alcoholism: Development, consequences, and interventions* (2d ed.). St. Louis: Mosby.

Snyder, S. H. (1986). *Drugs and the brain.* New York: Scientific America Inc.

Sobell, L. C., & Sobell, M. B. (1990). Self-report issues in alcohol abuse: State of the art and future directions. *Behavioral Assessment, 12,* 113–128.

Statman, J. M. (1993). The enemy at home: Images of addiction in American society. *Journal of Adolescent Chemical Dependency, 2(3/4),* 19–29.

Steinglass, P., Bennett, L. A., Wolin, S. J., & Reiss, D. (1987). *The alcoholic family.* New York: BasicBooks.

Stevens, J. (1987). *Storming heaven: LSD and the American dream.* New York: Atlantic Monthly Press.

Steven-Smith, P., & Smith, R. L. (1998). *Substance abuse counseling.* Upper Saddle River, NJ: Prentice-Hall, Inc.

Strickland, B. (1969). Philosophy-theory-practice continuum: A point of view. *Counselor Education and Supervision, 8(3),* 165–175.

Substance Abuse and Mental Health Services Administration (1993). *National household survey on drug abuse: population estimates, 1992.* (Publication No. SMA 93-2953). Rockville, MD.

Sullivan, W. P., Wolk, J. L., & Hartmann, D. J. (1992). Case management in alcohol and drug treatment: Improving client outcomes. Families in Society: *The Journal of Contemporary Human Services, 73(4),* 195–203.

Super, D. (1957). *The psychology of careers: An introduction to vocational development.* New York: Harper-Row.

Surgeon General (1979). *Smoking and Health.* A Report of the Surgeon General. U.S. Department of Health, Education, and Welfare. Washington, DC: U.S. Government Printing Office.

Surgeon General (1988). *The health consequences of smoking: Nicotine and addiction: Report of the Surgeon General.* U.S. Department of Health, Education, and Welfare. Washington, DC: U.S. Government Printing Office.

Szymanski, E. M. (1984). Rehabilitation counselors in school settings. *Journal of Applied Rehabilitation Counseling, 15(5),* 10–13.

Szymanski, E. M., & Parker, R. (1989). Relationships of rehabilitation client outcome to level of rehabilitation counselor education. *Journal of Rehabilitation, 55(4),* 32–36.

Taricone, P. F., Bordieri, J. E., & Scalia, V. A. (1989). Assessing rehabilitation needs of clients in treatment for alcohol abuse. *Rehabilitation Counseling Bulletin, 32,* 324–331.

Tate, D. G. (1994). The use of the CAGE questionnaire to assess alcohol abuse among spinal cord injury persons. *Journal of Rehabilitation, 60(1),* 31.

Telzrow, C. F. (1990). Management of academic and education programs in traumatic brain injury. In E. D. Bigler (Ed.), *Traumatic brain injury: Mechanisms of damage, assessment, intervention and outcome.* Austin, TX: PRO-ED, Inc.

Thomason, T. C. (1991). Counseling Native Americans: An introduction for non-Native American counselors. *Journal of Counseling & Development, 69,* 321–327.

Thomson, A. D., Jeyasingham, M. D., & Pratt, O. E. (1987). Possible role of toxins in nutritional deficiency. *Annals of the New York Academy of Science, 522,* 757–770.

Thoresen, C., & Ewart, C. (1978). Behavioral self control and career development. In J. Whiteley and A. Resnikoff (Eds.), *Career counseling.* Monterey, CA: Brooks-Cole.

Tice, C. J., & Perkins, K. (1996). *Mental health issues & aging: Building on the strengths of older persons.* Pacific Grove, CA: Brooks/Cole.

Tiedeman, D. V. (1961). Decisions and vocational development: A paradigm and its implications. *Personnel and Guidance Journal, 40,* 15–21.

Tishler, H. S. (1971). *Self-reliance and social security, 1870–1917.* Port Washington, NY: Kennikat Press.

Tracy, J., Josiassen, R., & Belleck, A. (1995). Neuropsychology of dual diagnosis: Understanding the combined effects of schizophrenia and substance abuse disorders. *Clinical Psychology Review, 15(2),* 67–97.

Trepper, T. S., Piercy, F. P., Lewis, R. A., Volk, R. J., & Sprenkle, D. H. (1993). Family therapy for adolescent alcohol abuse. In T. J. O'Farrell (Ed.), *Treating alcohol problems: Marital and family interventions* (pp. 261–280).

Trice, H. M., & Schonbrunn, M. (1988). A history of job-based alcoholism programs. In F. Dickman, B. R. Challenger, W. G. Emener, & W. S. Hutchinson (Eds.), *Employee Assistance Programs: A basic text* (pp. 9–47). Springfield, IL: Charles C. Thomas.

Trimble, J. E. (1995). Ethnic minorities. In R. H. Coombs & D. C. Ziedonis (Eds.), *Handbook on drug abuse prevention.* Needham Heights, MA: Allyn & Bacon.

Trimpey, J. (1989). *Rational recovery from addiction: The small book.* Lotus, CA: Author.

Uecker, A. E. (1970). Differentiating male alcoholics from other psychiatric inpatients: Validity of the MacAndrew scale. *Quarterly Journal of Studies on Alcohol, 31,* 379–383.

Urbano-Marquez, A., Estruch, R., Fernandez-Sola, J., Nicolas, J. M., Pare, J. C., & Rubin, E. (1995). The greater risk of alcoholic cardiomyopathy and myopathy in women compared with men. *Journal of the American Medical Association, 274,* 149–154.

USA Today. (March 12, 1997). Welfare-to-work not an easy road. 3A.

U.S. Department of Health and Human Services (1995). *Substance Abuse and Mental Health Services Administration (SAMHSA) substance abuse and mental health services statistics sourcebook.* Rockville, MD: U.S. Department of Health and Human Services.

U.S. Department of Health and Human Services (1996). *Drug use among U.S. workers: Prevalence and trends by occupation and industry categories* (SAMHSA document). Rockville, MD: U.S. Department of Health and Human Services.

U.S. Department of Labor (1970). *General Aptitude Test Battery.* Washington, DC: Government Printing Office.

U.S. Department of Labor (1979). *Guide for occupational exploration.* Washington, DC: Government Printing Office.

U.S. Department of Labor (1991). *Dictionary of occupational titles.* Washington, DC: Government Printing Office.

U.S. Department of Labor (1996). *Occupational outlook handbook.* Washington, DC: Government Printing Office.

Vandergoot, D., & Worrall, J. D. (1979). *Placement in rehabilitation.* Baltimore: University Park Press.

Van Thiel, D. H., Lipsitz, H. D., Porter, L. E., Schade, R. R., Gottlieb, G. P., & Graham, T. O. (1981). Gastrointestinal and hepatic manifestations of chronic alcoholism. *Gastroenterology, 81,* 594–615.

Vinacke, W. E. (1968). *Foundations of psychology.* New York: American Book Company.

Wade, J. C. (1994). Substance abuse: Implications for counseling African American men. *Journal of Mental Health Counseling, 16,* 415–433.

Wadsworth, R., Spampneto, A. M., & Halbrook, B. M. (1995). The role of sexual trauma in the treatment of chemically dependent women: Addressing the relapse issue. *Journal of Counseling and Development, 73,* 401–406.

Walker, M. L. (1991). Rehabilitation service delivery to individuals with disabilities. *OSERS News in Print, Fall,* 1–6.

Wallace, B. C. (1991). Crack cocaine: A practical treatment approach for the chemically dependent. New York: Brunner/Mazel.

Washton, A. M. (1987). Outpatient treatment techniques. In A. M. Washton & M. S. Gold (Eds.), *Cocaine: A clinician's handbook.* New York: The Guilford Press.

Washton, A. M., & Gold, M. S. (1987). Recent trends in cocaine abuse as seen from the 800-Cocaine hotline. In A. M. Washton & M. S. Gold (Eds.), *Cocaine: A clinicians handbook.* New York: The Guilford Press.

Watson, A. L. (1990). African Americans and substance abuse: Considerations for rehabilitation counselors. *Journal of Applied Rehabilitation Counseling, 21*(3), 55–58.

Watson, S. J., Trujillo, K. A., Herman, J. P., & Akil, H. (1989). Neuroanatomical and neurochemical substrates of drug-seeking behavior: Overview and future directions. In A. Goldstein (Ed.), *Molecular and cellular aspects of the drug addictions.* New York: Springer-Verlag.

Weed, R. O., Field, T. F. (1986). The differences and similarities between public and private sector vocational rehabilitation. *Journal of Applied Rehabilitation Counseling, 17*(2), 11–16.

Weed, R. O., & Field, T. F. (1994). *Rehabilitation consultant's handbook* (rev. ed.). Athens, GA: Elliot & Fitzpatrick.

Wegscheider-Cruse, S. (1981). *Another chance.* Palo Alto, CA: Science and Behavior Books.

Wegscheider-Cruse & Cruse, J.R. (1990). *Understanding co-dependency.* Pompano Beach, FL: Health communications.

Weil, M., & Karls, J. (1985). Historical origins and recent developments. In M. Weil & J Karls (Eds.), *Case management in human service practice.* San Francisco: Jossey-Bass.

Weinstein, S. P., Gottheil, E., & Sterling, R. (1997). Randomized comparison of intensive outpatient vs. individual therapy for cocaine abusers. *Journal of Addictive Diseases, 16(3).*

Weisner, T. S., Weibel-Orlando, J. C., & Long, J. (1984). "Serious drinking," "White man's drinking," and "Teetotaling:" Drinking levels and styles in an urban American Indian population. *Journal of Studies on Alcohol, 45,* 237–250.

Wesner, D., Patel, C., & Allen, J. (1991). A study of explosive rage in male spouses counseled in an Appalachian mental health clinic. *Journal of Counseling and Development, 70,* 235–241.

Wetli, C. V. (1987). Fatal reactions to cocaine. In A. M. Washton & M. S. Gold (Eds.), *Cocaine: A clinicians handbook.* New York: The Guilford Press.

White, B. (1997, March). *Back to the future? The lessons of history.* Paper presented at the annual spring meeting of the Illinois Alcohol and Other Drug Abuse Professional Certification Association, Arlington Hts., IL.

White, W. L., & Chaney, R. A. (1993). Metaphors of transformation: Feminine and masculine. (A Lighthouse Training Institute Monograph). Bloomington, IL: Lighthouse Training Institute, a division of Chestnut Health Systems.

Whitfield, C. L. (1987). *Healing the child within.* Pompano Beach, FL: Health Communications, Inc.

Widom, C. S. (1993). Child abuse and alcohol use and abuse. In S. E. Martin (Ed.), *Alcohol and interpersonal violence: Fostering multidisciplinary perspectives* (Research monograph no. 24, pp. 291–341). Rockville, MD: National Institutes of Alcoholism and Alcohol Abuse.

Willenbring, M. L., Ridgely, M. S., Stinchfield, R., & Rose, M. (1991). *Application of case management in alcohol and drug dependence: Matching techniques and populations.* Rockville, MD: U.S. Department of Health and Human Services.

Wilsnack, S. C., Wilsnack, R. W., & Klassen, A. D. (1986). *National Institute on Alcoholism and Alcohol Research Monograph No. 16, pp. 1–68).* Rockville, MD: National Institute on Alcoholism and Alcohol Abuse.

Wilson, J. Q. (1990). Against the legalization of drugs. *Commentary, 89.*

Winger, G., Hofmann, F. G., & Woods, J. H. (1992). *A handbook on drug and alcohol abuse: The biomedical aspects* (3d ed.). New York: Oxford University Press, Inc.

Wojakowski, D. (1997). *Substance abuse in the gay and lesbian community.* Available online: http://www.vub.mcgill,ca/clubs/lbgtm/info/substance.html.

Wolffe, K. E. (1997). *Career counseling for people with disabilities.* Austin, TX: PRO-ED, Inc.

Women for Sobriety, Inc. (1997a). *Women for Sobriety, Inc.* [Online]. Available: http://www.mcidapulse.com/wfs/.

Women for Sobriety, Inc. (1997b). Introduction/ history. In *Women for Sobriety, Inc.* [Online]. Available: http://www.meidapulse.com/wfs/wfs-history.html.

Women for Sobriety, Inc. (1997c). The New Life Program. In *Women for Sobriety, Inc.* [Online]. Available: http://www.meidapulse.com/wfs/wfs-chapters.html.

Women for Sobriety, Inc. (1997d). New Life Acceptance Program. In *Women for Sobriety, Inc.* [Online]. Available: http://www.meidapulse.com/wfs/wfs-program.html.

Wright, G. N. (1980). *Total rehabilitation.* Boston: Little, Brown and Company.

Wright, T. J., & Emener, W. G. (1992). Rehabilitation and placement: A focus on African Americans. *Journal of Job Placement, 8*(1), 17–22.

Yalom, I. D. (1970). *The theory and practice of group psychotherapy.* New York: Basic Books.

Yalom, I. D. (1985). *The theory and practice of group psychotherapy.* New York: Basic Books.

Zastrow, C. (1989). *Social work with groups.* Chicago: Nelson-Hall.

Zephier, R. L., & Hedin C. (1981, May). *Alcoholism among Indian students: Walking like you talk.* Paper presented at the National Indian Child Conference, Albuquerque, NM.

Zucker, R. A. (1994). Pathways to alcohol problems and alcoholism: A developmental account of the evidence for multiple alcoholism and for contextual contributions to risk. In R. Zucker, G. Boyd, & J. Howard (Eds.), *The development of alcohol problems. Exploring the biopsychosocial matrix of risk* (Research monograph No. 26, pp. 255–290). Rockville, MD: National Institute on Alcohol Abuse and Alcoholism.

Zuk, G. H. (1971). Family therapy. In J. Haley (Ed.), *Changing families: A family therapy reader.* New York: Grune & Stratton.

Zweben, A., & Barrett, D. (1993). Brief couples treatment for alcohol problems. In T. J. O'Farrell (Ed.), *Treating alcohol problems: Marital and family interventions.* New York: The Guilford Press.

Zytowski, D. G., & Warman, R. E. (1982). The changing use of tests in counseling. *Measurement and Evaluation in Guidance, 15,* 147–152.

Index